CALICO- N COTION

715 ASHBURY AVR

OCEAN CITY

399 - 7166

7th/8th

10A - 5P

# IMPROVING CARE FOR THE END OF LIFE

# IMPROVING CARE
## FOR THE **END** OF **LIFE**

*A Sourcebook for Health Care Managers and Clinicians*

Joanne Lynn, M.D.
Janice Lynch Schuster
Andrea Kabcenell, R.N., M.P.H.

The Center to Improve Care of the Dying
The Institute for Healthcare Improvement

*Foreword by Donald M. Berwick, M.D.*

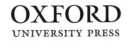

OXFORD
UNIVERSITY PRESS

2000

# OXFORD
## UNIVERSITY PRESS

Oxford   New York

Athens   Auckland   Bangkok   Bogotá   Buenos Aires   Calcutta
Cape Town   Dar es Salaam   Delhi   Florence   Hong Kong
Istanbul   Karachi   Kuala Lumpur   Madrid   Melbourne   Mexico City
Mumbai   Nairobi   Paris   São Paulo   Shanghai   Singapore   Taipei
Tokyo   Toronto   Warsaw

and associated companies in
Berlin   Ibadan

Library of Congress Cataloging-in-Publication Data
Lynn, Joanne, 1951–
Improving care for the end of life : a sourcebook for health care managers and
clinicians / Joanne Lynn, Janice Lynch Schuster, the Center to Improve Care of the
Dying, and the Institute for Healthcare Improvement ; foreword by Don Berwick.
    p.   cm.
Includes bibliographical references and index.
ISBN 0-19-511661-5
1. Terminal care.   2. Palliative care.   3. Death.   I. Schuster, Janice Lynch.
II. Center to Improve Care of the Dying.   III. Institute for Healthcare Improvement.
IV. Title. [DNLM:   1. Terminal Care—organization & administration.
2. Palliative Care—organization & administration.
3. Patient-Centered Care—organization & administration.
WY   152 L989i   2000]
R726.8.L96   2000
362.1′75—dc21        99-045308

Proceeds from the sale of this book go to:
Americans for Better Care of the Dying
PO Box 346
Marvin Center
Washington, DC 20037
(202) 895-9485
www.abcd-caring.org

9  8  7  6  5  4  3  2

Printed in the United States of America
on acid-free paper

To the hundreds of people who participated in the Breakthrough Series, for their commitment to making rapid change in improving end-of-life care. Their efforts and public spirit have paved a way for others to follow.

The lead authors also acknowledge the patience of their children, for whom death is oddly familiar in their daily lives: Nicholas and Christina Lynn; Conor, Meredith, and Alyson Lynch Fowler and Chad and Devan Schuster; and Ben Kuder.

# Foreword

A keystone is the center stone in an archway, without which the other stones tumble to the ground. Environmental scientists use the term "keystone species" to describe plants and animals whose presence powerfully supports or alters the flora and fauna in a given ecosystem. Trees, for instance, are the keystone species in a forest; bison are the keystone species in a grassland. Other species depend on the presence of the keystone species. When a keystone species disappears or is replaced by a stronger species, the entire ecosystem is transformed.

In a sense, care of the dying is both a "keystone" and a "keystone species" in the health care system. Failure to care well for seriously ill and dying people reflects the limitations that permeate the health care system—from gaps in clinician education to outdated financing structures. Excellent care for the dying can reflect a system's core strengths, as well.

As too many studies have shown, the health care system comes up short in treating pain, in communicating with patients and loved ones, and in helping dying patients live well despite disease. Yet many clinics, hospitals, nursing homes, and hospices have at hand the information and resources to make changes that improve end-of-life care, and to make them quickly. In so doing, clinicians and others could, in fact, alter the health care "ecosystem." Better end-of-life care would indicate the emergence of a stronger keystone species, one that enhances and strengthens the current environment, one that permits everyone to feel confident of receiving reliable, competent care. In the changed system, providers who specialize in care of the dying would demonstrate how to assess and treat pain, show ways to talk to patients and families about difficult subjects, address patient concerns about meaning and family, and develop programs and facilities that work in concert, not isolation.

Why am I so confident that change is possible? In a decade of working with health care providers and organizations to improve quality, I have seen important changes occur as a result of effective small-scale changes directed at improving patient care almost immediately. And most recently, through the Institute of Healthcare Improvement's Breakthrough Series on Improving Care at the End of Life, I have seen exactly how organizations large and small can make enormous changes in the care provided to dying patients. Led and encouraged by Joanne Lynn and a committed faculty team, forty-seven organizations representing a range of health care organizations collaborated for one year to improve end-of-life care in four areas: pain and other symptom management, advance care planning, family and meaningfulness, and continuity of care.

Through workshops and discussions with faculty and experts in end-of-life care, teams learned how to apply a rapid-cycle quality improvement model to change business as usual for dying patients and their loved ones. Groups learned from one another which strategies worked and which did not, where to find useful resources and relevant survey instruments, and how to approach old problems in new ways.

As people began to examine the usual care provided to most dying patients, they quickly discovered where improvement was needed and how simple tests of changes could lead to important changes in practice—and in principle.

For instance, one health care system was having trouble encouraging doctors to make earlier referrals for patients who could benefit from palliative and hospice care. In many cases, doctors simply did not consider their patients—even those with life-threatening illnesses—to be dying. As a result, patients in that community, as in so many others, had only a matter of days and weeks, rather than months, to enlist the full benefits of competent, integrated palliative and hospice care.

 Then the group decided to ask doctors a different question. Instead of asking doctors, "Which of your patients are dying?" the team began to ask, "Would you be surprised if this patient were to die this year?"

Changing the question changed the results. Doctors began to view patients in a different light, to recognize when patients were likely to benefit from end-of-life care and support, and to refer them for special support earlier.

Organizations that want to improve care of the dying can be encouraged by this story and by the other stories told throughout *Improving Care for the End of Life: A Sourcebook for Health*

*Care Managers and Clinicians*. By taking on seemingly basic issues, such as advance care planning and pain management, groups can become change agents, with a positive effect not only on care for the dying but on care for all patients.

Learning and applying the rapid-cycle model, which the Institute for Healthcare Improvement promotes through its Breakthrough Series and other events, is a straightforward process, one that this book explains. The model requires that groups target a specific area for change; plan changes based on good science, sound theory, and strong evidence; try several changes with small groups of patients; study the effects of the changes; and act accordingly. Using this model, one hospital was able to halve the time from pain assessment to medication delivery—going from three hours to just over one hour.

Many of the changes come from what common sense and compassion would have us do for other human beings. However, a common sense of purpose and direction—along with simple kindness—seem to have been lost in the chaos of mergers and acquisitions, downsizing and layoffs, budget cuts and price slashing, integrating and competing.

We need to refocus the energies of health care leaders on the experience of care itself, for the ultimate value of health care changes—the structures, the incentive, the investments, and the pressure—must in the end be assessed by the patients themselves, through their experience of our work.

Like many readers of this book, lay and professional, I feel a special sense of connection to end-of-life care as a species of care, keystone or not. Just a few years ago, my own father—a physician in practice for four decades—succumbed at age 84 to a long and difficult illness. As moved and grateful as I became at the dedication and tenderness of the many professionals who aided him, I became in equal measure enraged by a system of care—a totality—that could not sensibly hand his care across boundaries, that could not prevent eminently preventable complications, that could not keep him from having to wait, confused, in cold corridors and on anonymous stretchers. I became angry at a system—his system—that could not remember his name or his medications, even from one eight-hour shift to the next.

Now, having come into contact with the people whose work and aims are represented in this book, I know far better than I ever did before that lives need not conclude this way. I know now, with renewed confidence and precision, that we can, with strong will, sound ideas, and thorough execution, create and preserve forms of care for our final months and days that enhance dignity, assure comfort, and give meaning.

And if we can re-create the keystone of end-of-life care as a species, our success will echo. We will have learned how to think about systems, and new models of behavior, that can apply with equal effect in other troubled areas of health care. We have an ecosystem in jeopardy, and we who want to assure and enhance its future could hardly find a better place to start than to promise those approaching the end of life that they will be safe and respected while in our hands.

Donald M. Berwick, MD
Institute for Healthcare Improvement
Boston, Massachusetts, 1999

# Preface

This book aims to equip readers with the best available advice on how to make substantial improvements in the health care system so that it serves the seriously ill person who is coming to the end of life. Most of the examples here come from an extraordinary year-long collaborative on improving end-of-life care. Cosponsored by the Institute for Healthcare Improvement and the Center to Improve Care of the Dying, the project included more than four dozen health care organizations committed to changing practices for the sake of real quality improvement. As care for individuals improved, groups found that they were often able to improve their systems' usual functioning as well.

The Breakthrough Series teams tried changes in four critical areas: controlling pain and other symptoms; improving advance care planning; helping and comforting patients and families; and developing continuity of care. Almost all made real gains, and what they did will inspire and guide others. Their innovative projects provide a wonderful template for other organizations interested in improving the way people die in America's health care system.

This sourcebook features strategies that any manager of any health care system can try, almost immediately, to improve care—doctors in offices, nurse managers on hospital units, social workers for long-term care facilities, administrators of home care and hospice agencies, hospital chaplains, directors of volunteer services, and others.

This book describes the gains organizations have made in improving care, the changes they attempted and the successes they achieved. Each chapter offers step-by-step stories of successful efforts that are models of how to close the gap between what is known about good end-of-life care and what is actually done for patients.

In describing others' experiences, this book highlights ideas and how-to information so that others can begin to make the small changes that lead to real gains and improvement. While the focus is on ideas that worked, this book also includes a few that taught us much in their failings. Ultimately, we hope to provide the insight and inspiration to address this major public health problem by creating reliably good health care for everyone facing serious illness.

Throughout the book we signal ideas that could work and the level of evidence for them with a set of stars:

Key

★★★ Complete cycle (PDSA)—ideas tried and tested, with some evidence for usefulness

★★ Partial cycle (PD)—ideas tried, but evaluation not done or incomplete

★ Plan only (P)—Good idea, but little or no implementation (yet)

Part 1 of this sourcebook suggests quality improvement projects most organizations can attempt right now. These are based on the rapid-cycle breakthrough approach to quality improvement—the Plan-Do-Study-Act (PDSA) model, in which teams define problems, set goals, try changes, and see what happens. Throughout this book, readers will find examples of how Breakthrough Series teams used this model to improve not only their practices but also the lives of patients and their loved ones.

Part 2 focuses on changes patients and families often demand or would most benefit from—better and more reliable pain and symptom control, better advance care planning, and increased spiritual and psychosocial support.

Part 3 describes environments that encourage better practice. It describes the role and structure of palliative care services and their financing; ways to improve and integrate management information systems with clinical and financial systems; the human resources issues unique to this field; and opportunities for change in law and public policy.

Part 4 discusses opportunities for change in caring for patients with specific diseases: dementia and Alzheimer's, cancer, depression and delirium, and congestive heart failure and chronic obstructive pulmonary disorder.

The last chapter, "Getting Started," gives specific tips on how to get something done—by next Tuesday. We also provide a glossary, a compendium of resources (specific to each chapter as well as general), and a sampling of data collection instruments.

We are grateful for the opportunity to serve readers who are caring for seriously ill patients. We will appreciate your responses and suggestions, your stories, and the resources you find useful. We hope that when groups improve their own practices, they will share their programs, innovations, and successes with us by contacting the Center to Improve Care of the Dying and letting us share their stories with others. Please send them to the Center to Improve Care of the Dying, RAND, 1200 S. Hayes Street, Arlington, VA 22202–5012, or cicd@rand.org.

This book owes its existence to the Retirement Research Foundation of Chicago, Illinois, which gave a generous grant to enable us to work on it over two years. In addition, the Alfred P. Sloan Foundation of New York City has supported development of a companion book for patients, families and caregivers, the *Handbook for Mortals: Guidance for People Facing Serious Illness*, and that simultaneous work has enriched this book. The Oxford University Press and especially our editor, Joan Bossert, have been most supportive, flexible, and efficient. We also note with gratitude the guidance and commitment of James Levine, our literary agent.

Proceeds from the sale of this book will support Americans for Better Care of the Dying (ABCD), a national charitable organization dedicated to public education and policy advocacy on behalf of improving care for the last phase of life. Updates and reference information will readily be found on the Web site: http://www.abcd-caring.org. ABCD's monthly newsletter, *The Exchange*, which is available by subscription or on the Web, keeps pace with change and innovations in this field. We invite all readers to join ABCD to help raise a voice for good care at the end of life (P.O. Box 346, Marvin Center, Washington, DC 20052).

Just wanting to improve the way an organization provides end-of-life care puts health care managers and providers in excellent company. Some of the most prestigious and progressive hospitals, nursing homes, home care agencies, and hospices in America are undertaking the same task. And so too are some hospitals and home care agencies in the poorest and most disenfranchised communities in the country. All have found that improvement is possible. Although each approaches its problems differently, each has something to teach about improving end-of-life care.

Many people have been involved in writing and editing this book. Among us, we have cared for thousands of people who died. Also among us are some well-known leaders of quality improvement and managers of large care systems.

We are grateful for all those who so graciously contribute to help improve care for us all when we face the end of life.

# Acknowledgments

The Institute for Healthcare Improvement and the Center to Improve Care of the Dying renew their thanks to the American Hospital Association, the Nathan Cummings Foundation, Project on Death in America, the Alfred P. Sloan Foundation, the U.S. Department of Veterans Affairs, the Retirement Research Foundation, and the Robert Wood Johnson Foundation for their support of the Breakthrough Series and the writing of this book.

GRANT

# Contents

*The Core Team*

*Phil Higgins*, MS candidate, Center to Improve
Care of the Dying

*Andrea Kabcenell*, RN, MPH, Institute for
Healthcare Improvement

*Janice Lynch Schuster*, writer, Americans for
Better Care of the Dying

*Joanne Lynn*, MD, MA, MS, Center to Improve
Care of the Dying

*Casey Milne*, RN, BSN, CCM, CMC, Resource
Connectors, Ltd., and Center to Improve
Care of the Dying

*Lisa Spear*, Center to Improve Care of the
Dying

*Anne Wilkinson*, PhD, MS, Center to Improve
Care of the Dying


*Contributors*

*Felicia Cohn*, PhD, National Research Council/
Institute of Medicine

*Janet Heald Forlini*, JD, Abt Associates

*Nicole Makosky Fowler*, MHSA, Presbyterian
Senior Care (Oakmont, PA)

*Joan Harrold*, MD, Hospice of Lancaster County
(Lancaster, PA)

*Michelle Jacobs*, MPH candidate, Center to
Improve Care of the Dying

*Tom Nolan*, PhD, and Kevin Nolan, MS,
Associates in Process Improvement

*Christina Puchalski*, MD, Center to Improve
Care of the Dying


*Special Thanks to Many Others, Including:*

*Samira Beckwith*, ACSW, Hope Hospice and
Palliative Care (Fort Myers, FL)

*Paul Brenner*, Jacob Perlow Hospice
(New York, NY)

*Harvey Max Chochinov*, MD, PhD, University of
Manitoba (Winnipeg, Manitoba, Canada)

*June Dahl*, PhD, University of Wisconsin
(Madison, WI)

*Charlotte Eichna*, student intern, Center to
Improve Care of the Dying

*Betty Ferrell*, PhD, City of Hope (Duarte, CA)

*Ellen Fox*, MD, Department of Veterans
Affairs

*Stephen Franey*, FAACT (Portland, OR)

*Barbara Kreling*, Center to Improve Care of
the Dying

*Nancy Persily*, George Washington University
Medical Center

*J. Donald Schumacher*, PsyD, Center for Hospice
and Palliative Care (Cheektowaga, NY)

*Sherri Solomon*, RN, BSN, MPA, Hospice of
Michigan (Southfield, MI)

*Bill Thar*, MD, MPH, Franklin Health, Inc.
(Upper Saddle River, NJ)

*Susan Tolle*, MD, Oregon Health Services
University (Portland, OR)

*Vincent Jay Vanston*, MD, Mercy Health Partners
(Scranton, PA)


*Faculty: IHI Breakthrough Collaborative on
Care at the End of Life Series Planning Group*

*Joanne Lynn*, MD, MA, MS, Chair

*Andrea Kabcenell*, RN, MPH, Collaborative
Director

*Margaret Campbell*, MSN, CNS, Detroit
Receiving Hospital (Detroit, MI)

*Carolyn Cassin*, MPA, VistaCare
(Scottsdale, AZ)

*Richard Della Penna*, MD, Kaiser Permanente
(San Diego, CA)

*Perry Fine*, MD, University of Utah
(Salt Lake City, UT)

*Connie A. Jastremski*, MS, MBA, RN, SUNY
College of Nursing (Syracuse, NY)

*Timothy Keay*, MD, University of Maryland
School of Medicine (Baltimore, MD)

*Tom Nolan*, PhD, Associates in Process
Improvement (Silver Spring, MD)

*Thomas Smith*, MD, Medical College of Virginia/
Massey Cancer Center (Richmond, VA)

*Neil Wenger*, MD, UCLA School of Medicine
(Los Angeles, CA)

*Anne Wilkinson*, PhD, MS, Center to Improve
Care of the Dying

Albemarle Home Care/Albemarle Hospice (Elizabeth City, NC)

Allina Health System (Roseville, MN)

Balm of Gilead (Birmingham, AL)

Beth Israel Deaconess Medical Center (Boston, MA)

Cedars-Sinai Health System (Los Angeles, CA)

Clarian Health Partners (Indianapolis, IN)

Community Hospitals Indianapolis (Indianapolis, IN)

Community Memorial Hospital (Menomonee Falls, WI)

Coney Island Hospital (Brooklyn, NY)

Dartmouth-Hitchcock Medical Center (Lebanon, NH)

Department of Veterans Affairs Medical Center (Dayton, OH)

Elmhurst Hospital Center (Queens, NY)

Fairview Health System (Minneapolis, MN)

Franciscan Health System (Tacoma, WA)

✓ George Washington University Medical Center (Washington, DC)

Good Samaritan Regional Medical Center (Phoenix, AZ)

Gunderson Lutheran (La Crosse, WI)

✓ Hamot Medical Center (Erie, PA)

HealthPartners (Bloomington, MN)

Hope Hospice and Palliative Care (Fort Myers, FL)

Hospice at Greensboro and the Moses Cone Health System (Greensboro, NC)

Hospice of the Blue Grass (Lexington, KY)

Hospice of Michigan (Southfield, MI)

Hospice of Palm Beach County, Inc. (West Palm Beach, FL)

Hospice Care of Rhode Island (Pawtucket, RI)

Kaiser Permanente, San Diego (San Diego, CA)

M. D. Anderson Cancer Center (Houston, TX)

Massey Cancer Center at Virginia Commonwealth University (Richmond, VA)

✓ Mercy Health Partners (Scranton, PA)

North Kansas City Hospital (North Kansas City, MO)

On Lok Senior Health Services (San Francisco, CA)

Palliative Care Center of the North Shore (Evanston, IL)

Parkland Health and Hospital System (Dallas, TX)

Pediatric Advanced Cancer Team–Children's Hospital/Dana-Farber Cancer Institute (Boston, MA)

Queen Elizabeth II Health Sciences Centre (Halifax, Nova Scotia, Canada)

Saint Thomas Health Services (Nashville, TN)

San Diego Hospice (San Diego, CA)

Seton Medical Center (Austin, TX)

St. Joseph Hospital (Orange, CA)

St. Mary's Hospital Medical Center (SSM) (Madison, WI)

St. Mary's Health Center/SSM Health Care System (St. Louis, MO)

Strong Memorial Hospital (Rochester, NY)

UCLA Medical Center (Los Angeles, CA)

United Hospital (Allina Health Systems) (St. Paul, MN)

University of Utah Hospitals and Clinics (Salt Lake City, UT)

VA Medical Center (Gainesville, FL)

Wishard Health Services (Indianapolis, IN)

Wyoming Valley Health Care System (Wilkes-Barre, PA)

# PART I

## OVERVIEW

# Introduction

*Continuous Quality Improvement
for Better End-of-Life Care*

**1**

Our great-grandparents could only have imagined the "problems" improved public health and fantastic medical technology have created in our lives. To our predecessors, who had an average life expectancy of 46 years, our journey into old age would have seemed remarkable. And it is. Most of us will live well into our eighth decade, long enough to have had several careers, seen our children grown, and fulfilled many of our dreams and hopes.

Yet this journey is not easy. The diseases that kill us—often, congestive heart failure, chronic obstructive pulmonary disease, cancer, stroke, or dementia—occasion a prolonged time of disability and illness before death.

Living longer does not necessarily mean dying better; in fact, some of us suffer terribly while ill and dying, despite medication and services that can prevent and relieve many symptoms.

When people are seriously ill and dying, they often require ongoing, concentrated health care that includes psychosocial services and support. Patient and family needs may range from something as basic as understanding when to take medications, to something as complex as getting just the right home wheelchair delivered and paid for.

Research shows that patients and families do not ordinarily receive compassionate, humane care at the end of life. What is easy and routine is what usually happens—and in most health care settings, what happens is enough to heal the sick and cure the lame. Yet it does not comfort the dying.

It is not that health care professionals and society set out to create a terrible system, aiming to torment patients and families. Instead, the system is what developed while we tended to other urgent issues about cure and treatment. The health care

> We are what we repeatedly do. Excellence, then, is not an act, but a habit.
>
> —Aristotle

**Table 1.1 A Century of Change**

|  | 1900 | 2000 |
|---|---|---|
| Age of death | 46 years | 78 years |
| Leading causes of death | infection<br>accident<br>childbirth | cancer<br>heart disease<br>stroke/dementia |
| Usual place of death | home | hospital |
| Most medical expenses | paid by family | paid by Medicare |
| Disability before death | not usually | >4 years, on average |

system is tailored to handle emergencies and injuries, diagnostic tests, and surgery; but it is not designed to accommodate long periods of illness, to meet the needs of very frail elderly patients, or to address the diverse needs that dying patients have. The health care system is not designed to pay for or coordinate comprehensive medical and social services over the course of several years in a patient's life. Too many dying patients live and die in pain and experience distressing or uncomfortable symptoms. That such symptoms persist in an era that has seen the advent of so many effective treatments is an indictment of the status quo.

### The Temporarily Immortal and the Dying: Who's Who?

We talk about the living and the dying as if the difference were very obvious, as obvious as the distinction between men and women. But deciding who is "dying" is more subjective than that, more like the distinctions between "short" and "tall" or "thin" and "heavy," more a matter of perspective. We see death as if it were another country, and the dying as its residents, who enter on a particular date and time, and exit on another. Those not within the borders are safely excluded from that citizenry.

As long as we—patients, families, caregivers, clinicians—are pursuing a cure or even a "return to health," we see ourselves as being among the "living"—the "temporarily immortal." Once we accept that there is no cure, then we somehow join the "dying." Most of us would prefer to be counted among the dying for a short time at the end of life, not for years and years.

Many people with serious and eventually fatal illness continue to work and perform their social roles. Most do not look as though they are dying—and would not describe themselves that way, either. Different fatal illnesses result in very different courses to death. The point at which dying begins is often impossible to define.

The rather misleading way we think about the dying frames much of our public policy and health care. The Medicare hospice benefit, for instance, requires that patients have a "life expectancy of less than six months if the disease takes its normal course." Many laws about living wills, forgoing life-sustaining treatment, and advance directives use the term "terminal illness."

Estimating exactly when someone will die is very difficult to do, even for doctors who regularly work with dying patients. Although a disease such as cancer generally follows a predictable final phase, other diseases, such as dementia or heart disease, do not. In fact, most people who die of heart failure have a reasonable chance of living for another six months, even in what proves to be their last week of life. The SUPPORT investigators found that the median lung cancer patient still had a 50/50 chance to live for another two months one week before death—and a 20 percent chance on the day before death. For congestive heart failure patients a week before death, the median patient had about an 80 percent chance to live another two months; one day before death, that patient still had a 70 percent chance. In short, such patients do not seem discernibly different in their last few days than they were some months earlier.

When trying to label patients as dying (or not), organizations need to begin by redefining their terms. Rather than focusing on those who are clearly "dying," consider patients for whom increasing illness and disability will lead to death sometime in the next few years, and think about how to offer them the kinds of services that help patients live well while dying. We have come to use the "surprise" question, first used by Franciscan Health Services in Washington State. Ask clinicians, "Would you be surprised if this patient died in the next six months or so?"

This approach works well for defining the population for whom appropriate services include advance care planning, comfort care, and psychosocial support. However, defining the population in this way means there is no clear transition between "treatment" and "palliation." Some patients will need both ICU care and DNR decisions; some will want to be on transplant lists and tape an oral history for a family legacy.

Hospice: A Good Model— But Is It Enough?

For the last 25 years, people have found much help in hospice programs, which provide a comprehensive array of services to promote patient choice in end-of-life care and to attend to family needs. The hospice movement, which originated in England, gained popularity in America in the late 1970s; by 1981, the Medicare hospice benefit meant that hundreds of thousands of dying people could receive hospice care.

However, not everyone fits the hospice admission criteria that require patients to have a life expectancy of less than six months and to no longer participate in "curative" treatments. As a result, hospice serves about 23 percent of the people who die each year, for an average of about a month. The vast majority of dying patients— and, in turn, their families— do not have access to the health care and social support that hospice provides as a framework for peaceful dying.

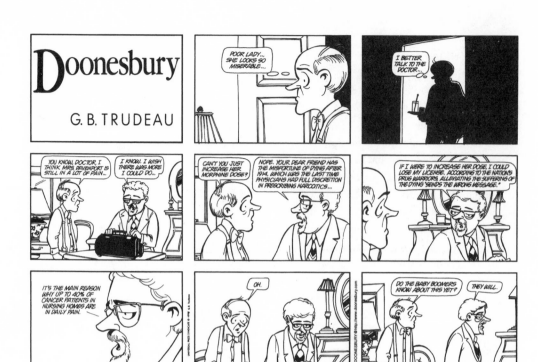

### The Breakthrough Series to Improve End-of-Life Care

The problems in end-of-life care, having received so much media attention that a Sunday "Doonesbury" featured the issue, have reached a crisis point—and a turning point. In 1996, the Institute for Healthcare Improvement (IHI) recognized that the end-of-life field might be ripe for substantial quality improvement using a collaborative approach: the Breakthrough Series. Experts in the field knew something about how to improve care, but there was a chasm between the best available knowledge and everyday practice.

Some organizations, true innovators in the field, had begun to respond to problems in care of the dying and were models for improvement. IHI leaders and faculty were convinced that improving care at the end of life would certainly achieve better clinical outcomes and, along the way, might reduce health care costs while improving patient and family satisfaction.

From July 1997 to July 1998, 47 health care organizations, including hospitals, hospices, home health agencies, long-term care facilities, Veterans Affairs medical centers, and community-based organizations, participated in the Breakthrough Series Collaborative on Improving End-of-Life Care.

Brainstorming sessions among leaders, experts, and faculty identified four target areas that could be improved immediately if an organization set out to do so:

- Improve pain and other symptom management
- Reduce the number of transfers and increase continuity of care
- Improve advance care planning
- Attend to the spiritual needs and opportunities for meaningfulness of patients and families

As the project got under way, participants and others found alarming problems in what they were doing as part of their "usual" care:

- One hospice discovered that half the patients being admitted had pain intensity levels greater than 5 (on a 0-to-10 scale).
- One hospital learned that it took 59 minutes from pain assessment to orders, and 110 more minutes from orders to administration—so hospital patients in pain were ordinarily waiting three hours for a response.
- One found that one-third of its attending physicians did not register to prescribe controlled substances and thus could not manage serious pain when patients were being discharged from the hospital.

The 47 organizations in the Breakthrough Series focused on quick changes, often starting by trying new programs or ideas on one or two or a dozen patients. They worked toward rapid breakthroughs, important improvements that could be done on a small scale "by next Tuesday." When these tests worked, they were tested with larger groups of patients, or in new settings. Organizations abandoned ideas that did not lead to improvement—and then came at the problem from a different angle.

Many participants found broad institutional support for their work—and others discovered that their work in improving end-of-life care had benefits for other units and providers in their systems. Some encountered unexpected obstacles. And others found that measuring change—and whether or not change amounted to improvement—was essential but largely uncharted territory.

Teams achieved many of their goals, often within just a few months. Examples are:

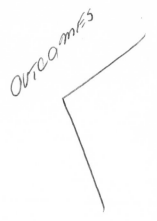
*Outcomes*

- Pain assessment was made a "fifth vital sign" and was assessed on 100 percent of shifts or visits.
- Dyspnea and other symptoms were monitored and treated by protocol.
- Advance care plans were documented for at least 80 percent of patients with serious illnesses.
- Comfort plans and hospice care were instituted earlier in the course of care.
- Families and patients experienced no episodes when pain or other symptoms felt "out of control."

By the end of the year, most were satisfied with the progress they had made, and many were committed to continuing their work to improve care. Here are some of the results. We'll tell their stories later; here we are just showing the kinds of gains made.

### Franciscan Health Systems

Compared to a control group of patients in a different site in the same care system (located in Washington State), a group targeted by Franciscan's Supportive Care Services had significantly fewer hospitalizations in the last year of life.

### Community Memorial Hospital

In September 1997, 13 out of 20 dying medical/oncology patients at Community Memorial Hospital in Menomonee Falls, Wisconsin, had their pain management goals met. By March, that number had increased to 100 percent.

### Veterans Affairs Healthcare System

When the project began, 15 percent of patients at Veterans Affairs Healthcare System in Dayton, Ohio, had documented

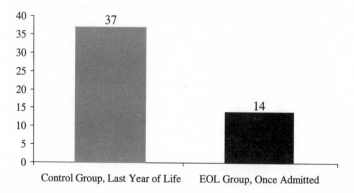

Figure 1.1 Number of Hospitalizations, Last Year of Life. Reprinted with permission of Franciscan Health System, Tacoma, WA.

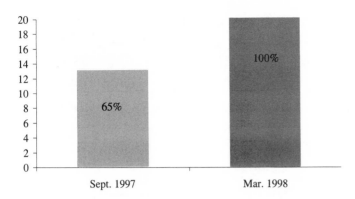

Figure 1.2 Patient's Pain Goal Achieved. Reprinted with permission of Community Memorial Hospital, Menomonee Falls, WI.

advance care plans; within 12 weeks, 90 percent of randomly sampled medical records had plans documented.

## Improvement around the Country

Today, many organizations are working to improve end-of-life care, committed to ensuring that all patients and families experience a "good death," a comfortable and meaningful period of time while living with serious, eventually fatal illness. These organizations include the Last Acts campaign of the Robert Wood Johnson Foundation, the Education for Physicians on End-of-Life Care (EPEC) of the American Medical Association, hospices and their professional associations, Americans for Better Care of the Dying, and multiple programs sponsored by the Department of Veterans Affairs.

Improvement in end-of-life care will ultimately come from many areas, from many approaches to change, and from the joint efforts of biomedical researchers, policymakers, health care professionals, and the public. Many strategies, in addition to quality improvement activities, will lead to significant improvements in end of life care. For instance:

- Biomedical researchers are trying to further understand the mechanisms of pain and other symptoms and to develop new ways to treat these problems.
- Alternative financing mechanisms have been proposed— for instance, the National Hospice and Palliative Care Organization hopes to revise the six-month prognosis rule for hospice admission to allow more access to hospice; and the Center to Improve Care of the Dying is undertaking a demonstration project, MediCaring, aimed at developing comprehensive ways to care for seriously ill patients with,

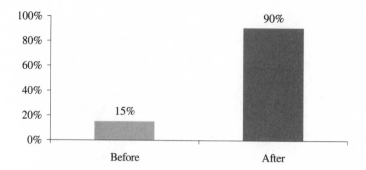

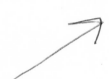

Figure 1.3 Advance Care Planning Documentation. Reprinted with permission of UA Healthcare System: Dayton, OH.

for example, congestive heart failure and chronic obstructive pulmonary disorders.

- Professional organizations are developing education programs, adding end-of-life issues to medical exams, and offering more continuing education courses addressing end-of-life issues.
- Grassroots, philanthropic, and consumer groups are pushing the health care industry, lawmakers, and society to look at "the American way of death" and to change it.

Most of us alive today—you, the reader, and the people you love—will die late in life of chronic illness; we will turn to the health care system for information, care, and support. We will be fortunate to live long and to be relatively healthy for a long time. We know that the care system does not function well, that most dying patients and their families suffer at the end of life. And we have an unprecedented opportunity to improve that system, to make a difference in how people die—not only in the next decade, but in the next year. Such opportunities to make a difference are rare—and if we do not take it now, we will find ourselves dying in the very system we allowed to drift.

### Innovators Need to Know

- Better end-of-life care demands a profound change in how we finance, design, and deliver health care for people with chronic and life-threatening illnesses.
- Categorizing the "dying" and the "living" prevents us from developing adequate systems of care for seriously ill patients.
- Rapid-cycle changes based on the Plan-Do-Study-Act quality improvement model can create real improvement in most organizations in less than a year.
- Many health care organizations have used the Plan-Do-Study-Act model to make significant strides in how they care for seriously ill patients.

# 2

# How to Make
# Improvement Happen

For most people, most of the time, what is easy and routine is what happens—until that easy routine comes apart. One case in point is how the health care system treats dying patients. In some instances, of course, it is not that the system is coming apart but that it was never developed. Readers seeking to fix or change this system may feel—for a while, at least—like loose cannons in their own organizations. This book shows how to test creative ideas and solutions with small groups of patients and, then, how to improve on those ideas to foster even more improvement. The model used is called the Plan-Do-Study-Act (PDSA) cycle; it is a practical and proven quality improvement tool. With this model, teams can start at virtually any point in the routine and change it for the better. This model is meant not to replace change models that organizations may already be using but to streamline and accelerate improvement. Most important, health care providers can apply the model in their daily routines to improve how they care for dying patients and families.

The PDSA model requires teams to set aims, measure changes, and decide whether or not they represent an improvement. The model has two parts that teams must use in order to make it work. The first part requires asking (and answering) three fundamental questions:

- What are we trying to accomplish?
- How will we know that a change is an improvement?
- What changes can we make that will result in improvement?

The second part requires taking action, using the PDSA cycle to test and implement changes in real work settings.

Whether you think you can, or whether you think you can't, you're right.

—Henry Ford

11

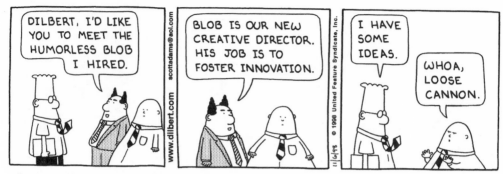

The questions are simple and straightforward, but answering them takes thought and analysis. The answers to these questions are the basis for improvement efforts. For instance, staff at Unique Hospice and Palliative Care Unit might think that they outperform the national average on pain management. After all, they reason, families and loved ones never complain. Even so, the group's Grade A Improvement team decides to examine the unit's performance, with the aim of showing that all patients on one unit are assessed for pain and that pain intensity levels will be at or below a 3 (on a scale of 0 to 10).

How will the group know that its change—reviewing charts for pain assessment and follow-up—is an improvement? Because the team has set a goal known to be part of good practice, for instance, that patient pain intensity levels will be below a 4. After reviewing five patients each week for one month on pain assessment, the team discovers that only three-fourths of patients have documented assessment and follow-up procedures and that more than half report pain intensity scores greater than 5. These data are very revealing to this team, who felt, like others, that no improvement was needed in their pain management program.

What changes can the team now do that will lead to improvement? The team begins a second improvement cycle and decides to measure "Pain as a Fifth Vital Sign." (This project is described in chapter 3.) Ongoing data collection will help them determine whether the team has reached its goal of 100 percent of patients being routinely assessed for pain and the appropriate intervention for pain relief being undertaken.

### Linking Plan-Do-Study-Act Cycles

The completion of each PDSA cycle rolls directly into the start of the next one. A team learns from the test (What worked

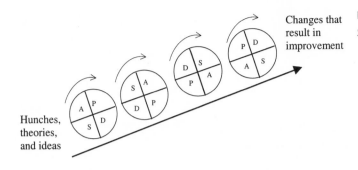

Figure 2.1 General Approach to Sequential PDSA Cycles.

Changes that result in improvement

Hunches, theories, and ideas

and what did not? What should be kept, changed, or abandoned?) and uses this information to plan the next test. By linking PDSA cycles in this way, teams refine the change until it is ready for broader implementation.

People are far more willing to test a change when they know the changes can and will be modified as needed, and quickly. Linking small tests helps overcome an organization's natural resistance to change. The phrase "It is only a test" is very reassuring to many.

Teams also find that they can test more than one change at a time, although each test ultimately leads to the same goal. The accompanying graphic shows the PDSA cycle as a dynamic process in which "hunches" can lead to results—as illustrated by the cycles showing how changes in family discussion, ventilator weaning, and sedation usage can point to improved family satisfaction with the intensive care unit (ICU).

## Setting Aims

Improvement requires setting aims. Without intent, there is no improvement. How can teams select their aims? One way is to review some of the "best practices" and "even better

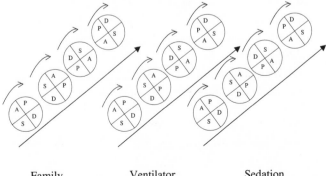

Family Discussion    Ventilator Weaning    Sedation Usage

Figure 2.2 Several PDSA Cycles to Tackle One Problem, Ventilator Withdrawal.

practices" presented in part II. If best practices for pain relief are not utilized at their organization, a team might want to select one or two ideas and use them as aims. Teams can also talk to patients and families and get a feel for what is lacking (or what is working) in the care and treatment they receive.

Set aims that will matter to patients and families; these are the aims most likely to motivate professional caregivers to improve practice.

Express aims in terms that can be quantified. For example, we want:

- A 30 percent reduction in patients reporting pain greater than 4 (out of 10)
- A 50 percent increase in those who state that their wishes are known and have been followed
- At least 90 percent of families reporting that they always know who to contact for emergencies

### Establishing the Team

Organizations that make change happen are those that value innovation and provide the time and other resources needed to test and learn from changes. An important assumption of rapid quality improvement is that "frontline" providers and others are familiar with the "nuts and bolts" of a particular care system—and that they already know a good deal about what might work better. Often, by encouraging frontline staff to solve long-recognized problems, teams find solutions.

With an aim in place, teams can begin to recruit others to help accomplish their goals. Obviously, teams need to have the right clinical and administrative people involved to make change happen. But this team will require support. Senior leaders and upper management will have to charter the team and approve of its aim, while many others need to endorse the improvement team's effort, creating organization-wide support for the endeavor.

Improving end-of-life care requires interdisciplinary action. The physicians, nurses, social workers, chaplains, pharmacists, administrators, and others who care for patients must work together to achieve improvement aims.

Teams need expertise of three types: system leadership, technical expertise, and day-to-day leadership. System leaders, such as vice presidents, need not be on the team, but they do need to care about and support the team's work. More than one

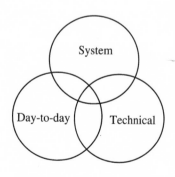

Figure 2.3 Essential Areas of Expertise in a Good Team.

person on the team may fit each dimension, and one individual may fill more than one role.

Improvement teams usually include the five to eight key participants in a care delivery issue. This number provides representatives from many disciplines, and enough people to share the work. However, there are not so many involved that meeting and decision making become difficult. Some programs seek ideas and input from patients and families, but including them on the team is usually not practical. Instead, teams have solicited ideas from patients by inviting 8 or 10 patients (or surrogates) to participate in a group discussion focused on improvements they would make in the organization's programs, services, and style.

The box to the right highlights the key reason for including different staff from all levels of the organization, and the skills and resources they can bring to improvement projects. Assisted living facilities, which may not have on staff all of the people needed to create change, might look to communities for links to pain clinics, hospice programs, or care managers.

## Establishing Measures

Measurement is an important part of the improvement process, allowing teams to quantify changes and determine whether or not a specific change actually leads to an improvement.

Measurement should provide answers to specific questions. For example, did instituting a protocol reduce the incidence of pain? Did establishing a set of advance care planning progress notes and procedures increase the percentage of patients who had discussed what they wished with their physician? Did the provision of written information and reminders prevent families from making unnecessary ER visits?

Improvement efforts require one or two key indicators documented over time. How much information will you need? Just enough to convince a benevolent skeptic. The data have to be credible, and on target, but not extensive. Avoid spending time building a large dataset; you really only need to know two or three things about each of a dozen patients. If you want to learn more about whether patient preferences are made part of treatment planning, you don't really need to collect reams of demographic and psychological profile data, only data focused on whether wishes were sought, documented, and respected.

The most convincing indicators are often those documented in a time series—percent of clinic patients each month who

---

### A Sample Quality Improvement Roster

*System Leadership—Vice President for Patient Services, Director of Palliative Medicine*

- Enough clout to institute change
- Authority to allocate the necessary time and resources
- Power in all areas affected by the change

*Technical Expertise— Physician—Champion*

- Knows the subject intimately
- Understands the care process
- Has expertise in improvement methods to help the team determine what to measure, assist in the design of simple, effective measurement tools, and provide guidance on the collection, interpretation, and display of data

*Day-to-Day Leadership— Nurse Manager, Pharmacist, Clinical Social Worker*

- Drives the project
- Assures that tests are implemented and data are collected ➡

---

have had an advance care planning discussion, or the average response time for pain relief on the oncology unit each week. Data plotted over time show the temporal relationship between changes made and the results, making a more convincing case that specific changes lead to improvement. Sometimes it is enough to measure "before" and "after," but that strategy won't let you evaluate whether it was the interventions or something else that had an effect.

Don't know where to start? Measures can have a positive or negative spin, depending on what a group wishes to show. Here are three sample "positive" measures:

- Each month, find the average days in hospice care for all patients with metastatic cancer.
- Each week, measure the percent of ICU families who say that patients' wishes were known and followed.
- Each week, find out the percent of patients whose pain intensity did not exceed their stated goal.

Other indicators may reflect poorly on what an organization is doing—but can demonstrate the need for change. Negative indicators might include the following:

- Each month, count the number of 911 calls made by outpatient hospice families.
- Each month, count the number of heart failure patients whose disease exacerbations lead to hospitalizations.
- Each week, count the number of dying patients who receive meperidine for pain.

### Establishing Registries

Teams need to find patients to target for quality improvement efforts. One way to do this is to establish a patient registry from which to cull data to track how care is affected by quality improvement efforts. The easiest place to start is with a list of patients. For example, groups with computerized patient databases might search for diagnoses, severity, or some other factor. Many teams find that the best way to assemble a registry is to talk to health care providers on a unit or in a specific discipline. For instance, groups involved in improving care for heart failure patients have asked cardiologists to review their patient panel and note whether it would be a surprise if a patient were to die within the year.

Teams can begin to make improvements to the system of care while a registry is being set up. Changes can be developed and tried with the patients identified. Refinements to the changes can be made based on discussions with caregivers, patients, and families. The learning can be expanded as additional patients are added to the registry. Over time, teams can gather evidence about whether a change is an improvement to the system.

## Developing Changes

In coming up with changes, remember this: All improvement requires change, but not all changes result in improvement. Be sure to focus on changes that are most likely to result in improvement. Ideas for change can come from a variety of sources: critical thinking about the current system, brainstorming, observing the process, a hunch, an idea from the scientific literature, or an insight gleaned from a different but analogous situation.

This book makes recommendations for change, based on general ideas about changes likely to work. Changes have proven merit and a basis in scientific or medical research. Many ideas are accompanies by stories from the efforts of other Breakthrough Series teams, describing the changes made and their effect on patient care. These stories and ideas are "rated" according to the accompanying key.

One way to decide whether an idea has merit is to ask frontline staff what they think of it. Their knowledge of the care process, with its inherent problems and feasible solutions, can be trusted as a screen for good ideas.

In the Breakthrough Series collaborative, teams found ideas for change from several sources. These included:

- A matrix of key changes that described current, best, and optimum practices in pain and symptom management, advance care planning, patient and family support, and continuity of care
- Recommendations or guidelines from key groups involved in end-of-life care (e.g., American Pain Society, American Geriatrics Society, and others)
- Published literature, including professional journals; Americans for Better Care of the Dying newsletter (*Exchange*) and Web site
- Conferences and listserv conversations

| Key |
| --- |
| ★★★ Complete cycle (PDSA)—ideas tried and tested, with some evidence for usefulness |
| ★★ Partial cycle (PD)—ideas tried, but evaluation not done or incomplete |
| ★ Plan only (P)—Good idea, but little or no implementation (yet) |

Teams selected areas in which they most needed to improve, then talked to their own staff for ideas and relied on some of the resources just described. Good ideas for improvement can be found everywhere—the challenge is for a team to select the ones that will be most effective in its organization.

## Testing Changes

### The Plan-Do-Study-Act Cycle (PDSA)

The PDSA model thrives on trial and error. The Plan-Do-Study-Act (PDSA) cycle is shorthand for testing a change—by planning it, trying it, observing the consequences, and then acting on what is learned from those consequences.

Teams need to be committed to doing all steps of the cycle. It is the only way to learn from the work.

**Step 1.** Plan a change
- State the objective of the test: What will the team do?
- Make predictions about what will happen and why.
- Develop a plan to test the change (Who will do what? When? Where? What data must be collected?).

**Step 2.** Do a change
- Carry out the test.
- Document problems and unexpected observations.
- Collect and assess data.

**Step 3.** Study a change
- Analyze the data.
- Compare the data to the team's predictions.
- Summarize what the team learns.

**Step 4.** Act on the next change
- Modify plans as needed, including
    Revise the action, or
    Select a new approach, or
    Extend the work into a new area, or
    Institutionalize the change.
- Prepare a plan for the next cycle.

### By Next Tuesday

Accelerating improvement means acting quickly. Most improvement efforts fail because so much time is spent considering, studying, and meeting that nothing ever changes. Organizations that want to improve can simply begin small-scale tests right away—today even! Running small-scale tests sooner improves patient care much more surely and quickly than does running large-scale cycles later. Even an ambitious and innovative change can be tested first on a small scale—for example, with only one or two physicians, with the next five patients, for the next three days. In general, make the strongest change that the team can do quickly, on the smallest sample that will be informative. When a team can show improvement, then expanding the scope will be much easier. But don't be timid about how substantial the change should be. Too trivial a change ruffles no feathers—but it inspires others to accept the status quo.

Each completed PDSA cycle, properly done, provides valuable information and forms the basis for further improvement. If a change that works on a small scale is improved in successive PDSA cycles, it can then be implemented with assurance on a larger scale.

Teams should ask, "What is the largest informative change we can make by next Tuesday?" This will not be the only change a team should make, and probably will not be the most important one, either. But by making an informative change "by next Tuesday," teams can break the inertia that keeps many improvement efforts from getting off the ground.

It is easy to become comfortable with the status quo. What is easy and routine is what happens. By showing practitioners that another way actually works better, you help them to see just how limited and suddenly archaic their routine practice has been.

### Using Storyboards to Demonstrate Progress

What to do with the data once it has been collected, analyzed, and interpreted? Teams need to promote their improvement efforts—sharing them within the organization, with other health care groups, and with the community—to achieve the support necessary to spread the improvements. Breakthrough Series teams show what they know by using storyboards (much like posters) that track progress in key areas. Teams can then tell their stories to colleagues, administrators, the community, and the public—and use simple graphs to demonstrate change and improvement. Storyboards tell the story of the work or project, how it was done, and what it accomplished (Rainey, 1998). In essence, storyboards are a paper "sound bite" that people can see, understand, and remember.

In presenting information via the storyboard, be sure to:

- Design it to be easily and quickly read and understood
- Include only critical information
- Keep it simple
- Tell the truth without fudging
- Make the goal or aim of the project clear and apparent
- Label axes on graphs; give the number of responses and the date

In Breakthrough Series programs, teams follow a basic outline for what to include on their storyboards:

- Organization name and location
- Aim
- Measures
- Changes
- Results

### Spreading Change: From One to Many

When a team improves care for a group of patients or in one unit, the entire organization is likely to want to spread the change further: from cancer to cardiac patients, from one unit to another, or even from one hospital to another within the system.

For dissemination to occur, organizations need:

- A leader who is responsible for the spread of change
- Change that is in accord with the organization's strategic mission for the year
- A well-proven change to spread
- Resources to initiate change in other areas

Breakthrough Series teams have been able to spread enthusiasm for changes from one area to another—from pain management to dyspnea management, and from oncology to the intensive care unit. The opportunity to use this method in multiple areas is compelling.

### Innovation as a Way of Life

When teams begin to use the PDSA model for change in one practice area, they often discover other areas ripe for improvement. Improvements in advance care planning, for

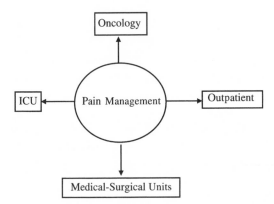

Figure 2.4 Spread the Word: Improvement throughout the Care System.

example, can lead to the need for better spiritual support and increased continuity of care. Most teams learn to tackle many areas at the same time because it makes sense to do so.

There are other spin-offs of this work as well. Better pain management for patients in the last phase of life will undoubtedly lead to better pain management for all patients—from those with postoperative pain to those with chronic pain. Better family support will lead to better communication in the ICU for all families.

Teams with a method for making improvements will make it a way of life in all practice areas, especially if managers support and encourage improvement and innovation.

*Taking Action: Parkland Health &*
*Hospital System*

Parkland Health & Hospital System in Dallas, Texas, is a 997-bed public hospital serving Dallas County and is affiliated with the University of Texas Southwestern Medical School. Three physicians in Hematology-Oncology, a nurse case manager, a nursing unit manager, a chaplain, and the vice president for patient services made up the team. They focused on improving care for oncology patients at the end of life, based on observations that appropriate palliative care referrals were occurring only a few days before death—which was, to this team, too late. Here is what they did:

**1.** They Set Their Aim

Increase by 50 percent the number of medical oncology patients receiving palliative services (pain management, social and spiritual support, primary care, and hospice referral) prior to the last month of life.

Figure 2.5a Palliative Services prior to the Last Month of Life. Reprinted with permission of Parkland Health and Hospital System, Dallas, TX.

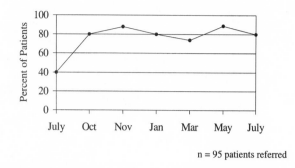

n = 95 patients referred

### 2. They Established Measures

A change is an improvement if there is a substantial increase in something important, for example:

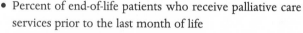

- Percent of end-of-life patients who receive palliative care services prior to the last month of life
- Mean length of time from palliative care referral until death for these patients
- Percent of palliative care patients who achieve their pain management goals (self-determined) or
- Percent of patients and families who are very satisfied with their care

The team felt that all standards should be met, not just increased use of palliative care services. The services had to result in improved experiences for patients.

### 3. They Developed Changes

The team wanted to establish more accessible palliative care, with the goal of enabling hospital staff to provide appropriate pain and symptom management and to get needed referral services. After learning about other palliative care services, Parkland decided to create a clinical position for a case manager to coordinate all palliative care. In this way, the referral process would be standardized, a bottleneck that slowed referrals would be removed, and access to needed information would be greatly enhanced.

### 4. They Tested Changes

The team wanted to establish a standard way of getting people into palliative care and coordinating their care. All of these changes were tested first on a small number of patients. As the team saw positive results, they increased the number of staff

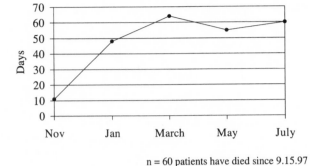

n = 60 patients have died since 9.15.97

Figure 2.5b Average Number of Days Receiving Palliative Services prior to Death. Reprinted with permission of Parkland Health and Hospital System, Dallas, TX.

participating in the project and thus increased the patients receiving palliative services. We have organized a small series of changes into each of the "tests" outlined below.

**Test 1:** Establish a palliative care referral process.

The team designed and tested a process that included who should be referred, procedures for making the referral, and standard palliative care orders.

**Test 2:** Assign a case manager to coordinate palliative services.

The case manager is responsible for finding and receiving consults, coordinating services for patients, maintaining weekly contact with the patients not admitted to hospice, and serving as a liaison between outpatient clinics and hospice providers. This person is the "glue" that holds the care together, who speeds and smooths all transitions. As a result, social work referrals increased 50 percent and pastoral care referrals increased 15-fold (from 6 to 94 percent of patients).

**Test 3:** Train nursing staff in pain assessment.

Once staff members learned about uniform pain assessment and were consistently able to assess patients' pain levels, it became easier to manage pain using palliative care consults and standard orders for pain. Eventually, outpatient clinic nurses also tried out routinely making follow-up phone calls to patients at home to assess pain levels and response to medication changes. They found that most patients continued to have serious pain and that virtually all of them could get this pain under control with one or two phone calls.

**Test 4:** Use multidisciplinary team conferences weekly to plan and modify care.

Multidisciplinary team meetings allow all members of the care team to see the spectrum of needs and respond in a coordinated manner.

**Test 5:** Establish a referral model (algorithm) to increase access and continuity between primary care and oncology.

Specific rules and procedures about who should be referred and when were used to help primary care and oncology physicians improve access to appropriate care.

**5.** They Chalked Up Successes

Parkland staff reported positive results in all four domains targeted by the Breakthrough Series:

- *Continuity*: Eligible patients receiving palliative services increased from 40 percent to 80 percent.
- *Advance care planning*: Average number of days receiving palliative care services prior to death increased from 13 to 58 days.
- *Family support*: Patients or families stating that they were very satisfied with services increased from 40 to 100 percent.
- *Pain management*: Pain management goals are being achieved (there was a 50 percent increase in patients who state that they reach their pain goal), but no change in pain levels is visible as yet.

## Troubleshooting: Ways to Avoid Common Traps

All teams encounter the same pitfalls, and some fall right in. The key is knowing what the problems are. Teams that recognize when they are stuck can often climb right back out.

*Problem 1: Studying the Problem Too Long without Acting*

Teams that spend more than four weeks collecting baseline information are stuck. If discussions about data collection dominate team meetings, the team has fallen into an information abyss.

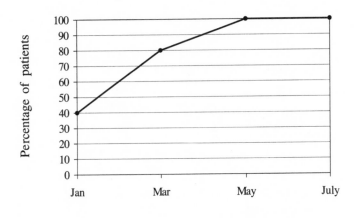

Figure 2.6a Patient/Family Satisfaction. Reprinted with permission of Parkland Health and Hospital System, Dallas, TX.

n = 6 patients surveyed
17 family members surveyed

*Solution: Collect Just Enough Data*

- Use simple sampling techniques, such as "every fifth patient" or "on every Tuesday and Thursday afternoon," for data collection that is good enough.
- Use one or two indicators of the results. For example, including family satisfaction with care may be enough to show that a new communication strategy is working. It would not likely be worth the effort to add 10 more measures just to determine whether a change is an improvement.
- Use available resources. Use paper and pencil methods rather than waiting for the information system to generate

|  | July 1997 | September 1997 | November 1997 | January 1998 | March 1998 | May 1998 | July 1998 |
|---|---|---|---|---|---|---|---|
| Patients received Palliative Services prior to the last month of life | 40% | 80% | 87% | 80% | 76% | 88% | 80% |
| Average number of days receiving services before death | * | * | 13 | 48 | 62 | 55 | 58 |
| Patients receiving Hospice Services | * | * | 63% | * | 70% | 60% | 81% |
| Patients receiving Pastoral Care Consultants | * | * | 6% | * | 77% | 94% | 100% |
| Patients goals for Pain Management met | * | * | 76% | * | 67% | 71% | 71% |

*N = 95 patients*        *\* Not Measured*

Figure 2.6b Palliative Care Service Accomplishments September 1997 to July 1998. Reprinted with permission of Parkland Health and Hospital System, Dallas, TX.

the data needed, or use that electronic data if it has what the team needs! Sometimes teams use the electronic data to get the "denominator"—and another source to get the numerator (for instance, the percentage of patients discharged from the hospital with heart failure who receive supportive care services).

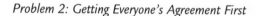

- Integrate data collection with the daily routine. Making pain a fifth vital sign is an excellent example of building a key measure into everyday practice. So is charting on a flow sheet that can be used for data collection, or keeping a check sheet to mark off events (such as referrals to palliative care).

- Use a related measure as a "proxy." If the team cannot measure continuity directly, measure how many different providers see the patient in one day or one week, or the numbers of families who report not knowing who to call in with questions about patient care.

*Problem 2: Getting Everyone's Agreement First*

The entire nursing staff need not agree to treat pain differently. Start with the staff members who will be trying the new assessment approach. In health care, we sometimes seek consensus around changes before agreement is needed or warranted, missing the opportunity to try new approaches. Participants need not agree "for all time," only for a while. Most people can make this commitment just to be cooperative.

*Solution: Start with Small Groups and Gradually Add People Working on the Change*

- Find innovative staff members—the champions—who are interested in testing changes first.
- Have them design and test the changes on a small scale.
- Measure the results and make them visible.
- Gradually bring in successive groups of participants to try the change. For example, recruit another medical group, another nursing unit, or another clinic.

*Problem 3: Educating without Changing Structures or Expectations*

The most common tool for change in health care is an education program. It is also the least effective if done without other system changes. Education is very useful for helping people adopt new changes that they are motivated to adopt, but education alone does not create lasting change. If your massive education campaign leads to no real behavior changes, you are going nowhere.

### Solution: Focus on Powerful Changes

- Choose changes that cause a direct improvement in behavior. Implement a protocol, change a referral pattern, establish specific criteria, or standardize a previously erratic pattern of care.
- Use the right words. When describing the change, be sure to use words such as "revise, improve, implement, establish," not "continue, educate, study, recruit."
- Create prompts for correct behavior. Make it easy to participate—distribute a pain protocol card or an alternative therapy kit, and make these available to everyone.
- If the organization really needs an education program, include education about the PDSA model for change, and integrate education with implementation.

### Problem 4: Tackling Everything at Once

A team may be eager to tackle it all—pain management, advanced care planning, and meaningfulness and spiritual support—aiming to improve every problem in patient care at once. However, starting changes in each area simultaneously takes a tremendous amount of staff time and requires tolerance of uncertainty and disruption in many areas at once. If team members feel that they cannot pay attention to all the changes the team wants to make, then the team has taken on too much.

### Solution: Focus and Sequence the Changes

- Focus on one area first.
- Choose the change that will be the "easiest." The easiest is likely to be the one with a strong champion, senior leadership support, and popular appeal. Be sure it is a real change, preferably one that will improve patient or family experience, not just education or data collection.
- Let senior leaders know what you need to make progress and ask for help.
- Select subsequent changes based on what the team is already accomplishing. For example, working on advance care planning may naturally lead the team to find ways to improve bereavement support.

*Problem 5: Measuring Nothing—or Everything*

Having no data is a problem. Unfortunately, good work will not stand on its own merits. If the team cannot describe the effect of the changes it has made, it will not be able to continue with the good ones—or recognize the bad ones. And, as mentioned above, teams need to avoid the comfortable niche of measuring so much that they don't have time to make much happen. We find it a useful rule of thumb to allocate energy this way: "If you have five units of energy to spend on making improvement, use four on change and one on measurement." Be sure not to use much less on change or much more on measurement.

*Solution: Just Enough Data (again)*

- See problem 1 above!
- Track at least one indicator over time. Measure it at least monthly.
- Use "subjective" data. Ask two or three physicians every month how the pain protocol is working out for them. Ask one or two patients every day how they feel about the planning discussion. Especially as an interim step, these responses will be useful for identifying problems and will also spur you to further (useful) data collection.

*Problem 6: Failing to Build Support
for Replication*

If a team has great results for a few patients, but no one else adopts the changes, it has not made much headway. Early in the process, team members need to tell others about what they're doing—to make colleagues curious to know more—so that others will be more willing to try the team's changes. In this way, teams do good work for their patients while laying the groundwork for further improvements.

*Solution: Promote the Project and
Engage Senior Leaders*

- Announce the improvements being made, including aims and schedule.
- Post results where staff can see them. For example, post a chart showing the percentage of patients on the unit

with pain less than 4 out of 10 and update the data each week—or each day.

- Promote the topic in newsletters and paycheck stuffers and on bulletin boards.
- Engage senior leaders. Update the senior leader sponsoring the team's work on changes and results and what he or she could do to promote the change. Promotion examples include putting the project on the senior management meeting agenda, mentioning the work at board meetings, writing an article or letter about it, or inviting leaders to attend team meetings or visit patients involved in the intervention.
- Train others to follow the team's lead. Be sure to provide adequate training to the staff members who are beginning replication of the changes.
- Talk to leaders about their own experiences with end-of-life care—good and bad—to remind them of how important this work is.

## Problem 7: Assuming That the Status Quo Is OK

In health care, we have come to accept some very troubling practices. Think, for instance, about patients in the last phase of life who receive futile CPR or doctors who keep prescribing meperidine. Some aspects of the status quo never set off the alarms that they should. If a team cannot think of anything to improve about the way it cares for dying patients, team members are not looking critically at the status quo. Sometimes, under scrutiny, the status quo actually becomes shocking. Sometimes, just measuring the dysfunction in the status quo is so embarrassing that it motivates a readiness to change.

## Solution: Think about How It Could Be

- Find the horrible stories. Ask two or three nurses or physicians to tell a terrible experience in end-of-life care and identify the arrangements in the organization's systems or routines that allowed the catastrophe to happen.
- Find the ideal. Ask staff members what would be their ideal for care at the end of life, and discuss what would have to change to make this happen in the organization.
- Ask the patients how it could be. Interview two or three families of patients who died in the system and ask what they thought of the care provided: What was helpful? Upsetting? Good? Bad? What could have made it better?

Improving practices within an institution is generally regarded as good management. The use of continuous quality improvement techniques (CQI), however, begins to make innovation look like research, and therein lies a problem.

The primary purpose of ethical review is to assure that a research design uses ethical methods and otherwise conforms to ethical standards. External oversight is provided by committees (often called IRBs, or institutional review boards) that are usually comprised of peers from the scientific, professional, and medical communities and laypeople representing community perspectives.

Research and quality improvement share many characteristics. In CQI endeavors, patients are subject to the efforts to correct, enhance, or otherwise change those practices. This process may involve changes a patient will not notice, such as a new flowchart on which to record vital signs. Or the process may involve noticeable changes that are not burdensome or that a patient might welcome, such as a new practice of having attending physicians' names and phone numbers at the bedside. However, the process may entail changes that result in practices contrary to a patient's expectations—for instance, visits from additional staff members or participation in advance care planning discussions.

Patients whose lives are touched by CQI endeavors are not usually regarded as research subjects. Improvement teams may not have any obligation to obtain the informed consent of their subjects, or even to notify their subjects of the changes being implemented and evaluated, even when some risk to patients

Table 2.1 Characteristics Typical of CQI and Research

|  | CQI | Research |
| --- | --- | --- |
| Develop hypothesis | X | X |
| Gather data | X | X |
| Analyze data | X | X |
| Validate hypothesis | X | X |
| Randomize/control study |  | X |
| Immediate practice change | X |  |
| Enrich knowledge base |  | X |
| Immediate behavior change | X |  |
| External auditing |  | X |
| Applies to larger group |  | X |
| Careful, systematic study |  | X |

is possible. External review is not usually sought. However, to assure that the "good intentions" being examined are not merely the whim of the improvement team, the endeavor should be grounded in the values shared across a community of peers.

## Making and Keeping Promises: Satisfaction Guaranteed?

At first glance, this new approach to change and improvement may seem daunting—or it may appear to be too far from the kinds of change institutions usually practice. But because care of the dying is known to be so poor, and has been so for many years, teams might find solutions just by taking a fresh look at an old problem. One way to do this is to consider making promises to patients and families, promises about how a patient dying in the health care system can expect—and therefore demand—to be treated.

### Making Promises: A Vision of a Better System

A better health care system for the end of life would follow through on these seven promises:

**1.** Good medical treatment:

You will have the best of medical treatment, aiming to prevent exacerbations, improve function and survival, and ensure comfort.

- Patients will be offered proven diagnosis and treatment strategies to prevent exacerbations and enhance quality of life, as well as to delay disease progression and death.
- Medical interventions will be in accord with best available standards of medical practice, and evidence-based when possible.

**2.** Never overwhelmed by symptoms:

You will never have to endure overwhelming pain, shortness of breath, or other symptoms.

- Symptoms will be anticipated and prevented when possible, evaluated and addressed promptly, and controlled effectively.

- Severe symptoms—such as shortness of breath—will be treated as emergencies.
- Sedation will be used when necessary to relieve intractable symptoms near the end of life.

**3.** Continuity, coordination, and comprehensiveness:

Your care will be continuous, comprehensive, and coordinated.

- Patients and families can count on having certain professionals to rely upon at all times.
- Patients and families can count on an appropriate and timely response to their needs.
- Transitions between services, settings, and personnel are minimized in number and made to work smoothly.

**4.** Well-prepared, no surprises:

You and your family will be prepared for everything that is likely to happen in the course of your illness.

- Patients and families will come to know what to expect, and what is expected of them, as the illness worsens.
- Patients and families will receive supplies and training needed to handle predictable events.

**5.** Customized care, reflecting your preferences:

Your wishes will be sought and respected and, whenever possible, followed.

- Patients and families will come to know the alternatives for services and will expect to make choices that matter.
- Patients will never receive treatments they refuse.
- It is usually possible for patients to die at home if they so desire.

**6.** Use of patient and family resources
(financial, emotional, and practical):

We will help the patient and family to consider their personal and financial resources, and we will respect their choices about the use of their resources.

- Patients and families will be aware of services available in their community and the costs of those services.

- Family caregivers' concerns will be discussed and ad-dressed, and respite and home aide care will be considered as part of the care plan when appropriate.

**7.** Make the best of every day:

We will do all we can to see that you and your family will have the opportunity to make the best of every day.

- The patient is treated as a person, not a disease.
- The care team attends to the physical, psychological, so-cial, and spiritual needs of patient and family.
- Families are supported before, during, and after the pa-tient's death.

This sourcebook is full of examples of how others improved practice by reconsidering what they were doing, having a vision of how to do it better, and promising themselves, if no one else, that they would do a better job.

### Innovators Need to Know

- The PDSA model provides a framework for beginning changes on a small scale and increasing their scope as they prove successful.
- Look to frontline staff for ideas on what to improve.
- Recruit a team that can provide day-to-day leadership, has the necessary technical expertise, and has the support of system leadership.
- Groups must collect the data to know when a change is actually an improvement.
- Most groups can do something to improve care "by next Tuesday."
- Barriers to change can be overcome.
- Consider an external ethics review for some CQI projects.

### Resources

*ABCD Exchange*, monthly newsletter from Americans for Better Care of the Dying, features new and innovative programs and ideas: http://www.abcd-caring.org.

Institute for Healthcare Improvement
135 Francis St.
Boston, MA 02215
Phone: 617-754-4800
http://www.ihi.org

*The Fifth Discipline: The Art and Practice of the Learning Organization*, by Peter Lenge. New York: Doubleday, 1990.

*The Improvement Guide: A Practical Approach to Enhancing Organizational Performance*, by G. J. Langley, K. M. Nolan, T. W. Nolan, C. L. Norman, and L. P. Provost. San Francisco: Jossey-Bass, 1996.

*A Whack on the Side of the Head: How You Can Be More Creative*, by Roger Von Oech. New York: Warner, 1990.

*Innovations*, on-line journal on end of life care http://www.edc. org/last acts/

# PART II

## IMPROVED PATIENT CARE THROUGH IMPROVED PRACTICE AND SYSTEMS

The good news about end-of-life care is that any health care organization in the country can take immediate steps to improve how it cares for dying patients and those who love them. These important changes need not wait for one more study, meeting, survey, or signature—health care providers who understand how to use the rapid-cycle model can begin using it this week (or by the time they've finished this book!). Each chapter in this section explains why particular changes are needed and how improvement teams can use the Plan-Do-Study-Act model to achieve them.

Although pain is a frequent problem for patients, it often goes untreated or undertreated. The reasons for this problem are complex, yet some solutions—such as making pain a fifth vital sign or asking patients to set their own target levels for pain intensity—are straightforward. Chapter 3 describes ways organizations can better prevent, assess, and treat pain.

Shortness of breath, or dyspnea, is a common symptom at the end of life, occurring as part of the disease or in the course of ventilator removal. Dyspnea, like pain, is frequently untreated. Chapter 4 describes ways to make its treatment routine and patient comfort a priority.

In a live-for-today society, people find it hard to make plans for the future; serious and complex illness makes advance care planning an even more daunting task for most people. By expanding popular notions of what advance care plans are and should be (beyond the useful but limited living will or the idea that advance plans are simply about "pulling the plug"), health care providers can help patients and families anticipate problems, talk about alternatives and preferences, and map a treatment plan and goals for living well. Chapter 5 describes steps patients, families, and health care providers can take to improve advance care planning.

Serious and complex illness often raise issues of meaningfulness, purpose, and spirituality. Chapter 6 discusses ways to support patients and families and their relationships with one another. Some families appreciate simple gestures, such as being given a pager so they can take a rest while keeping vigil in an ICU; some appreciate visits from hospital chaplains or other spiritual leaders; still others benefit from grief and bereavement programs.

The concluding chapter in this section focuses on ways to improve continuity of care, so that patients do not feel like numbers or diseases or billing codes because organizations do not treat them as if they were. Basic steps, such as preventing in-hospital transfers during the final hours of life, can do much to promote comprehensive care.

# Preventing, Assessing, and Treating Pain

**3**

One need not have read a professional journal lately to know that people are dying in pain. Like the security guard in "Frank and Ernest" (next page), too many health care providers do not hear or have learned to ignore patients' pain.

Several recent studies have demonstrated that pain is undertreated. The Study to Understand Prognoses and Preferences for Outcomes and Risks of Treatments, or SUPPORT (SUPPORT Principal Investigators, 1995), collected data on 9,105 very sick hospitalized patients and, after identifying problems in their care, tried and failed to correct them. SUPPORT researchers found that more than half of the patients who were awake at all in their final days were in serious pain. In a five-state study (Bernabei et al., 1998) of 13,625 nursing home cancer patients over the age of 65, fully one-quarter of those who reported daily pain received no analgesics. Most of the rest received doses that were inadequate or too weak, and performance worsened as patients were older.

Poor pain management is not limited to nursing homes and hospitals. A survey of 3,200 American, British, and Canadian oncologists pointed to serious shortcomings in oncologists' ability to offer optimal pain relief and to recognize depression in their patients. Although 95 percent said they felt competent to manage pain, more than half said that more than 20 percent of their patients die in pain. An analysis of practice patterns found that 25 percent of those surveyed do not routinely provide optimal pain relief. Half said they did not feel competent to manage a dying patient's depression. The survey also found that up to 25 percent of oncologists do not like taking care of dying patients (Emanuel and Emanuel, 1998).

Life's sharpest rapture is the surcease of pain.

—Emma Lazarus

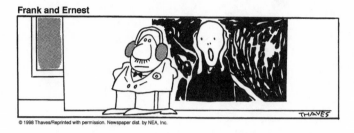

### In This Chapter

Good pain management may even extend life—contrary to the widely held belief that aggressive pain management hastens death. In fact, untreated pain can lead to depression, apathy, and the loss of a will to live. The shortcomings in treating patient pain mean that a wide variety of changes will lead to improvements in patient care. This chapter features easy-to-replicate programs from Breakthrough Series groups, instruments for assessing pain and measuring improvement, and good ideas on how to do a better job—by next Tuesday.

This chapter describes many successful changes, as well as ideas that seem worth trying based on what we know about pain management. Subjects include:

- Defining pain
- Describing patient and provider rights and responsibilities
- Using patient self-reports
- Measuring pain as a fifth vital sign
- Using clinical practice guidelines
- Making pain management an institutional priority
- Setting standards for pain control
- Giving health care providers handy resources and offering ongoing educational programs
- Reviewing prescribing practices for opioids
- Improving practices in nursing homes and assisted living facilities

First, here is a review of current, best, and "even better" practices. The remainder of this chapter focuses on activities that directly affect care and activities that can improve the way an institution or organization improves pain management.

Throughout this sourcebook, activities are marked according to the following key.

## Table 3.1 Use of Analgesics by Nursing Facility Residents with Cancer

| Analgesic use | Daily pain group | No pain |
|---|---|---|
| | (n = 4,003) | n = 9,610) |
| Nonnarcotic only | 659 (16%) | 2,297 (24%) |
| Weak opiates (e.g., codeine) | 1,293 (32%) | 870 (9%) |
| Strong opiates (e.g., morphine) | 1,029 (26%) | 390 (4%) |
| Any analgesic | 2,984 (74%) | 3,557 (37%) |

Reprinted with permission from Bernabei et al., 1998, p. 1879

---

### Key

★★★ Complete cycle (PDSA)—ideas tried and tested, with some evidence for usefulness

★★ Partial cycle (PD)—ideas tried, but evaluation not done or incomplete

★ Plan only (P)—Good idea, but little or no implementation (yet)

---

## Know Current Practices, Emulate "Best" Practices, and Strive for Optimum Practices

Most dying patients, in most settings, most of the time, are in pain or suffer other symptoms. In making baseline measures, many Breakthrough Series teams were surprised to find just how poorly their programs were doing—but this poor finding challenged groups to do better.

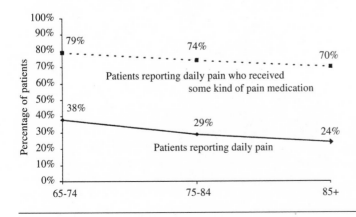

Figure 3.1 Nursing Home Residents Receiving Pain Medications, by Patient Age. Reprinted with permission, Bernabei et al., 1998.

The current state of pain management in most institutions in the country is far from ideal. In contrast, best practices enable clinicians to assess and alleviate most pain and other symptoms. When best practices are used, patients and families come to expect relief from suffering, not agony. By aiming for best and optimum practices, improvement teams can set goals for their patients, hospital wards or units, and institutions.

The following case study shows how one organization pinpointed institutional barriers to effective pain management, then used Plan-Do-Study-Act cycles to improve practice.

### ★★★ St. Mary's Health Center

Nurses, a physician, a pharmacist, a case manager, and a chaplain were on the team for St. Mary's Health Center in St. Louis, Missouri, which aimed "to improve patient satisfaction by improving the assessment and treatment of pain on in-patient medical/surgical units." The team chose this aim after finding that St. Mary's had no standard process to assess or manage pain. The team planned to create a standard that would improve assessment and reduce the response time.

Once the group had its plan, it set goals:

- Assess the intensity of pain for all patients within 30 minutes of arrival in the unit.
- Reduce response time to less than 30 minutes between assessment and orders to administration of pain medications for 80 percent of patients with pain greater than 3 (on a 0 to 10 scale).
- Have 80 percent of patients report satisfaction with how the hospital staff managed their pain.

The team decided to try several changes:

- Add a pain assessment tool that included location, intensity, and a target level to all admission forms.
- Standardize the time frame for completing pain assessment.
- Adapt and distribute an equianalgesic chart.
- Put a pain ruler and face scale at each bedside.

Within a year, the St. Mary's team had data that reflected its success. The accompanying charts compare baseline measures to six months after the intervention began.

Other organizations might want to try some of St. Mary's starting points—for instance, to reduce the time from orders to medication administration—as a place to begin their own pain improvement projects. Groups might consider helping patients and providers define and recognize pain and to define

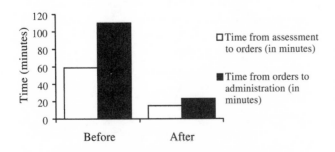

Figure 3.2 Faster Pain Relief. Reprinted with permission of St. Mary's Health Center, St. Louis, MO.

Even Better "Best" Practices

- Pain, depression, dyspnea, and anxiety are assessed on a specified schedule (admission, change in status, and periodically) 100 percent of the time.
- All appropriate modalities are used, often on time-limited trials—including opioids, nonsteroidal anti-inflammatory drugs (NSAIDs), adjuvant analgesics, physical therapy (applications of heat and cold), massage therapy, behavioral techniques, hypnosis, steroids, neuroablative procedures, stimulants, and so on.
- Skilled consultants are readily available to patients in all settings (including ICU, hospital, nursing home, and home).
- Settings are created in which patients and loved ones expect competence, control, and comfort.
- During transfers between units or sites, patients are never left in pain.
- There are routine care reviews and feedback opportunities for quality improvement, public education, and accreditation.

Patient Name: _____ Room #: _____ Home Phone: _____ Medical Record: _____ Date of admission: _____

| Diagnosis: _____ | Admitting MD: _____ | Teaching OR | IF Teaching? |
|---|---|---|---|
| Type of Admission:  OOS   In patient  (circle one) | Non Teaching  (circle ONE) | MD name _____ | |

| Date:<br><br>Reviewer: | Have your pain needs been met to your satisfaction during this hospitalization?<br><br>Yes        No<br><br>Comments: | During this hospitalization have you experienced any unpleasant side effects from your pain medicine?<br><br>Yes        No<br><br>Comments: | If Pain Noted with score > Patient's Target:<br><br>Time Interval (in minutes)<br>Admin.<br>Assessment to Orders | Time Interval (in minutes)<br><br>Orders to Admin. Of Rx | One Hour Post<br><br>Numeric Pain Level<br><br>(0-10) |
|---|---|---|---|---|---|
| Admission Pain Assessed (5th VS) completed within 30 min.of arrival (Y/N) | | | | | |
| Presence and/or Absence Pain Noted (Y/N) | | | | | |
| Location of Pain Noted (Location/N) | | | | | |
| If Pain Noted, Pain Scale Utilized (Y/N) | | | | | |
| Numeric Pain Level (0-10) | | | | | |
| Patient's Target Level | | | | | |
| Date:<br><br>Reviewer: | | | | | |

Figure 3.3 Admitting Pain Assessment. Reprinted with permission of St. Mary's Health Center, St. Louis, MO.

patient and provider rights and responsibilities in terms of pain management.

## ★Define Pain

Severe, unrelieved pain takes a terrible toll on a patient's physical and emotional well-being, compromises his or her quality of life, and can become very stressful for the family and loved ones. In a society that tends to equate suffering with strength—professional ballplayers may be the worst role models for this attitude—admitting to being in pain can be seen as a weakness. Patients and families have their own ideas about pain and their own reasons for not wanting to talk about it. Some fear, for instance, that worsening pain means worsening disease. A useful rule of thumb is that pain is whatever a patient says it is.

Breakthrough Series teams, and pain experts around the country, know that one step in the improvement cycle is to get doctors and nurses to talk to patients about pain. These conversations help patients realize the importance of reporting when they are in pain, understand different treatments for pain, and expect that pain will be relieved. These conversations can comfort patients and families, letting them know that their final months or hours need not be overwhelmed by pain.

Patients may not fully understand how pain can affect all aspects of daily life. Posting the accompanying list in waiting areas or in examination rooms can help them pinpoint their problems and symptoms and may prompt them to ask clinicians for help.

Some patients have trouble rating pain on a 0-to-10 scale. Clinicians can overcome this difficulty by providing patients with a frame of reference. Explain that a 0 or a 1 means no pain. A 3 means a patient might be able to watch an hour of a favorite television show or read a newspaper without paying much attention to being in pain. A 5 means that a patient might be able to watch part of a show or glance at a magazine but is too distracted by pain to find much pleasure in any activities. Any score over a 5 means that a patient is on the verge of being—or is already—consumed by pain and that the pain intensity is creating a medical crisis. Explain to patients that waiting until pain is severe and intense before mentioning it to a doctor or nurse is like waiting until a fever is 106 before calling the doctor. Such a delay can make it even more difficult to control a patient's pain—but it is a mistake many patients and providers make.

### What Can Pain Do to You? It Can Make You:

- Less able to function
- Tired and lethargic
- Lose your appetite or have nausea
- Unable to sleep or have disrupted sleep
- Experience less enjoyment and more anxiety
- Depressed, anxious, or unable to concentrate on anything else
- Feel a loss of control
- Limit contact with family and friends
- Be less able to enjoy affection
- Have a changed appearance
- Feel that you are a burden to families
- Suffer more
- Want to die

*Source*: AHCPR, Management of Cancer Pain

## ★Define Patient and Provider Rights and Responsibilities

Some organizations write and post statements about pain management that explicitly describe patient rights and responsibilities, along with what to expect from health care providers. Such statements put into real, concrete terms what an institution believes it should do for patients and demonstrate a commitment to pain management. People are likely to trust and rely on organizations that make patient comfort a top priority.

### Rely on Patient Self-Reports

Having patients report their pain intensity levels, and helping them to set goals for pain management, is critical to good pain management. However, patients may need guidance before they can describe or rate their pain intensity level. Organizations have an array of standard pain assessment tools from which to choose, as well as newer versions that meet patients' linguistic or expressive abilities. Using these starting points, teams can begin to apply the rapid-cycle model.

### ★★★Standardize Pain Assessment Protocols

*Coney Island Hospital and Kaiser Permanente, San Diego*

Coney Island Hospital is an acute care facility that serves a diverse patient population in Brooklyn, New York. Its Breakthrough Series team aimed to improve pain management through the use of a standard pain intensity scale of 0 to 10. First, the team established baseline measures by informally surveying staff. Nurses, as it turned out, had misconceptions about the use and dosing frequency of pain medications. Almost all patients in a particular unit were on "PRN" (which means "as needed") pain medications, and these patients often waited until their pain intensity levels were very high before seeking relief. Based on these findings, the Breakthrough Series team tried a pain management intervention that offered education and training sessions for professionals and for patients.

Following the training sessions, the team introduced a simple flow sheet for two units to use to document both pain intensity levels and changes in those levels once pain medication was given or increased. In this way, the team found that pretreat-

---

## Statement on Pain Management

All patients have a right to pain relief. Health care providers will:

- Inform patients at the time of their initial evaluation that relief of pain is an important part of their care and respond quickly to reports of pain.
- Ask patients on initial evaluation and as part of regular assessment about the presence, quality, and intensity of pain and use the patients' self-report as the primary indicator of pain.
- Work together with the patient and other health care providers to establish a goal for pain relief and develop and implement a plan to achieve that goal.
- Review and modify the plan of care of patients who have unrelieved pain.

*Source*: From *Building an Institutional Commitment to Pain Management, The Wisconsin Resource Manual for Improvement*, Wisconsin Cancer Pain Initiative, University of Wisconsin.

ment pain intensities for 46 patients were over 7; after treatment, the intensity level dropped to below 5.

The Coney Island team made comprehensive pain assessments part of its change strategy. Other groups may do the same by asking patients about the location of their pain, its nature, its time and course, its duration, and how different treatments have affected it. Simply saying that a patient's pain intensity is a 7 may be accurate—but is not adequate.

Like Coney Island, when the Breakthrough Series team from Kaiser Permanente in San Diego, California, began its project, patient charts had no standardized pain measure. The team began to use a pain flow sheet and assessment tool for outpatients who were dying. Patients were given a pain ruler and then were asked to respond to a questionnaire about their pain. The team made follow-up telephone calls to assess patient pain intensity levels. In this project, 88 percent of patients received appropriate callbacks, and 45 percent of these calls led to changes in the pain management regime. Following the telephone calls and additional visits, 84 percent of patients reported that their levels of pain intensity were acceptable.

*TELEPHONE*

Groups can readily encourage patients to think about their own needs for pain control: At what level is pain unacceptable? What is the patient's own goal? What is the lowest intensity level at which a patient will ask for relief? By setting their own standards for pain management, patients can define their own pain scales. Keep in mind, though, that patients are likely to underestimate or underreport pain, that they do not expect much relief from pain, and that they will be satisfied with any attempt to relieve their suffering. *Do more than what low patient expectations require!*

### ★★★Use Culturally Appropriate Pain Assessment Methods

*On Lok Senior Health Services*

San Francisco's On Lok Senior Health Services, the original model for the Program for All-Inclusive Care of the Elderly (PACE), serves a culturally and ethnically diverse patient population of frail elders. When its Breakthrough Series team found that standard pain scales did not work well for its patients, the team developed its own tools, including an assessment that gauged the patient's emotional state, nonverbal cues, and mobility. The questionnaire asked patients about their desire for comfort, their current status, and their goals for the future.

(The appendix includes copies of On Lok's assessment tools on page 288.)

Goals for patients nearing the end of life included:

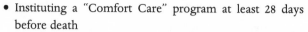

- Instituting a "Comfort Care" program at least 28 days before death
- Providing pain assessment and management to 100 percent of patients
- Offering psychosocial and spiritual support to 80 percent of patients
- Having 90 percent of patients' families participate in a family conference

To measure improvement, On Lok staff followed progress notes in medical records:

- Reviewing all deaths each month
- Identifying deaths caused by chronic illness
- Documenting the date the comfort care plan was begun
- Looking for evidence of pain management, psychosocial and spiritual support, and counseling

Because the average On Lok participant is in the program for three years, staff often found it difficult to acknowledge when a patient was nearing the end of his or her life. To help interdisciplinary staff recognize this phase of life, the On Lok team offered training sessions that included a focus on observing changes in patients (such as decreased or difficult mobility, slow or guarded behavior, and withdrawal from usual interactions).

The accompanying charts demonstrate On Lok's success: 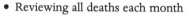 Within months of starting this project, the percentage of patients with pain intensities greater than 4 decreased from 60

|  | Before EOL project | After one year of project | % change |
|---|---|---|---|
| % of chronic illness deaths with comfort care plans | 59 | 78 | 32 |
| Duration of comfort care plans (average days) | 13.6 | 54.9 | 304 |

Figure 3.4 Improved Comfort Care Plans at On Lok Senior Health Services. Reprinted with permission of On Lok Senior Health Services, San Francisco, CA.

Table 3.2 Achievement of Aims, On Lok Senior Health Services

| | Before EOL project | After one year of project | % Change |
|---|---|---|---|
| % of chronic illness deaths with comfort care plans | 59 | 78 | 32 |
| Duration of comfort care plans (average days) | 13.6 | 54.9 | 304 |

percent to 20 percent. Within one year, pain assessment and management for dying patients went from 33 percent to 86 percent of patients, and the length of comfort care plans increased from 13.6 days at the start of the project to 54.9 by its conclusion.

## ★Tools in Translation

### St. Vincent's Hospital

New York City's St. Vincent's Hospital translated pain scales into 16 different languages, including Japanese, Chinese, Pakistani, Polish, Greek, and Spanish. One Breakthrough Series team, Wisconsin's United Hospital, translated the pain scale into Hmong. All of these translations can be ordered, and some can be downloaded, from the Mayday Pain Resource Center (see resources at the end of this chapter).

*CULTURE*

## ★★★Give Patients a Frame of Reference

### St. Mary's Medical Center

Patients may not have a frame of reference for their pain and so may find it hard to report or describe it. The team at St. Mary's Medical Center in Madison, Wisconsin, tried several approaches to educate patients about pain management and, at the same time, to heighten provider awareness of the need to ask patients about pain intensity levels. St. Mary's wrote and distributed two patient education pamphlets, developed three algorithms on pain management for health care workers, posted a large 0-to-10 scale in patient rooms, and developed a vital sign sheet with a graph for reported pain intensity and acceptable levels.

The group reviewed five charts and surveyed five patients each week. At the end of a 16-week study, St. Mary's had achieved some of its pain management goals. As documentation improved, so did patient satisfaction.

## ★★Make Pain a Fifth Vital Sign

Making pain a fifth vital sign is a relatively straightforward way to improve pain management. The American Pain Society first promoted the phrase as a way to increase awareness of pain treatment. Simply by requiring routine pain assessment—along with pulse, blood pressure, respirations, and heart rate—organizations make pain management a priority. Teams that try this approach need to simultaneously develop (or use) protocols for managing any pain intensity level greater than 3 (on a 0-to-10 scale).

In 1999, the U.S. Department of Veterans Affairs (VA) launched an ambitious program called "Pain as a Fifth Vital Sign" in all of its medical facilities and in all patient encounters with its health care system. The VA system sees about 3.5 million patients annually, so the effect of this program is likely to be widespread.

The VA notes in its tool kit on pain assessment, "Implementation of 'Pain as the Fifth Vital Sign' is a mechanism for identifying unrelieved pain. Screening for pain can be administered quickly for most patients on a routine basis. As with any other vital sign, a positive pain score should trigger further assessment of the pain, prompt intervention, and follow-up evaluation of the pain and the effectiveness of treatment."

Despite the VA's excellent model, providers are likely to encounter colleagues who have trouble adopting this strategy and who may argue:

- *"We already have too many things to check—alcohol, drugs, birth control, smoking."* That's true. But it is also true that this is important, treatable, and commonly missed. It's not much to measure patient pain levels once a day in the hospital; patients with no pain require no follow-up. Those with unacceptable scores do.
- *"But pain isn't really a number like blood pressure or heart rate,"* or *"I don't trust patient reports."* Occasionally, this is a problem. However, to patients, pain is very real. The numbers make asking about it more efficient, so that better assessment can be effectively targeted. And absolute numbers are less important than knowing whether or not

the patient is disabled from pain and how pain levels change from day to day.

By anticipating barriers and objections, teams can develop approaches and responses that encourage other health care providers to join in—or, at the very least, to try the idea.

### ★★★Use Clinical Practice Guidelines

Hundreds of expert panels, individuals, and organizations have developed guidelines on everything from managing urinary incontinence to treating HIV/AIDS patients. Guidelines, sometimes called clinical pathways, are available; these highlight best practices in treating the array of problems patients face at the end of life. The federal government has launched a new Web site, http://www.guidelines.gov, from which one can download carefully selected guidelines. In addition to guidelines developed by federal agencies, professional organizations (e.g., the American Pain Society) and international groups (e.g., the World Health Organization) have developed their own. The Joint Commission on Accreditation of Healthcare Organizations (JCAHO) is revising its standards to incorporate pain assessment and treatment. These materials—and others developed by regional and local organizations—point the way to improved pain management.

Improvement teams may want to try various guidelines. In selecting one, keep in mind these common attributes of good guidelines:

- They provide genuine guidance.
- The patient population is clearly defined.
- The guidelines are based on evidence.
- They are clear and flexible.
- Exceptions to recommendations are described.
- Recommended actions can be measured.
- The information provided can actually be used.
- The material is current (Davis, 1999).

Is there evidence that guidelines work or improve patient care? Researchers in Washington State recently reported that the use of guidelines improved "usual pain outcomes." The accompanying sidebar describes results of a study using clinical practice guidelines to improve management of cancer pain.

In a study of 81 cancer patients, researchers at Washington State's Swedish Medical Center found that the use of a treatment algorithm for pain management, based on guidelines from AHCPR, improved "usual pain" outcomes. The study's Cancer Pain Algorithm addresses pain assessment, analgesic drug choice decisions, and reassessment. The decision tree includes side effect treatment protocols, equianalgesic conversion ➡

charts, and a primer for intractable pain.

Researchers followed patients for three months, taking pain measurements at five intervals: at baseline; at two weeks; and at one, two, and three months after the start of the intervention. Pain outcomes were "usual" and "worst" pain as measured by a Brief Pain Inventory. Pain outcome tools included:

- An average pain intensity score from a Daily Pain Diary
- Pain "character" using descriptive words and a ranking scale
- Pain interference with seven different activities
- Pain location
- A composite score based on intensity, character, relief, location, and interference

Patients whose care was facilitated by use of the pain algorithm had statistically superior results in reduction of "usual pain." Control group patients had an initial decrease in pain intensity but finished the study with a slight increase in usual pain scores. Patients in the algorithm group, however, experienced a steady decrease in usual pain scores (Du Pen et al., 1999). (Figures 3.5, 3.6)

### ★★★ Make Pain Management an Institutional Priority

Patient and provider education alone will not be sufficient to create widespread change in an institution's pain management practice. Institutional change tends to come on the heels of institutional commitment, a public statement or promise that pain management is a top priority.

One pain management consultant (Super, 1996) has reported on a quality improvement project she and her colleagues undertook at an urban medical center in Portland. When the project began, patients had an average pain intensity level of 6.3 on a 0-to-10 scale. In an effort to reduce this intensity level, 850 nurses participated in 23 mandatory four-hour classes; more than 100 physicians, social workers, pharmacists, and administrators also participated. After this huge educational effort, the mean pain score dropped to 5.7—still a poor level.

The administration decided to make pain management improvements an institutional objective. Patient documentation was revised to include baseline assessment and routine reevaluation of pain intensity. At this point, the mean pain rate fell to 3.2. Signs were posted in every patient room to tell patients and families to expect pain relief and to report unrelieved pain. The mean rate continued to fall, and in 18 months it had reached 2.3!

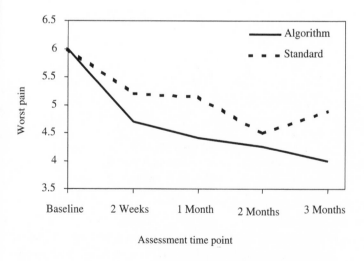

Figure 3.5 Worst Pain Scores: Algorithm versus Standard Care. Reprinted with permission, DuPen et al., 1999.

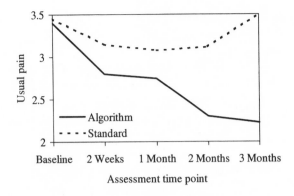

Figure 3.6 Usual Pain Scores: Algorithm versus Standard Care. Reprinted with permission, DuPen et al., 1999.

### ★★★Balm of Gilead Center

During the Breakthrough Series, the team from Cooper Green Hospital, a public hospital serving Jefferson County, Alabama, created the Balm of Gilead Center in Birmingham to provide hospice services to poor and indigent community members. As it worked to make pain management an institutional priority, the team:

- Established pain as a fifth vital sign, measuring it every time other vital signs were checked.
- Set a standard for pain management. Any ratings over 3 on a 1-to-5 scale required that pain treatment protocols begin.
- Distributed a pain ruler for all staff to carry in their pockets.
- Posted pain scales at all patient bedsides.
- Computerized a tracking system to follow pain intensity reports in patient records.

Patients actually began to use the pain intensity rulers to communicate about other problems. When asked to point to the number that represented her pain, one patient pointed to one number and said, "My pain is here," and then pointed to another number and said, "And my anxiety is here."

### ★Set Pain Control Standards

Organizations that are committed to improved pain management must establish—and enforce—institutional standards. There are several ways to do this; some have been tested in PDSA cycles, and some have not. Most seem like reasonable ideas that could be "tested" with a small number of patients.

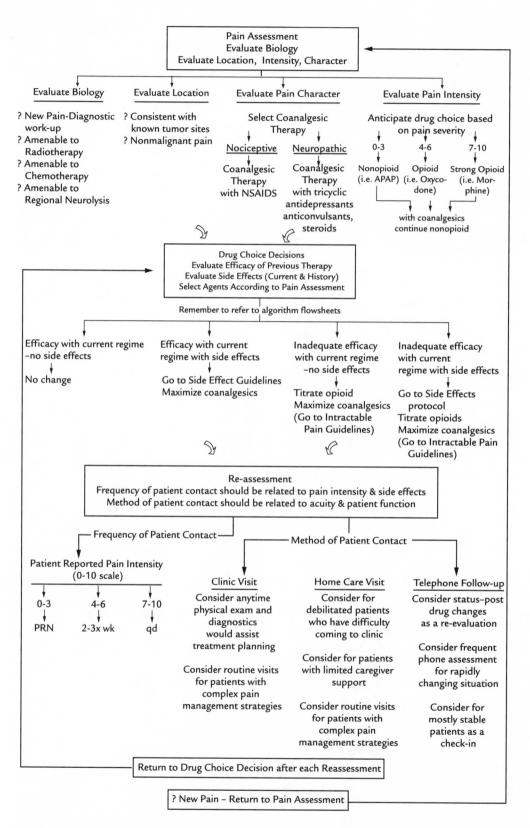

Figure 3.7 Pain Management Algorithm. Reprinted with permission, DuPen et al., 1999.

★★★Continuously Monitor Pain Treatment until
   Acceptable Intensity Is Reached

*North Kansas City Hospital*

The team at Missouri's North Kansas City Hospital set a broad aim: to routinely assess and control patient pain intensity. The team tried several changes, such as focusing attention on pain assessment on all nursing units, encouraging patient self-reports, and increasing staff monitoring of medical records for pain treatment.

The team also decided to monitor the pain intensity levels for cancer patients in the oncology unit for at least a 24-hour period to assess the duration of pain control achieved through interventions. Data were separated into five categories for pain treatment: patient-controlled analgesia (PCA), continuous epidural infusion (CEI), other types of acute pain control, palliative care pain control, and home health patient pain control.

To measure the effect of changes, four nursing units collected data on two patients each week; pain management services collected data on all continuous epidural patients and on 30 patient-controlled analgesia pump patients per month. The pain level for all oncology patients was to be less than or equal to a score of 3 (on a 0-to-10 scale) following the pain treatment, and 24-hour monitoring of pain control was measured for two oncology patients each week.

The team aimed to have 95 percent of patients reporting pain below an intensity of 3 on a 0-to-10 scale. During the initial project, about 65 percent of patients rated pain at or below 3. The team decided to set a new aim for the current fiscal year: 95 percent of patients will report pain at or below a self-defined tolerance level. During the third fiscal quarter, the team reported that 78 percent of patients were at or below their own pain goal. In cases where pain was not relieved, the team focused on talking with patients and families and working with pain management experts.

Through the quality improvement project, the team learned that process change can be made easier by including it as part of a major quality improvement effort. Physicians in the various units responded to data the team provided and became involved in day-to-day pain management for patients. Eventually, the team helped establish a department-wide pain indicator to meet Joint Commission on the Accreditation of Healthcare Organizations standards for performance improvement. The team said that it successfully raised awareness among nurses on the importance of pain management and has since adopted pain as a fifth vital sign.

The team also found that it was difficult to develop simple, easy-to-follow data collection forms; during the project year, the group revised the forms four times, only to find that some forms still lacked one or more of the necessary elements.

Patients were not always willing to participate in pain treatment, telling nurses they expected to be in pain and, as a result, refusing medication. The team found that ongoing patient and family education programs are essential to changing this perception.

Thanks to the team's efforts, the hospital's board of trustees and the formal subcommittees on pain management, oncology care, and palliative care now receive routine reports on pain management and control.

### ★★★Develop Follow-up Procedures

*Kaiser Permanente, San Diego*

Hospice staff from the Kaiser Permanente-San Diego team identified several problems: At admission, more than half of the patients admitted to the hospice had significant, uncontrolled pain. There were no standard methods for pain assessment or for follow-up on pain management. To improve this situation, the team began to hold biweekly meetings, creating for the first time a sustained effort between hospice, continuing care, and oncology professionals.

The group focused on three aims for end-of-life patients visiting oncologists' offices:

- Meet patient pain level goals 80 percent of the time.
- Make follow-up calls within three to five days when the patient's pain is greater than the patient's pain goal, and do this for 100 percent of cases.
- Record pain intensity for all visits for dying patients.

The team changed what had become routine by:

- Giving patients a pain questionnaire and ruler
- Assessing depression and anxiety
- Making follow-up telephone calls

At the first follow-up phone call, most patients who had been in pain still reported problems—but nearly all could be managed over the phone by a nurse. By the end of the project:

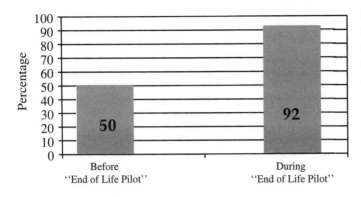

Figure 3.8 Pain Control upon Initial Hospice Assessment. Reprinted with permission of Kaiser-Permanente, San Diego, CA.

- 92 percent of patients had pain controlled upon hospice admission.
- 90 percent received appropriate follow-up.
- 94 percent had pain intensity documented.

The team was so successful that the project is now being expanded throughout the department and southern California Kaiser Permanente plans.

### ★★★Try a Range of Innovations

#### United Hospital

The Breakthrough Series team at United Hospital in Minneapolis, Minnesota, aimed to have 90 percent of the group's cancer patients report a pain intensity of less than 5 on a 0-to-10 pain scale. The team studied a pilot group and found that 50 percent of oncology patients were in significant, uncontrolled pain (level greater than 5) prior to hospice admission. To do this, the team tried several tactics, including the distribution of equianalgesic cards and the development of a pain liaison nurse program. Each week, staff reviewed four randomly selected charts on the oncology unit and on the four critical care units.

Changes tested included ongoing pain management education, use of multilingual pain scales, addition of pain assessment to the Nursing Admission History Form, and development of a pain protocol (standing orders) for oncology. This protocol includes substantial adjustment of doses without further physician input—an approach that seems key to rapid responses.

The pain management liaison nurse performed several roles: distributing pain management information to nurses at the bedside, increasing resources for pain management on each unit, and encouraging interest in pain management among colleagues.

### ★Require Certain Providers to Be Registered to Prescribe Controlled Substances

Some hospitals found that very few of their physicians had registered to prescribe controlled substances—even among physicians who had many patients likely to need these medications! Think about the physicians who work with your end-of-life patients (e.g., geriatricians, oncologists, general internists). Are they registered or authorized to prescribe controlled substances? If not, the institution may be willing to make such registration a requirement for maintaining hospital staff privileges.

### ★Review Prescribing Practices for Opioid Drugs

One striking opportunity for improvement is in opioid drug prescribing practices. The most glaring issue for many Breakthrough Series teams was the use of meperidine. One hospital calculated the morphine equivalent dosages for all of its repeated dose prescriptions. Half were for meperidine, the only opioid that is routinely contraindicated because of its short duration of action and because one of its metabolites is a central nervous system stimulant (often causing delirium and agitation). Although physicians' commitments to historical prescribing patterns are strongly held, a pharmaceutical committee embarked on a program of changes to prevent this misuse. Similar pharmacy-based and often automated approaches could nearly halt incorrect conversions from one delivery system or drug to the next (e.g., when changing from an IV to oral morphine).

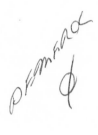

### ★Improving Pain Management in Nursing Homes and Assisted Living Facilities

Severely disabled and institutionalized people present challenges for health care providers in assessing pain and response to treatment, in preventing and managing side effects, and in confronting difficulties in informed consent. Nursing homes and assisted living settings face many challenges in managing pain for frail elderly patients and those with dementia. Some facilities may not have licensed personnel available at all times and thus may require unusual arrangements for opioid storage and administration. Many facilities have residents who cannot report pain or advocate for relief.

Assessing pain in demented patients or in those who cannot communicate can be difficult; few of these patients with chronic pain cry out, moan, sweat profusely, or have rapid heartbeats. Most just reduce activity and withdraw from others. The only way to relieve their pain is to have an attentive and consistent caregiver who notices that the person is in pain and then observes the patient's response to treatment.

Some professional and lay caregivers are reluctant to give opioids to demented patients. In some instances, caregivers fear inducing delirium. Others say that by experiencing some pain, the patient remains more alert.

How might nursing homes assess their pain management performance? Simple measures might be:

- Does the facility require routine pain assessments?
- When pain is identified, does anyone respond? If so, how quickly?
- Does the response to serious pain (e.g., pain over a level 3 on a 0-to-10 scale) include opioid drugs on a regular schedule?
- Are the rates of acetaminophen, combination drugs, and opioids all within a reasonable range? For instance, if opioid use is virtually nonexistent, and acetaminophen and combination drugs are often ordered "as needed" or in high doses, the institution has a pain management crisis.

## Resources

American Chronic Pain Association
P.O. Box 850
Rocklin, CA 95677-0850
Phone: 916-632-0922

This membership-based organization provides support for those suffering from chronic pain, has over 800 local chapters, and provides written educational materials.

Mayday Pain Resource Center
City of Hope National Medical Center
1500 Duarte Road
Duarte, CA 91010
Phone: 626-359-8111, ext. 3829
E-mail: maydaypain@smtplink.coh.org

Key Recommendations
for Managing
Chronic Pain in
Older People
*American Geriatrics Society*

- Pain should be an important part of each assessment of older patients; along with efforts to alleviate the underlying cause, pain itself should be aggressively treated.
- Pain and its response to treatment should be objectively measured, preferably using a validated pain scale.
- Nonsteroidal anti-inflammatory drugs (NSAIDs) should be used with caution. In older patients, NSAIDs have significant side effects and are the most common cause of adverse drug reactions. (The new Cox-2 agents may have a better side effect profile.)
- Acetaminophen is the drug of choice for relieving mild to moderate musculoskeletal pain.
- Opioid analgesic drugs are effective for relieving moderate to severe pain.
- Nonopioid analgesic medications may be appropriate for some patients with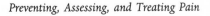

Key Recommendations
for Managing
Chronic Pain in
Older People
(*Continued*)

neuropathic pain and
other chronic pain
syndromes.

- Nonpharmacologic
  approaches (e.g.,
  patient and caregiver
  education, cognitive-
  behavioral therapy,
  exercise, etc.), used
  alone or in combination
  with appropriate
  pharmacologic
  strategies, should be an
  integral part of care
  plans for most chronic
  pain patients.
- Referral to a
  multidisciplinary pain
  management center
  should be considered
  when pain management
  efforts do not meet the
  patient's or the health
  care provider's goals.
- Regulatory agencies
  should review existing
  policies to
  enhance access to
  effective opioid
  analgesic drugs for older
  patients in pain.
- Pain management
  education should be
  improved at all levels for
  all healthcare
  professionals.

*Source*: American Geriatrics
Society, 1998.

This is a resource for health professionals and the public that covers information about pain management.

National Chronic Pain Outreach Association
7979 Old Georgetown Road, Suite 100
Bethesda, MD 20814-2429
Phone: 301-652-4948
Serves as a clearinghouse of information related to chronic pain and provides written materials.

PharmInfo Net
Internet address: http://www.pharminfo.com
The Pharmaceutical Information Network is provided by VirSci Corporation, a company not associated with any pharmaceutical company. A broad range of information and educational materials is available.

There are Indigent Drug Programs available through a number of drug companies. In order to access these programs, a physician must apply to these programs on behalf of the patient. Certain states have Pharmaceutical Assistance Programs, which are operated by state governments. To get a listing of the companies and states with these programs, contact Cancer Care for a copy of *Helping Hand: The Resource Guide for People with Cancer* at this Web site: http://www.cancercare.org/hhrd/hhrd.htm.

# 4

# Managing Dyspnea and Ventilator Withdrawal

"Dyspnea" is a medical term that means shortness of breath—but that does not fully describe the terrible anxiety and suffering that struggling to breathe causes for patients and families. The World Health Organization (1998) describes dyspnea as an "unpleasant awareness of breathing." Patients feel breathless or have trouble breathing. No wonder, then, that untreated dyspnea contributes to suffering and anxiety.

Severe dyspnea is associated with chronic respiratory failure and with the final course of many illnesses. Anxiety can lead to or worsen dyspnea. Patients sometimes experience dyspnea during ventilator withdrawal. For patients who have been on ventilators during an earlier exacerbation of disease, advance care planning should address future ventilator use and withdrawal. Health care providers need to talk to patients and families about what to expect, under what situations to initiate and withdraw the ventilator, and how dyspnea will be treated.

The National Hospice Study (Greer et al., 1984) found that 70 percent of cancer patients had dyspnea in the last six weeks of life; other studies have shown that between 29 and 74 percent of dying patients have dyspnea. As death approaches, symptoms may worsen; in one study of seriously ill patients, more than half were reported to have severe dyspnea in the last three days of life (Lynn et al., 1997).

Dyspnea is often left untreated, not because we lack effective treatments but because many physicians resist using opioid drugs or sedative hypnotics for dyspnea, fearing that their use will lead to respiratory depression and death. Although patients who have been on opioid drugs for a few days or more are fairly resistant to respiratory depression, many physicians continue to

Just because dying is natural doesn't mean it's easy.
—Dan Tobin, MD

59

see the potential for respiratory depression as an absolute barrier to treatment. "Opiophobia" (Campbell et al., 1999) describes some physicians' absolute refusal to use opioids for fear that doing so may hasten death. In fact, in the dying patient, there is no way to prove whether or not the opioid hastened death. As dying progresses, with or without the opioid, several physiologic changes that indicate imminent death are the same as signs of opioid toxicity.

In Britain and elsewhere, patients with chronic symptomatic dyspnea are routinely given opioids in doses that relieve symptoms; their physicians do not feel that this practice shortens life. Indeed, the benefits of restful sleep and reduced anxiety may help these patients to live well a little longer.

Although law and medicine have taken some liberties with the original religious doctrine, many practitioners and most courts (including the U.S. Supreme Court, in *Washington et al., Petitioners No. 96-100, v. Harold Glucksberg et al.*, 117 S.Ct. 2258 [1997]) rely on "double effect" to assess whether opioid use (as well as other treatments with some risk of causing death) is justifiable. The double effect reasoning holds that if a patient is suffering enough to warrant the risk of opioid use, and if the intent was only to relieve that suffering, it is acceptable to have risked causing an earlier death. In other words, if the alternative is to leave the patient in misery, and if the treatment is aimed at relieving suffering rather than at causing death, then treating with opioids is acceptable, even if doing so may hasten death.

### In This Chapter

Several Breakthrough Series teams aimed to reduce and relieve dyspnea, primarily by training clinicians and establishing competencies and by studying and reducing practice variations. This chapter provides information and protocols for ventilator withdrawal, including ways to prevent dyspnea during this process. It also includes strategies for assessing and treating dyspnea and for using the Plan-Do-Study-Act model as a way to improve patient care.

Can an organization promise its patients that anytime they are feeling short of breath or suffocating, prompt relief will be provided? Yes. If clinicians who care for these patients are confident in their ability to relieve dyspnea and can promise them that sedation will be promptly available to avoid a sense of suffocation near death, such promises can be made. Readers should note that the strategies that have proven effective for pain management—such as writing standing orders or authorizing nurses to act independently—are not as effective in improving management of dyspnea. This chapter offers guideposts for organizations and individuals who are certain that change is necessary—and possible.

Physicians should be able to treat patients with dyspnea with opioid drugs and close observation. When using opioids to treat dyspnea, the dose must be titrated to the patient's responses; hypersomnolence will precede significant respiratory depression and signal the clinician to adjust the opioid dose. In the unusual event that a patient experiences respiratory depression after initiating or increasing the dose of opioid, close observation until the effects decrease is usually sufficient. Narcotic antagonists are almost never necessary, although they are available.

### ★★★Hospice Care of Rhode Island

The team from Hospice Care of Rhode Island focused on improving dyspnea management for two reasons: Families reported that dyspnea was one of the most troublesome symptoms, and nurses identified managing dyspnea as an opportunity to improve their practice. Hospice Care of Rhode Island provides care for approximately 1,000 dying patients each year, with a daily census of about 375 patients.

The team aimed to reduce dyspnea by half in patients admitted to the inpatient hospice unit, while providing care that was consistent with patient preferences for avoiding dyspnea and sedation.

The team's first step was to establish uniform assessment for dyspnea, a process that included development of a dyspnea assessment tool for patients unable to rate their dyspnea. The team proposed dyspnea management competencies for nursing staff. Competencies included:

- Communicating with patients and families about goals for symptom management
- Contacting physicians about treatment goals and plans, including the type of treatment to be used and its route of administration
- Recognizing when dyspnea is severe or distressing to patients
- Understanding and using a uniform assessment tool
- Interpreting when patients are satisfied that dyspnea is under control
- Reassessing treatment management on a regular basis

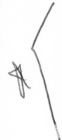

## Principles of Dyspnea Management
*Hospice Care of Rhode Island*

- Dyspnea is burdensome for patients and loved ones.
- All patients' status will be monitored based on patient self-report, if possible. Since dyspnea, like pain, is a subjective experience, patient report is paramount to treatment decisions.
- Assess the patient's dyspnea.
- Key to determination of severe dyspnea is not only its severity, but the patient's perceived suffering. For example, a patient with chronic obstructive lung disease may have severe symptoms that are not perceived as bothersome.
- Acute dyspnea in a dying patient shall be treated as a medical emergency; prompt relief of symptoms is mandatory. ➡

As part of its clinician education program, the team developed principles of dyspnea management, which are highlighted in the following box.

Graphs from Hospice Care of Rhode Island show just how dramatic improvements can be in managing dyspnea. In a five-month period, the Breakthrough Series team reduced rates of unrelieved dyspnea per shift from more than 50 percent to less than 5 percent.

### ★★★Assess Dyspnea

Like pain, dyspnea often goes unrecorded and untreated. Programs that care for the dying need to make the assessment of dyspnea a routine part of patient care. Assess dyspnea by asking patients:

- How severe are symptoms?
- Is it acute or chronic?
- What level of exertion leads to symptoms?
- What are the patient's goals and priorities—what is the level of comfort required and the level of consciousness the patient wants to try to maintain?
- Does the patient feel that he or she is suffering?

Some dying patients are unable to report distress because of changes in consciousness from either acute or chronic illness. In these patients, dyspnea may be untreated because it is not

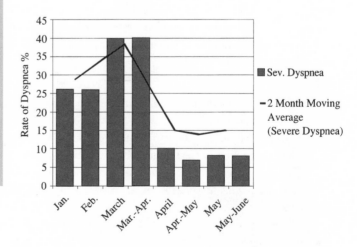

Figure 4.1 Episodes of Severe Dyspnea. Reprinted with permission of Hospice Care of Rhode Island.

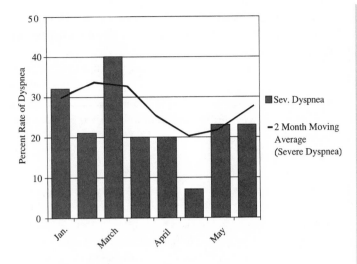

Figure 4.2 Severe Dyspnea in the Last 48 Hours. Reprinted with permission of Hospice Care of Rhode Island.

Principles of
Dyspnea Management
(*Continued*)

To measure its progress in controlling dyspnea, the group used three indicators:

- Severe dyspnea defined as greater than 3 (on a 0–10 scale), not relieved during eight-hour nursing shift
- Several episodes of severe dyspnea in patients who had more than 24 hours in hospice
- Severe dyspnea in the last 48 hours of life in patients with more than 24 hours in hospice

  Reprinted with permission of Hospice Care of Rhode Island

recognized. However, a number of behaviors signal distress, such as:

- Tachypnea (rapid breathing)
- Tachycardia (rapid heartbeat)
- Restlessness
- Accessory muscle use (labored voluntary muscle efforts in the neck and chest)
- Flushing or cyanosis
- A look of fear
- Grunting at the end of each breath
- Nasal flaring

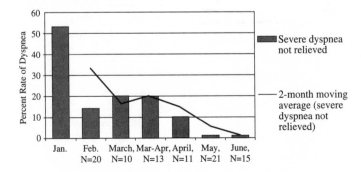

Figure 4.3 Rates of Dyspnea Not Relieved by End of Shift.
Reprinted with permission of Hospice Care of Rhode Island.

To improve management for patients with dyspnea, the team from Hospice Care of Rhode Island wrote guidelines and standing orders.

## ★★★Treat Dyspnea by Improving Management of Ventilator Withdrawal

Dyspnea is one of the many symptoms that occur when patients are weaned from ventilators; others include pain, anxiety, and excessive secretions. The decision to remove life support is difficult for families and health care providers. The goal during this process is to maintain patient comfort. Terminal weaning differs from traditional weaning because the process continues, regardless of the patient's vital signs, and comfort measures are used despite their effect on vital signs.

### UCLA Medical Center

UCLA Medical Center has a policy for terminal weaning that requires informed consent by the patient or surrogate, collaboration among all members of the health care team, and discussions with families to describe the process and alternative methods. The policy also recommends that other professional staff, including social workers and chaplains, be notified of the family's wishes and be available should the family request help. Patients and families are assured privacy, time to grieve, and quick access to all caregivers.

## ★★Implement Appropriate Ventilator Withdrawal Techniques

The withdrawal of mechanical ventilation is a terminal care process that the patient is not expected to survive. Ventilator withdrawal should be a humane procedure focused on the comfort of the patient and the family.

A small number of case reports and descriptive studies describe the usual practices used during ventilator withdrawal. These studies have investigated the use of analgesics or sedatives, the method for reducing ventilation, and decisions about extubation. Providers must choose a method of sedating the patient before weaning him or her. Faber-Langendoen (1994) surveyed 273 critical care physicians involved in ventilator management during terminal weaning. Of these, 74 percent ordered morphine and 54 percent ordered benzodiazepines.

## Analgesia or Sedation

Analgesics or sedatives during ventilator withdrawal are intended to reduce dyspnea, anxiety, fear, or pain; the drugs of choice have been opioids and benzodiazepines. Morphine is the preferred opioid because it reduces pain, dyspnea, and anxiety and contributes to reducing excess lung water (Brody et al., 1997). Some patients—those who have severe neurological injuries or damage and who are incapable of experiencing distress, including those who have been pronounced dead by neurologic criteria—will require no analgesia.

In a prospective study of patient responses during rapid terminal weaning in an unconscious patient sample (Campbell et al., 1999), the investigators reported that many patients (35 percent) required no analgesia/sedation at any time during this procedure. There were no significant correlations between the amount of morphine used and the duration of survival afterwards. Additionally, when comparing those who received morphine and those who did not, there were no differences in length of survival. The average dose of morphine in those who required analgesia was 5.5 mg/hr.

## Paralytic Agents

A few clinicians favor the use of paralytics during ventilator withdrawal, although this practice is difficult to justify. Those who prefer it argue that continuing the paralytic drug gives the patient a comfortable appearance and precludes any sign of respiratory struggle, which could upset the family. However, the potential negative effects for the patient outweigh this positive effect for the family.

Paralytics are used to minimize oxygen consumption and regulate ventilation, but they have lost their therapeutic rationale in the situation of ventilator withdrawal. Furthermore, patients are unable to show discomfort, making it impossible for clinicians to determine whether adequate analgesia/sedation is being provided before, during, or after the ventilator withdrawal process. Paralytics do not confer any sedation or analgesic effects. Finally, if the patient is conscious, paralysis prevents physical interaction with loved ones.

## Withdrawal Methods

There are three distinct methods of ventilator withdrawal:

- Terminal extubation
- Immediate t-bar placement
- Terminal weaning

*Terminal extubation* entails the rapid cessation of mechanical ventilation and removal of the artificial airway, followed in many cases by the administration of humidified air or oxygen. Immediate t-bar placement is a one-step ventilator cessation with continued airway support. Terminal weaning is a stepwise reduction of ventilatory support, leaving the artificial airway in place during the withdrawal of ventilation. Some patients have their airway tubes removed after t-bar or wean if airway comfort can be predicted. There is little empirical data to support one method over another, particularly with regard to analysis of patient experience.

Terminal extubation has been criticized because it can lead to marked respiratory struggling and significant distress that is profoundly disturbing to patients, family members, and health care professionals (Gilligan and Raffin, 1995; Strother, 1991). Furthermore, distress from airway compromise cannot be easily reduced with analgesia or sedation (Carlson et al., 1996). The only clear circumstance in which terminal extubation is an appropriate withdrawal method is for the patient who is brain-dead and incapable of experiencing distress from airway compromise.

Terminal weaning affords precise titration of medications and careful adjustment of the process itself to ensure patient comfort. The process can be accomplished rapidly, over minutes to hours, or in a more protracted fashion of several hours, depending on the patient's circumstances. Preliminary results from a prospective study of patient responses during ventilator withdrawal suggest that an immediate cessation of ventilation by placement on a t-bar can be accomplished without patient distress in the face of severe neurological insults (e.g., global anoxic encephalopathy) in which the patient has only brainstem activity. A rapid terminal wean afforded comfort for patients with some cortical activity and the possibility of experiencing distress (Campbell, 1998).

The decision to extubate could be handled as a secondary decision following the withdrawal. Airway problems can develop after extubation and are potential sources of distress to patients, families, and caregivers. One investigation reported no distress in patients terminally extubated; however, 28 percent of patients in that sample had gasping/labored respirations that may have been indicative of distress (Faber-Langendoen, 1994). On the other hand, family members may especially want for their loved one to be free of tubes before he or she dies and to be able to give a kiss or caress that would be hard to do with a tube in the loved one's mouth. It is worth asking family members before presuming to know the best plan.

Extubation may be relevant for patients who will experience distress from the endotracheal tube. The adequacy of the gag and cough reflexes, volume of pulmonary secretions, duration of intubation, and patient consciousness should be considered when determining whether extubation should be performed (Campbell and Carlson, 1992).

### ★★Queen Elizabeth II Health Sciences Centre

The Breakthrough Series team at Queen Elizabeth II Health Sciences Centre in Halifax, Nova Scotia, aimed to improve family satisfaction with patient care (in the ICU) and particularly with the management of pain, dyspnea, and sedation whenever life support is withdrawn and to achieve consistency in patient care. One of its most important activities was a study of variation in practice for ventilator cessation: Everyone involved had his or her own method.

In general, wide practice variation signals an opportunity for improvement. Usually, having as many ways to do something as there are people doing it is a sign that no one has really thought the process through and that no practice pattern will be implemented well by all.

The variation in practice survey asked nurses to respond to a given scenario; it was not a study of actual practice variation. Through responses to the scenario, however, the team measured the amount of sedation nurses recommended and their preferences for weaning and titration of FiO2 at the time life support was withdrawn. The Breakthrough Series team found that 65 percent of nurses wanted single-step reduction in FiO2, while 31 percent preferred a graded reduction. The amounts of morphine and lorazepam nurses recommended using varied 2widely. Based on the survey results, the team developed a sedation algorithm and a ventilator withdrawal checklist.

In addition to the practice variation study, the Breakthrough Series team tried several changes, which it measured by:

- Tracking intensity levels or scores for dyspnea, pain, and sedation
- Conducting family satisfaction surveys during three separate periods
- Making a quality-of-death review

### ★Seton Healthcare Network

As part of its palliative care program, the Seton Healthcare Network in Austin, Texas, has developed the following guidelines for ventilator withdrawal.

1.  Does the patient have a living will or a durable Power of Attorney for health issues?   Yes
    No

    If yes, is the proposed decision to withdrawal life support in accordance with the   Yes
    wishes expressed in the living will or the durable Power of Attorney?   No
    Copy on the chart.   Yes

2.  Has the referring doctor been notified?   Yes

3.  Has the second staff physician's opinion to withdrawal life support been obtained?   Yes

4.  If the patient is capable, has he/she been involved in the decision making process?   Yes

5.  If the patient is not capable or unconscious, has the next-of-kin/substitute decision   Yes
    maker been involved in the decision making process?

6.  Has the ICU doctor communicated the plan of care to the family?   Yes

    If No, why? e.g, *unable to reach*   No
    _____

7.  Has the discussion been documented on the chart by:
    Physician _____   Yes
    Nurse _____   Yes

8.  Has the Do Not Resuscitate Order been written?   Yes
    When
    _____

9.  Has the patient and/or family had the opportunity to speak to a spiritual resource   Yes
    person?   Declined

10. Are there any particular religious/cultural practices to be followed at the time of   Yes
    death? List:   No
    _____
    _____
    _____

11. Where appropriate, have other consulting support services been notified?   Yes
    Not Required

12. Have COMFORT MEASURES been implemented?   Yes

13. Has all other active treatment been withdrawn?   Yes

_____        _____
Physician's Signature                  Nurse's Signature
                                        Date _____
                                                Yyyy/Mm/Dd

Figure 4.4 Withdrawal of Life Support Checklist. Reprinted with permission of Queen Elizabeth II Health Sciences Centre, Halifax, Nova Scotia.

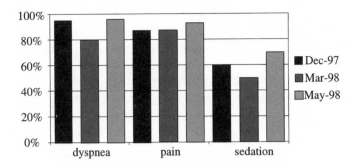

Figure 4.5 Percentage of Patients with Acceptable Symptom Scores at the Time of Discharge from ICU. Reprinted with permission of Queen Elizabeth II Hospital, Halifax, Nova Scotia.

Methods of weaning that 75 ICU nurses were most comfortable with.

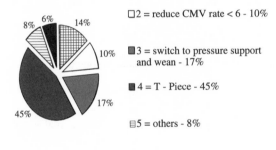

1 = extubate - 14%

2 = reduce CMV rate < 6 - 10%

3 = switch to pressure support and wean - 17%

4 = T - Piece - 45%

5 = others - 8%

6-2 or more answer - 6%

Figure 4.6 Variation in Practice with Mechanical Weaning. Queen Elizabeth II Hospital, Halifax, Nova Scotia.

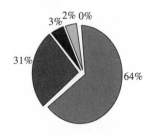

1 = no change = 0%

2 = reduce FiO$_2$ to 21% of area = 64%

3 = gradual reduction of FiO$_2$ to 21% = 31%

4 = any other choices = 3%

5 = 2 choices =2%

Figure 4.7 Weaning FiO$_2$ during Withdrawal of Life Support (Nurse Preferences). Queen Elizabeth II Hospital, Halifax, Nova Scotia.

Preparation: Prior to Withdrawal

- Discontinue all medications/tests/treatments not directed toward comfort care.
- Remove unnecessary lines and tubes.
- Maintain one IV access site for administration of analgesia and sedation.
- Determine noninvasive monitoring needs.
- Discontinue unnecessary alarm systems, including internal defibrillator devices or pacemakers.
- Assemble equipment and medication necessary for comfort and pain control.
- Provide quiet atmosphere and unlimited visiting.
- Ensure that caregivers who are uncomfortable with the process can withdraw from the case.
- Notify the chaplain.

Withdrawal

- The attending physician and chaplain are encouraged to be present.
- Raise head of bed, if possible.
- Clear the airways of secretions if necessary for patient comfort.
- Administer and maintain appropriate levels of sedation/analgesia for signs of dyspnea and distress.
- Reduce ventilator settings to provide minimal support or remove the patient from the ventilator.
- Extubate the patient and, if indicated, place on oxygen as a comfort measure.

**Innovators Need to Know**

Because so many dying patients will experience dyspnea, treating and controlling it is critical to improving their care. Patients who know that dyspnea will occur are (for good reason) afraid—and organizations that can promise to relieve this symptom will do much to relieve patient fear and anxiety.

- An institutional commitment to relieving dyspnea is critical to improving treatment.
- Providers need continuing education that dispels "opiophobia."
- Patients and providers need to talk about dyspnea and discuss the benefits and risks associated with treatment.

- Providers can meet clinical competency standards for dyspnea management.
- Standing orders that limit variations in practice also enable providers to respond more quickly to patient needs.
- Patients, families, and providers need to discuss the likelihood that a patient will be placed on a ventilator and whether or not the patient wants a trial on the ventilator.
- To have such a discussion, the care system has to be able to deliver profound sedation if that is the only way to avoid death by suffocation.
- Any physician who can start a ventilator should be required to know how and when to stop it.

### Resources

*Symptom Relief in Terminal Illness*, by the World Health Organization. Geneva: WHO, 1998.

*Forgoing Life-Sustaining Therapy: How to Care for the Patient Who Is Near Death*, by M. L. Campbell. Aliso Viejo, CA: American Association of Critical Care Nurses, 1998.

# Beyond the Living Will

*Advance Care Planning for All*
*Stages of Health and Disease*

**5**

Many people believe that having a living will is a safeguard against unwanted medical treatment. Although living wills are useful, they do not guarantee that physicians and families will know what to do in a medical emergency, that wishes will be honored, or that patients will die with dignity and in comfort. Achieving these goals requires a continuous process in which patients and clinicians converse about changes in treatment goals, medical status, or preferences. One "advantage" of life-limiting diseases is the opportunity they afford to plan for future medical treatment and to make important decisions ahead of time, such as when to remove a feeding tube or forgo a ventilator. A disadvantage, however, is the way in which the health care system responds routinely to urgent situations.

For example, when a patient's heart stops, physicians and nurses will usually try to restart it. This process ensures that the moment of death will not be peaceful or prayerful; instead it will be a blur of hasty actions and strong measures. Although some patients will benefit from such measures, others—who will need a clinician's recommendation about the benefits and burdens of such attempts—will not. This latter group must note and plan for the measures they want taken. Otherwise, attempts at resuscitation are automatic.

One good reason for making advance care plans and directives is the opportunity to get the best responses to urgent situations. Another reason is that patients may want to direct certain aspects of care based on their particular values and priorities. Finally, some people want to make plans to protect their families from having to make troubling decisions for them. These three aims can be achieved when patients, families,

This decision is mine. I have
lived a full life
And these are the eyes that
I want you to remember.
—"Try Not to Breathe," REM

and clinicians take time to consider what is likely to happen as the condition progresses and which treatments should be used—or not—when complications occur.

Beyond the basic benefits of advance care planning just described, federal law mandates that patients in institutions that receive Medicare or Medicaid funding be given information about state laws governing advance directives. The Patient Self-Determination Act of 1991 also requires institutions to educate staff and community members about the availability of advance directives. Finally, the law prohibits facilities from discriminating against patients based on whether they have an advance directive.

For several years, institutions and organizations nationwide have worked to improve advance care planning for all people, regardless of their health status—yet advance care planning still needs work. In some cases, the challenge will be to get physicians to talk to patients about the likely course of a disease and the decisions that must be made as it progresses. For others, the challenge may be to make sure patient wishes are known and accessible. Regardless of the particular challenge an organization faces, the ideas and strategies developed by other organizations may prove helpful.

### In This Chapter

Breakthrough Series teams tried several change strategies, and this chapter describes those strategies as well as particularly innovative or successful programs tested by other groups. This chapter highlights:

- Setting institutional goals
- Taking specific steps
- Making patient wishes known and accessible
- Involving the community
- Creating opportunities for advance care planning
- Educating health care providers
- Addressing cultural differences

### ★★★Gundersen Lutheran Medical Center

The team from Gundersen Lutheran Medical Center, anchored by a facility based in La Crosse, Wisconsin, included an advance practice nurse, an oncologist, and a clinical ethicist. Since the early 1990s, Gundersen, along with other major health care systems in the La Crosse area, has worked on community-wide programs to improve advance care planning. Staff from Gundersen and Franciscan Skemp health care developed an initiative called "Respecting Your Choices," which used patient and family education, community outreach, education for non-medical professionals, standard training sessions, and standard methods for documenting and tracking advance directives. At the end of a two-year period, a retrospective study of 540 decedents found that 85 percent had completed an advance directive (compared to a national average of 15 percent) and that, of these, 95 percent were in the medical record. In 98 percent of the deaths, treatment was forgone, as patients had directed.

The team decided to refine the usual approach to advance care planning by writing a script physicians could use when talking to patients. In these cases, advance care planning conversations began with the question, "What makes you happy at this stage of your illness?" The script helped clinicians guide discussions about end-of-life decision making by touching on goal setting, resources, emotional issues, and communication. As a result of such discussions, some patients changed the course of their care and treatment.

For instance, following one round of chemotherapy, a 73-year-old woman with advanced cancer talked to the team's advance practice nurse. The woman had suffered severe symptoms during previous treatment, and her family did not want her to pursue another round of chemotherapy. The patient, however, said that she "had never been a quitter" and felt that she needed to try chemotherapy "one more time." She told the nurse that if the chemotherapy made her sick again, she would stop the process, realizing that doing so would lead to her death.

After the chemotherapy, the woman was rehospitalized with a high fever, pneumonia, and increased lethargy. When her oncologist recommended more chemotherapy, the advance practice nurse stepped in to discuss the patient's wishes, sharing notes from the earlier conversation. The oncologist agreed to end the treatment; the patient was admitted to hospice and died comfortably at home three days later.

This woman and others cared for by members of the Gundersen Lutheran team benefited from the team's aims to improve advance care planning and to provide opportunities for patients and families to find meaningfulness in the face of serious illnesses.

Changes tested included:

- Identifying patients with metastatic cancer early after diagnosis
- Communicating patient responses to the advance planning discussion to doctors and other health care providers
- Expanding use of the script to more physicians

The team measured its progress by tracking:

- Hospice length of stay (LOS), with an aim of increasing the median LOS from 19 days to 36 (greater than the 1995 national hospice median of 29 days)
- Patient and physician perception that the interview was helpful
- For patients in the intervention group, compared with a control group, an improved quality of life

Gundersen's project achieved several tangible results:

- The number of participating physicians increased from one to eight.
- Almost all patients (95 percent) reported that the interview process itself was meaningful.
- Patients felt that they benefited from improved communication with loved ones and with health care providers.
- Patients became more involved in the process—and expected their health care team to be involved as well.
- Of the 42 patients in the pilot intervention, the first 9 who died had a median length of stay in hospice of 32 days—close to the team's goal of 36 days.

Next steps will be monitoring the program's effect on the median length of hospice stay; studying the value of the tool itself, as well as the process; finding additional ways to use the interview instrument in patient-provider interactions; and expanding the use of interventions with other patient populations.

### ★★Review the Current Advance Care Planning Process

Widespread change in advance care planning requires that health care facilities and systems change current practices in counseling patients, recording plans, and transferring records of plans made. To this end, organizations can set many goals for advance care planning. Here are a few goals that are reasonable, based on what others have achieved.

- Patients and families report no surprises as the disease progresses—patients and families are prepared for and have anticipated events that would otherwise have been unexpected or frightening.
- All seriously ill patients have a conversation about advance care planning with a health care professional who is skilled at advance care planning—and all in-patients and seriously ill patients have documented advance care plans in their medical records (unless they are unwilling to do so).
- All health care professionals working with seriously ill patients learn to discuss, document, and implement advance care planning.
- All emergency medical services come to an agreement with area hospitals and facilities on advance care planning standards and protocols.
- The documented preferences of all patients are followed, unless there are very good reasons to overrule (e.g., if it is mandatory to protect public health).
- Representatives from relevant community organizations (e.g., churches, senior centers, law offices) participate in community-wide programs to encourage advance care planning.
- Seriously ill patients and their families rarely resort to calling 911, because they are prepared to work with plans, supplies, and resources at home.

### ★★★Dayton Veterans Affairs Medical Center

The Breakthrough Series team from the Dayton (Ohio) VA Medical Center aimed to increase to 95 percent the number of veterans, among those diagnosed with congestive heart failure, chronic obstructive lung disease, or lung cancer, who participated in advance care planning discussions. To measure progress, the Breakthrough Series team tracked advance care planning documentation by reviewing 50 randomly selected charts each week.

Among the changes tested, the team:

- Redesigned a video on advance care planning for patients and families
- Revised and distributed a patient education booklet
- Developed discussion guidelines for providers and for follow-up

---

Considering Plans for
Future Health Care:
Holistic Health Care
Planning Script
(*Continued*)

3. If you have to choose between living longer and quality of life, how would you approach this balance?
4. Are there any special events or activities you are looking forward to?
5. What needs or services would you like to discuss?
6. Do you want information about anything related to your present or future care?
7. What sustains you when you face serious challenges in life?
8. Do you have any religious or spiritual beliefs that are important to you?
9. In what way do you feel you could make this time especially meaningful to you?
10. What do you hope most for those closest to you?

Facilitator Impression and Recommendations:

Updates:

---

- Initiated an advance care planning clinic
- Revised the center's policy and bylaws on advance care planning and on hospice/palliative care, requiring them in certain circumstances
- Developed computer software to aid in advance care planning
- Initiated a bereavement support group

In a 12-week period, documentation of advance care planning discussions and follow-up increased from approximately 15 percent of charts to almost 90 percent.

The group established a clinic for advance care planning. In the course of a year, more than 150 patients and families have attended the clinics, which provide, in one hour, the following elements:

- An introduction and overview of advance care planning, including basic definitions, terminology, and review of handouts
- A 30-minute video, adapted and personalized for the Dayton VA's use, followed by a question-and-answer session
- Emphasis on the patient's right to control the decision-making process, to ask questions and have needs met
- Time to stay and complete forms
- An opportunity to take material home, including the video, in order to encourage other family members to become involved

★★Use or Adapt Comprehensive Advance Care Planning Forms

Planning is far more than what most patients and many providers believe it to be—that is, it is far more than just "pulling the plug" or turning off a machine. Instead, advance care planning

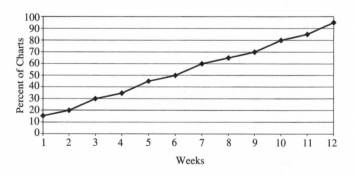

Figure 5.1 Documentation of Advance Care Planning. Reprinted with permission of VA Healthcare Systems, Dayton, OH.

can and should include discussions and document plans that address the "ifs" and ambiguities of living with chronic illness, such as:

- Role of the family, including their interests and well-being, and their authority to revise advance care planning documents
- CPR/DNAR (cardiopulmonary resuscitation and "do not attempt resuscitation" orders)
- Respirator
- Hospital transfers and placement issues (including home)
- How assets and benefits are to be used
- Treatment options
- Pain management
- Hydration issues
- Artificial nutrition
- Blood transfusions
- Organ and tissue donation
- Medical device donation
- Plans for cremation or burial, funeral or memorial services

★★Make Patient Wishes Known and Accessible

Some states have developed quick ways to make sure patient wishes are known by all health care providers who are treating them, or who may treat them, such as emergency medical services (EMS) crews. Among strategies being used in various areas are:

- DNR orders, sometimes printed on a particular brightly colored paper or put in a special form, and then posted on medical records and in prominent places in the home
- Wrist bracelets indicating a patient's DNR (do not resuscitate) wishes
- Prescription medicine vials containing emergency information, to be carried in glove compartments and stored in freezers, where EMS personnel have been instructed to look for them

Many organizations are working to make sure patient wishes are known and accessible. The project in La Crosse, Wisconsin, described above, is one example of such an endeavor. Three other projects, one involving a physician order, one entailing community-wide education, and one featuring a simplified planning document, have also been successful.

## What Makes an Advance Care Plan Complete?

- Plans that are more specific and detailed than a basic "do not attempt resuscitation" or a "do not intubate" order
- Ongoing discussions—in which clinicians balance frankness and sensitivity—and revisions that reflect changes in patient health or preferences
- Designation of proxy, if possible
- System that assures transferral across health care facilities and hospital units
- Completion and accessibility of all legal documents to clinicians, surrogate decision makers, and health care proxies
- Steps to put plans into action (bracelets for the emergency medical service staff, medications at home, family training, and so on)
- Discussion about who will make decisions and how they will be made, how the decision-making process will work

### ★★★Oregon's POLST—Physician Orders for Life-Sustaining Treatment

Oregon uses the POLST document, developed by a multidisciplinary task force of the Center for Ethics in Health Care at Oregon Health Sciences University with representatives from across the state, to help health care providers honor patients' treatment wishes. The POLST document underwent revisions after extensive pilot testing. Printed on shocking pink card stock, the one-page document is attached to the front of medical records in hospitals and nursing homes. Individuals living at home are encouraged to post the form in a prominent place where any EMS personnel who come to the patient's aid can see it. The POLST was originally designed to resolve problems in respecting DNR orders when patients were transferred from nursing homes to hospitals and was intended to prevent unwanted transfers or hospitalizations. Chapter 7 features more information about the usefulness of the POLST document (Tolle et al., 1998).

### ★★Georgia Health Decisions

*Critical Conditions: Make Your Final Health Care Decisions* is the slogan developed by Atlanta-based Georgia Health Decisions (GHD) to encourage Georgians to participate in meaningful advance care planning with families and health care providers. Following a pilot project in eight communities, the program will eventually be used statewide for intense public education and end-of-life planning.

"We learned one thing in Georgia, based on focus groups," said Beverly Tyler, executive director. "People have a false sense that they innately know what loved ones would want. In fact, unless they have been through a serious illness, people think the only decision to be made is whether to pull the plug or not."

### ★★Florida Commission on Aging with Dignity and "Five Wishes"

Thanks to efforts by the Florida Commission on Aging with Dignity, any adult can use a booklet titled "Five Wishes" to guide his or her thinking about how they want to be treated, should they have a life-threatening illness or become unable to voice their decisions. The booklet provides an easy way to record one's wishes. It meets all the requirements of the law in 33 states and the District of Columbia. In one year, more than 250,000 Floridians received copies; within a few weeks of its release on the Web, it was downloaded more than 15,000 times. The final version improves upon the usual legal language of living wills by encouraging comments on the many ways in which a person might choose to be treated. Subjects covered include:

- Medical treatment wanted (or not)
- Desired level of comfort
- How patient wants to be treated
- What patient wants family to know
- Health care proxy

A copy of the "Five Wishes" booklet is included in the Resources section at the back of this book. See page 328.

## Recognize Opportunities to Address Advance Care Planning

There are many settings in which advance care planning can and does occur, such as:

- Senior centers
- Community-based care settings
- Home health agencies
- Hospice
- Clergy
- Elder law attorneys
- Geriatric care managers (most are nurses or social workers)

In the context of this book, advance care planning revolves around dying patients. However, advance care planning can occur at many points, which the following chart illustrates.

### ★★Elmhurst Hospital Infectious Disease Clinic

People with HIV/AIDS may need to make permanency plans for minor children who survive a parent's death. Asking people to develop these plans is difficult—but essential. Staff members at Elmhurst Hospital Infectious Disease Clinic in Queens, New York, address advance care planning at several points during the course of a patient's illness:

Table 5.1 Putting Advance Care Planning into Action

| Health status examples | Recommended content of discussions | Action items | Communication strategy |
|---|---|---|---|
| Healthy | Surrogate<br><br>Outcome states<br><br>Atypical beliefs or preferences | May complete durable power of attorney document<br><br>Should include preferences regarding long-term artificial hydration and nutrition | "Is there anything I should know about you that might affect what medical treatment you would want?"<br><br>"If you become too sick to tell me what you want done, who would you like me to speak with?" |
| Diagnosed with a serious illness | Surrogate<br><br>What is important for you/what are your goals<br><br>Adverse outcomes<br><br>Time-limited trials<br><br>Likely outcomes | Same as above<br><br>MD discusses prognoses and outcomes with and without recommended treatments<br><br>MD talks to surrogate | "You will recover almost completely from this stroke. We are going to treat you to reduce your risk of another stroke. However, it is important to plan ahead. Do you have any thoughts about your medical care if we ever did not expect a good recovery?"<br>"Unlike what you see on TV, CPR is rarely effective when you have a serious illness, such as stroke." |
| Limited life expectancy on the basis of disease or of age alone. | More explicit conversation about outcomes and courses with treatment options | Same as above<br><br>State specific preferences and formulate contingency plans for urgent complications (CPR, shortness of breath, fever, etc.) | "Mrs. M, your breathing is really a problem for you almost all of the time now. Tell me a little about what you think will happen."<br>"Mrs. M, you want medical care to focus on comfort, and you want to stay at home. Is that correct? If you do get short of breath, and it does not respond to usual treatments, we will use morphine to keep you from feeling breathless. The chances are that you would die in such an episode, but you would be comfortable. Have I understood you correctly? Let me tell you a little more about hospice . . ." |

*Source:* Teno & Lynn, 1996

- At the first appointment for care in the clinic
- During the first episode of illness
- When the patient recognizes the need for home care services and accepts them
- When weight loss or frequency of episodes makes the illness grave

## Educate Clinicians and Community Leaders about Effective Advance Care Planning

Advance care planning is a process of documenting discussions and decisions about a patient's current choices for future medical care and treatment. The process encourages understanding and reflection on the meaning of the disease and its significance in one's life. Advance care planning can address predictable events associated with specific diseases—such as the use of tube feeding for Alzheimer's patients—and prevent such events from escalating into medical emergencies or family crises.

Advance care planning addresses the unique issues patients and families face—for instance, by allowing them to state the course of treatment they would prefer in specific medical situations or the person they would want to make decisions for them if they were incapacitated.

Successful advance care planning depends on clinicians who:

- Understand what makes an advance care plan "complete"
- Seek, discuss, and document patient choices, develop contingency plans, and discuss these plans with families or proxy
- Are willing and able to put specific elements of the plan into effect (e.g., certain emergency medications in the home, or "do not attempt resuscitation" orders placed prominently in the home)

When working with seriously ill and dying patients, clinicians must understand:

- The diagnosis, prognosis, and disease process and how it will change over time
- Health care options, including home care and community-based care options
- What is possible and routine given the patient's diagnosis and circumstances
- Any ambiguities about prognosis or preferences

### ★★M. D. Anderson Cancer Center

Houston's M. D. Anderson Cancer Center serves approximately 400 inpatients and 2,000 outpatients daily and provides indigent hospital care for Texans with cancer.

The Breakthrough Series team aimed to improve advance care planning for its gynecologic cancer patients. The goal was for 75 percent of these patients to participate in a Gynecology Advance Planning (GAP) consult and to have an advance care planning note in their charts. The preprinted note provided a prompt for physicians to cover important end-of-life issues and documented the content of the physician discussion. The physician intervention was followed by conversations with support personnel trained to help patients with end-of-life planning, dubbed "GAP consults" by the team.

To encourage this process, physicians and others participated in a "breaking bad news" workshop, which was based on a model first described in 1992 by Robert Buckman. A physician at M. D. Anderson tailored Buckman's model to the specific needs of gynecologic cancer patients; the workshops featured didactic sessions and role-play.

In a survey of patient satisfaction with physician discussions, physicians received high marks for sensitivity and truthfulness and lower marks on time spent with patients and listening. During the GAP consults, patient concerns focused on faith and spirituality (83 percent), family issues (75 percent), and medical concerns (58 percent).

Convincing clinicians and others to include advance care planning notes proved to be a challenge. The same procedure is now being piloted in the gastrointestinal center. The "breaking bad news" workshops have been well received, and that process is continuing with residents and fellows.

### ★★★University of California at Los Angeles

The UCLA Breakthrough Series team developed a tool that encourages doctors to talk openly to patients about their illness, its progression, and their preferences. The one-page Care Plan Discussion Document (CPDD), written and refined over several months, can be completed in a few seconds once the issues have been discussed (see below).

The CPDD asks providers to note several aspects of the care being provided to a dying patient and includes material helpful for medical social workers. The tool aims to stimulate discussions earlier in the course of the illness and provide a structured

Table 5.2 Effect of Care Plan Discussion and Document.
Reprinted with permission of UCLA Medical Center, CA.

| Control Group | Intervention |
|---|---|
| 8 patient charts | 19 patient charts |
| No discussions of prognosis or preferences on medical records | 11 completed CPDD; of these: |
| | 7 discussed prognosis |
| | 4 discussed preferences |
| | 5 discussed resuscitation |
| 2 discussed/wrote DNR orders | 5 completed DNR orders |

method to document that conversations have occurred. The multiple-choice form addresses the following questions:

- What is the goal of admission?
- What is the chance of surviving one year?
- Has the prognosis been discussed?
- What does the patient think of this prognosis?
- What are the patient's wishes for care?
- Which treatments would the patient undergo to prolong life?

★★*Community Hospitals of Indianapolis*

Hoping to enable patients to make advance care plans long before they arrived in an acute care setting, Community Hospitals of Indianapolis developed a four-hour training program for parish nurses and pastors designed to:

- Increase the comfort level of parish nurses and pastors in end-of-life discussions and planning
- Provide a mechanism for the community at large for training about end-of-life issues
- Begin a way to affect end-of-life care before patients arrive in acute care settings

Previous attendees receive information about upcoming sessions. The group has also developed a resource guide on end-of-life issues for parish nurses and pastors. The guide features print and Internet resources about state regulations regarding advance directives, social services information, and other materials. The success of this program inspired another large health care system to tailor the materials for sessions in its communities.

## ★★Address Cultural and Ethnic Differences about Advance Care Planning

Cultural and ethnic differences affect the willingness of different ethnic and minority groups to engage in advance care planning. For many Asian Americans, family decision making takes priority over individual expression about treatment preferences. Among many African Americans, including those who have witnessed mistreatment and misinformation in the health care system and those who recall the Tuskegee syphilis study, there is a distrust of the health care system.

Two Breakthrough Series teams—New York City's Coney Island Hospital and the Balm of Gilead Center in Birmingham, Alabama—tried to improve advance care planning for poor patients and for minority groups.

Coney Island Hospital provides acute care to poor and underserved patients, who have often come to the hospital in emergency situations. Conversations about end-of-life care proved to be emotionally charged, and many families resisted participating, often because they felt that doing so meant giving up hope for the patient. Health care team members were uncomfortable with discussing choices and did not always know how to approach patients and families without eroding hope.

In looking at ways to improve care, Coney Island identified the following problems in its current care:

- Patients admitted to the hospital had not had an opportunity to express preferences for end-of-life care.
- Patients and doctors often had no prior relationship.
- Serial discussions about advance care planning were not documented on patient charts.
- Language and cultural barriers complicated conversations.

Coney Island tried many changes:

- Renewed staff training regarding how to designate a health care proxy and how to complete documents
- Identification of advocates who were able to initiate discussions with patients and complete documents, often in

their native language; later, patient advocates were called in through consultation to assist in gathering and verifying information

- Creation of a script to encourage discussions of treatment choices

A similar approach proved successful for the Balm of Gilead Center at Cooper Green Hospital, a public hospital. The Breakthrough Series team aimed to develop an approach to advance care planning that would encourage these patients to participate, rather than feel alienated by the process. The group planned to address potential barriers in very specific ways:

- A designated layperson would be used to interview patients, so they would feel less distrustful of authority or the system.
- Advance care planning would be offered and encouraged as something "for all of us," regardless of health status, thus addressing superstitions about discussing—and thus causing—death.
- By focusing on unhurried, patient-centered listening, staff members would keep patients from feeling overwhelmed or manipulated by the process.
- By guiding patients through the form step-by-step, staff members could adjust for reading skills and comprehension level without embarrassing or intimidating the patient.

The group developed and tested a script that is very conversational and is meant to put the patient at ease. An excerpt follows:

Let me tell you about the project I'm working on. Cooper Green Hospital is very interested in encouraging all of us to think ahead about our health care to make sure that we are the ones who get to make the decisions about how our care will be handled down the road. I'm talking to lots of people—hospital staff, inpatients, outpatients, even people in the community—about this, and I wonder if I could talk to you, too. As I said, I'm having the same conversation with all sorts of people—so this has nothing to do with your current illness or any concerns about your condition. By the way, what is your understanding of your illness and what you can expect?

Figure 5.2 Cooper Green Hospital Health Care Proxy. Reprinted with permission of Cooper Green Hospital, Birmingham, AL.

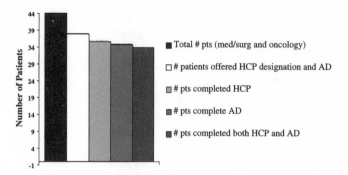

■ Total # pts (med/surg and oncology)

☐ # patients offered HCP designation and AD

▨ # pts completed HCP

◪ # pts complete AD

▨ # pts completed both HCP and AD

## ★★Steps to Improve Advance Care Planning

Some organizations have managed to improve advance care planning despite limited resources and funding. For instance, New York's Coney Island Hospital found a volunteer who led a focused effort to improve advance care planning on one unit. Through his efforts, 13 health care proxy documents were completed in a two-month period.

Other ways to improve advance care planning include:

- Naming a health care proxy on all hospital consent forms, such as surgical consent forms
- Asking health insurance companies to ask enrollees to designate a health care proxy on the enrollment form
- Including the health care proxy on computerized databases and systemwide networks
- Starting a community living will project, a coalition of organizations to focus on living wills and increase public awareness of advance care planning
- Referring home health care patients to a social worker for end-of-life assessments and planning
- Establishing practices that enable doctors to write a patient's CPR preferences at the time of admission (e.g., over the phone)
- Establishing a timeframe within which Do Not Attempt Resuscitation orders will be explicitly discussed and the discussion documented in a patient's chart, after hospital or nursing facility admission
- Having a standardized location in the patient's record for documenting plans for emergency and end-of-life care (in addition to the advance directive), such as a vinyl pocket or a particular line on the problem list that refers to specific notes inside
- Distributing patient education brochures on advance care planning or making available instructional videotapes

- Implementing computerized reminder system on patient charts for outpatient clinic visits

## Innovators Need to Know

The activities undertaken by these and other groups demonstrate that given the opportunity, individuals and clinicians can have meaningful discussions about the difficult territory of death and dying, that advance care planning can affect patient care, and that the tools and information to direct such plans are available. Most groups in the Breakthrough Series found that they could quickly address problems in advance care planning and make a significant difference in how it was done. Use them as a model to begin improvements!

- Useful advance care planning requires an ongoing dialogue between the patient, his or her loved ones, and the health care team.
- Make advance care planning a routine part of health care; discuss it with all patients, the sick and the well, young and old, and keep the conversation going. Tailor the conversation to the patient's health status and clinical circumstance.
- Revise forms to reflect specific changes likely to occur during the course of a chronic fatal disease.
- Make a special effort to address the unique needs and concerns of underserved populations, such as the poor and minorities.
- Involve other community organizations in education efforts, including the local media, bar association, worship communities, and other health care organizations.
- Include advance care planning elements in computerized databases and systemwide records (e.g., generate reminders to staff).
- Encourage insurance plans and managed care organizations to promote advance care planning efforts among their beneficiaries.

## Resources

For more information about living wills, contact:
Choice in Dying
1035 30th Street NW
Washington, DC 20007

Phone: 800-898-9455
Phone: 202-338-9790
Fax: 202-338-0242
http://www.choices.org

To order "Five Wishes," contact:
Florida Commission on Aging with Dignity
P.O. Box 1661
Tallahassee, FL 32302-1661
The document is free, although the group requests a $4 donation. You may download it from the Web at http://www.agingwithdignity.org. It is also reprinted in the Resources section starting on page 327 at the back of this book.

For more on the POLST Document, contact:
Oregon Health Sciences University
Center for Ethics in Health Care, L101
3181 SW Sam Jackson Park Road
Portland, OR 97201
Phone: 503-494-4466
Fax: 503-494-1260
Order a sample via e-mail: ethics@ohsu.edu.

For an excellent "values questionnaire" to help guide patients through advance directives and issues about future health care, contact:
Vermont Ethics Network
City Center-89 Main Street
Drawer 20
Montpelier, VT 05620
Phone: 802-828-2909
For information on how to complete an ethical will, visit http://www.ethicalwill.com.

# Relationships, Spirituality, and Bereavement

## Supporting People in Difficult Times

Health care providers are beginning to realize that meeting the emotional and spiritual needs of dying patients and their loved ones can be as important as providing good medical care. As a Gallup study (1997) reported, "Those who are dying are more than objects of medical attention. They remain human beings with the wide variety of needs they experienced over the course of their life—practical, emotional, spiritual, as well as medical." Health care professionals can alleviate patient suffering by helping them to find meaning despite illness and by offering opportunities for inpatients and nursing home residents to participate in spiritual and religious rituals.

Studies indicate that most Americans want to talk about their spiritual lives when confronted with the end of their physical lives. A national survey (Gallup, 1997) demonstrated the importance people place on human contact and prayer at the end of life.

- A majority said human interaction would be important to them if they were dying:
  - 55 percent would want someone with whom to share their thoughts and fears.
  - 54 percent would just want someone with them.
  - 47 percent would want someone holding their hand or touching them.
  - 50 percent would want the opportunity to pray alone.
  - 50 percent would want to have someone praying for them.

- People seek comfort from family and friends:
  - 81 percent turn to family.

> We are here on earth to do good to others. What the others are here for I don't know.
>
> —W. H. Auden

- 61 percent turn to close friends.
- 36 percent said that a member of the clergy could be comforting.
- 30 percent said a doctor could be comforting, and 21 percent said a nurse could.

By addressing patient and family fears and concerns, providers can promote a better quality of life for patients, alleviate their anxiety, and provide the human contact sometimes lacking in today's medical system. Spirituality is one way to help people find hope and meaning in the midst of suffering.

Organizations offer a range of supportive services, such as chaplain referral activities to increase caregiver confidence, community outreach programs, and bereavement support and counseling. These services have been the mainstay of hospice programs for many years, and hospices are usually willing to share what they know with others.

When emotional and spiritual needs go unmet, clinicians and patients miss the opportunity to make informed decisions, to talk to families, to resolve financial and legal issues, or to make the most of the time they have.

Spirituality includes the search for ultimate meaning and purpose in life. Each person specifies the definition to fit his or her own beliefs and experiences. Expressions of spirituality include religion, music, art, nature, and other spiritual beliefs. There are spiritual aspects to many relationships people have. As people approach death, they often struggle with existential questions, such as "Why me? Why now? Why this? How will my loved ones survive my death? What will happen to me when I die? What's next?" Although spiritual questions such as these have no easy answers, clinicians can support patients and their loved ones along their spiritual journey, as the patient and family try to come to peace with these issues.

One doctor has written, "Just because dying is natural doesn't mean it's easy" (Tobin and Lindsey, 1999). Many dying patients question both their physical health ("Why is my body doing this? What does this symptom mean?") and the universe and their role in it. Health care providers who are prepared to guide and counsel patients in a compassionate, caring way through the difficult transitions at the end of life fulfill one of medicine's important roles to comfort the sick.

## In This Chapter

This chapter describes the changes different systems tried—from urban and rural public hospitals to community-based hospices—to provide more holistic patient care by supporting

## Patient and Family Needs

- Being held and comforted by loved ones
- Being listened to—sharing their hopes, dreams, fears, and anxiety with loved ones and caregivers
- Having the opportunity to pray or meditate, participate in sacred rituals, listen to music, and spend private time with family and friends
- Receiving blessings from family, friends, and clergy
- Making peace with God, family, and friends
- Seeking forgiveness from God, family, and loved ones
- Being at peace with themselves and with others

human relationships, spirituality, and meaning in life both for patients and for health care providers. Changes described include:

- Incorporating chaplains and clergy on the health care team
- Offering diverse complementary therapies to patients and families
- Providing "hospitality" carts to families keeping vigil in ICUs
- Improving caregiver confidence through education and telecommunication
- Training clinicians in communications skills
- Recruiting and training volunteers to interact with patients and families
- Assessing patient suffering and ways to cope with it
- Discussing what helps patients and families find meaning in life
- Establishing and offering bereavement services for patients, families, and staff members

Unlike the experiences of groups working to improve dyspnea or continuity, groups that tried to improve in this area found that even the most basic change could lead to improvement. This is a sad commentary, reflecting the very poor state of human affairs in medical care. Yet it is also a powerful reason to improve—now.

### ★★★Fairview Health Systems

Many Breakthrough Series participants made changes to address patients' emotional and spiritual needs while providing medical care. Among the successes achieved were those by Fairview Health Systems, a Minneapolis-based system of hospitals, nursing homes, and home health and hospice care. The Fairview team included hospice, geriatrics, and home health care program staff.

The team tried many changes, often working to blend traditional medical care with alternative healing methods. For instance, an ICU nurse who was also a Hebrew cantor sang to a frail elderly patient who was in isolation and on a ventilator. The patient's high anxiety often triggered alarms. However, as the cantor/nurse intoned psalms, his breathing rate quieted, his anxiety level went down, and he slept peacefully.

Other seriously ill and dying patients at Fairview have been comforted by a harpist trained in performing for—and working with—very sick patients. As the harpist plays, patient pulses,

---

**Best Practices to Enhance Supportive Care**

- Hospice care that routinely includes family and spiritual concerns and that offers education and counseling about what to expect as the disease progresses and as the patient nears death
- Grief counseling programs for bereaved families and loved ones, regardless of place of death (e.g., ICU, nursing homes)
- Programs that support family caregivers and respect patients' spiritual search for meaning and religious rituals

Even better practices would enhance best practices several steps, by:

- Entering the experience in terms of human life, spirituality, and meaning, rather than in terms of medical and physiological issues. In this context, professional caregiver habits become secondary to patient and family living patterns and preferences.
- Using episodes of serious illness as opportunities to talk about death and dying and loss, about what gives ultimate meaning in life, and about setting priorities on values and goals in one's life
- Creating rituals to mark passages in life
- Reassuring families by explaining what is happening and counseling them
- Learning how to provide care that accepts death as part of life while prolonging and enhancing the quality of life and relieving suffering

breathing, and anxiety improve. The harpist has played for families keeping vigil for loved ones in the ICU.

The Fairview team's Plan-Do-Study-Act cycle aimed to increase patient comfort by reducing pain, dyspnea, anxiety, and depression by half. Changes tested included guided imagery exercises and meditation as an adjuvant to pain treatment; imagery and therapeutic massage to reduce anxiety among families in the pediatric ICU; and harp music for pain and anxiety among pediatric patients and their families. Grant money enabled the team to provide music and massage therapy in its nursing homes and hospice.

To measure the effect of changes, the group asked nurses, chaplains, and social workers to carry out a test on one or two patients and report the results to the end-of-life study team. The team worked with other health care providers to use therapies that they might not have tried previously.

In many situations, patient symptoms improved. As a result, the end-of-life team offered a two-day conference at which 70 participants learned more about using complementary therapies at the end of life. Orders to initiate complementary therapies were added to the standard palliative care plan, which is now available in four of Fairview's hospitals. In addition, the group has assembled 13 palliative care kits that are available on several nursing units. The group wrote a booklet titled "Journey through the Dying Process," which Fairview printed and is distributing systemwide.

With foundation money, the Fairview team continues work begun during the Breakthrough Series. Staff plan to:

- Hold seven community meetings to enhance awareness of end-of-life issues and to discuss ways to develop community-wide strategies to improve end-of-life care
- Provide comprehensive training to physicians and other health care practitioners about end-of-life care
- Expand bereavement support groups beyond the current programs
- Offer additional support groups for grieving children

Through this process, the Fairview team learned that patients and families want to try complementary therapies—but found that professionals had to volunteer their services. The team developed a list of providers within the Fairview system who can provide complementary therapies. The team plans to develop ways to improve access to complementary therapies, pay for these services, and centralize requests.

## Palliative Care Kit Contents
### Fairview Health Systems

This kit will be used for many patients. Some of the items will be given to the patient or family; other items should remain in the kit to be reused.

Prayer book: to meet a variety of spiritual needs
- The book includes a variety of poems, prayers, and scripture.
- Refer to the table of contents and ask the patient and family if they have any requests or topics listed that would be helpful to them. These can be read silently by the patient or aloud by the patient, family, or caregiver.
- The book should remain in the kit.

Anointing oil: to be used for blessings and other rituals
- There is an instruction sheet that accompanies each vial of oil that will assist you in how to use it.
- Any remaining oil in the vial should be given to the family.

CD player/tape player and CDs/tapes: to provide music therapy
- Music therapy can ease stress and help relieve pain. Play the tapes, or ask the family to bring in some music the patient enjoys.
- All tapes and CDs should remain in the kit.
- (Only a few kits have a CD or tape player included; it will be clearly marked if it is supposed to have a player included.)

Potpourri/sachet: to provide aromatherapy
- Aromatherapy is intended to relieve pain and alleviate tension.
- Put some potpourri/sachet in the small blue dish to add a soothing fragrance to the room. Only a small amount is needed.
- Close the bag and save the fragrance for future use.

Lotions: to provide massage therapy
- Massage therapy can help both muscle pain and stress-related conditions. Use the lotions to have the family provide a simple massage to the patient's hands.
- For massage, apply lotion, then simply gently rub the back of the patient's hand, working lotion into the thumb and fingers. Then turn the hand over and massage the palm, extending the massage to the fingers. This routine allows the family to hold the patient's hand while taking part in the patient's care.
- The patient and family can keep the lotion, if they choose.

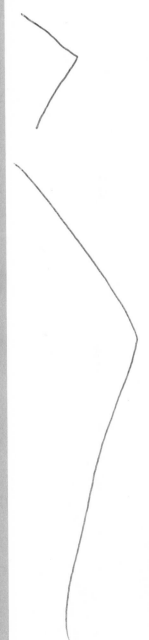

### ★★★Promote Patient and Caregiver Confidence
### in the Care System

Faced with life-limiting illness and an array of medical, social, emotional, and mental concerns, families may feel very uncertain about how to care for a loved one at home. Just the logistics—making sure someone can open the door for a home health aide, for instance, or get to the pharmacy to fill a late-night prescription—can daunt even the best-organized family. Families—and patients—can quickly come to doubt their ability to deal with the illness at home or may question the commitment of the health care system to respond when needed.

Caregivers can feel more confident when they know that they can always reach a health care professional who is familiar with the patient's needs, when they understand symptoms and their treatment, when they know more about disease progression, and when they have time to "recharge."

### ★★★*Hospice of Michigan: "Caregivers as Colleagues"*

With its Breakthrough Series project, "Caregivers as Colleagues," the Hospice of Michigan aimed to improve patient and family confidence. More than 20 teams statewide care for the Hospice of Michigan's daily census of more than 900 patients. For its Plan-Do-Study-Act cycles, the group aimed to decrease caregiver anxiety and increase caregiver confidence. To measure the effects of changes, the team:

- Compared control and study patient groups and caregiver anxiety level in each group
- Looked at unplanned hospital admissions, 911 calls, and ER visits
- Tracked increases in caregiver confidence following interventions

The team tested each intervention with about 10 patients. During the first Plan-Do-Study-Act cycles, family caregivers were given a pager, which hospice staff could use to contact caregivers who were not present in the home during a hospice visit. More important, carrying the pagers allowed caregivers to feel that patients or family members could easily reach them. During the second cycle, participating families were asked to pay for the pager, although some were given financial assistance.

Other changes tested were:

- Giving caregivers telephone stickers listing ~~the hospice~~ number. Families reported putting the stickers in many locations.
- Making a second visit to patient and caregiver within 48 hours of the initial hospice admission to explain medication management. The Breakthrough Series team found that a significant barrier to teaching caregivers about medications was the emotional state of patients and families during the admission. By separating the intake visit from the caregiver education visit, the team helped caregivers better understand medications and patient care. During this visit, nurses also monitored the accuracy of dosing.
- Assigning hospice social workers to broker services within hospice and the community. These individuals, called "doulas," offered a link between patients and families and the larger community. The doula and caregiver worked together to define needs and resources and set a schedule for completing various tasks. Caregivers agreed to complete certain tasks described in a written care plan—and study showed that most completed all tasks.

The team learned several things during its study cycles. For instance, when its changes were successful, the team found it easy to spread the word and encourage others to try those changes. The team also learned that health care providers cannot always assume to know what would be best for caregiv-

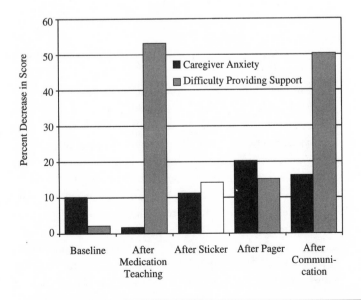

Figure 6.1 Decrease in Anxiety and Difficulty Providing Support. Reprinted with permission of Hospice of Michigan, Southfield, MI.

Figure 6.2 Unplanned Events per 100 Patient Days, by Intervention Tried. Reprinted by permission of Hospice of Michigan, Southfield, MI.

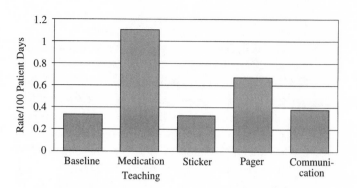

ers and instead must ask about caregivers' needs. The group was surprised to find that caregivers do not necessarily want or need more communication with health care providers. The team found that caregivers did want information about hospice visits—but only when calls came at the "right time." One way to resolve this was to have the case manager set up a communication schedule with the family caregiver.

## ★★Improve Clinicians' Communication Skills

Delivering bad news is a difficult task but one that doctors and others can learn to do with compassion, empathy, and respect. To help physicians develop the communication skills necessary for such conversations, many organizations sponsor provider training programs. Some Breakthrough Series teams took this a step further by training community representatives to talk with patients and families.

### ★St. Thomas Health Services: "The Packet"

As many innovators discover, not every health care provider is ready for change or understands quality improvement in end-of-life care. The Breakthrough Series team from St. Thomas Health Services in Nashville, Tennessee, encountered a physician who was reluctant to engage in any of the team's change cycles. However, one day he called the team leader to ask for "the packet," something to help him talk to dying patients. The team quickly wrote and began to distribute a collection of documents they titled "The Packet: Communication Guide for Care of the Patient with Life Threatening Illness," which featured checklists to guide clinicians through the steps involved in providing good end-of-life care. The checklists are a "care map" to protocols and policies and describe the role of each care team member. The requesting physician's "packet" was assembled in a day.

With "The Packet," the team aimed to improve communication between physicians and patients or their surrogates. To measure initial success, the team planned to track increased patient/family/physician/caregiver satisfaction with care, although the patient may have died. As the project continued, the team found that families gave consistently high satisfaction ratings—even when communication was poor, pain was not controlled, and other factors were less than ideal. It changed its measures to include:

- Increased end-of-life ethics consults
- Data collection about elements of a good and bad death
- Decreased costs of dying, without an increase in mortality rates
- Increased patient comfort, competency, confidence, and satisfaction

The checklist encouraged continuity of communication among providers and with patients—helping everyone to sing from the same sheet. Information in "The Packet" became the basis for a communications flowchart now used as a teaching instrument. The focus on communications created the expectation that doctors would discuss end-of-life issues with patients, gave nurses more direct authority in communicating with patients and clinicians, and highlighted the need to focus on spirituality. The appendix includes several checklists from "The Packet."

### ★Dartmouth-Hitchcock Medical Center: Learning to Pronounce Death

Finding that many clinicians did not appreciate the emotional significance of the pronouncement of death to family members or the basics of good communication with families, Dartmouth-Hitchcock Medical Center in Lebanon, New Hampshire, developed a pocket card to guide clinicians through the steps of pronouncing a patient dead.

### ★★★Provide Direct, Practical Support to Families and Loved Ones

Sometimes the act of listening to patients and families comforts them. Volunteers from the community or local clergy are often willing to listen—and often have more time to do so than do physicians—and to visit or call patients.

**Quick Reference Card for Pronouncement of Death**
*Dartmouth-Hitchcock Medical Center*

- Recognize the extreme emotional significance of the actual pronouncement of death to family members in room.
- Establish eye contact with family member(s) present.
- Introduce self to family.
- Examine patient for absence of breath sounds and heart sounds.
- Note time of death.
- After confirmation of death, verbally acknowledge patient's death to family.
- Communicate condolences verbally (i.e., "I'm sorry for your loss") or nonverbally.
- Determine legal next-of-kin from chart face sheet.
- Ask legal next-of-kin about autopsy, organ donation, funeral home name (family can call it in later).
- Nurse/secretary will contact Deceased Patient Coordinator to help complete the paperwork.
- Notify attending MD of death.

### ★★★ Wishard Health Services

Wishard Health Services in Indianapolis focused on improving family support. The group tested changes within eight major areas: family and loved one support, staff education and training, staff support and self-care, community involvement, patient education, facility modification/hospitality, hospice development and palliative care service, and physician/medical student education.

One change involved training "family consolers" or "rovers," volunteers trained to provide resources, information, and comfort to families of patients dying in the ICU. Experienced bereavement counselors trained volunteers. Among the measures used for the program were the number of families seen, conversations held, staff contacts, consolers involved, and patient deaths in the ICU.

For families keeping vigil, a door tag with an end-of-life logo is posted to notify staff that a patient is near death and to alert them to modify care. In addition, staff stock a hospitality cart for the room, offer shower facilities, and provide or assist with meals, parking, and toiletries. The group set up a "relaxation room" for ER and ambulance services staff.

As the project progressed, the team found that a primary barrier to success was a lack of knowledge about hospice, palliative care, and end-of-life options. The team believed that this situation was made worse by staff who were unwilling or afraid to try anything other than what they were used to doing. In a short survey of ICU staff and junior medical students, 50 percent of the former said that they were in any way familiar with hospice and palliative care services; 63 percent of the students said they were. As a result, the group developed a staff education program that included a monthly presentation on end-of-life issues; a quarterly summary of the Breakthrough Series team's work, which was sent to more than 850 doctors and others; and quarterly classes on chronic illness and death by violence.

### ★★★ Mercy Health Partners

Mercy Health Partners of Scranton, Pennsylvania, aimed to decrease the sense of loneliness and isolation felt by dying patients who have little family or social support. Pastoral companions, who participated in several training sessions on the needs of dying patients, were assigned to be present for patients.

Measures were the number of patients enrolled, the number of visits made by pastoral care volunteers, the number of hours spent with patients, and comments from patients and family members about the visits.

Outcomes demonstrated success—from 57 visits with 16 patients in March, to 128 visits with 25 patients in June. Patients commented, "I don't always feel like talking, but I am glad you stop and pray for me." The Breakthrough Series team reported no negative comments on the program from either staff, families, or patients. The team learned that because patient needs are so individual, no methodology could be developed, and that the only important agenda was the patient's. To journey with a dying patient, the team found, requires a special kind of presence, and companions had to be willing to engage in reflection and to learn from the experience.

The group plans to expand the program so that it provides round-the-clock coverage, and it will also expand the volunteer base. Between February and December 1998, 941 patients were seen, 2,525 visits made, and 705 hours spent with patients. Today, almost 30 volunteers participate in the program, which has been expanded to offer evening and weekend coverage. Three or four volunteers come in daily, coordinating schedules to cover more units. Many of the original volunteers were Catholic, and the team is working to recruit volunteers from other denominations as well.

### ★★★Assess Patient and Family Perceptions of Suffering

Measuring the extent to which patients and families suffer can guide providers in how to meet each person's needs. One Breakthrough Series team studied ways to evaluate suffering and looked at strategies that seemed to help patients and families cope.

### ★★★Health Partners

Based in Minneapolis, Health Partners is a nonprofit family of health care organizations and plans that provides health care services, insurance, and HMO coverage to more than 800,000 members. The team aimed to relieve suffering at the end of life by asking patients about their level of suffering and their ability to cope with this suffering and by offering interventions focused on reducing patient suffering and/or increasing coping skills.

The goal in identifying suffering was to reduce that level by half. The study occurred in home and skilled nursing facilities.

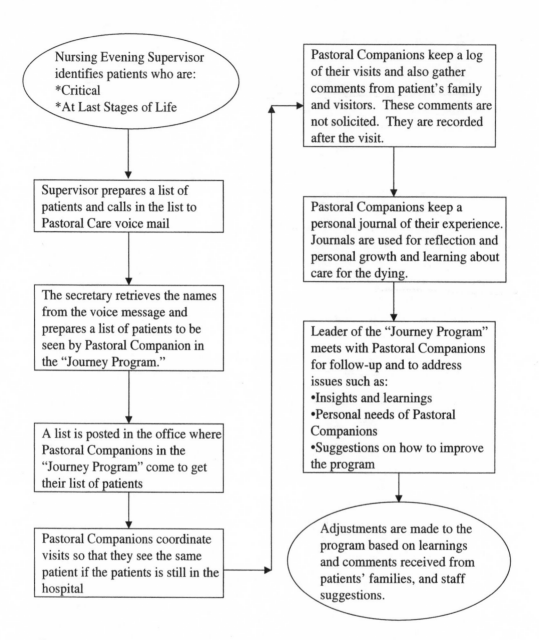

Figure 6.3 "Journey Program" Process for Patients in the Final Stages of Life. Reprinted with permission of Mercy Health Partners, Scranton, PA.

Specific changes included:

- Developing and implementing a standard of care that included developing a comprehensive, easy-to-use "comfort assessment" to assess pain, suffering, and coping ability
- Developing a "comfort index" tool to identify gaps between patients' coping abilities and levels of suffering
- Cataloging strategies patients used successfully to relieve suffering

As one clinical nurse specialist said, "The suffering assessment helped us shape the care plan. We found after using it that the patient's needs were quite different than we had expected. We were able to accomplish a lot with the patient in a very short period of time." After completing the assessment, one hospice patient said, "It's the first time I've slept since I got the diagnosis."

To measure suffering, the group developed several forms for ranking three different categories of suffering: physical, spiritual, and personal/family. The group tracked variables before and after the intervention and also used qualitative reports on what patients use to reduce suffering and cope with their illness.

Measures included many patient self-reports, such as:

- Pain (0-to-10 scale)
- Physical, spiritual, and personal/family suffering (0-to-10 scale)
- Ability to cope with suffering (0-to-10 scale)

How much are you suffering due to your symptoms?

    0  1  2  3  4  5  6  7  8  9  10
    No Suffering              Extreme Suffering

How much are you suffering due to unfinished business?

    0  1  2  3  4  5  6  7  8  9  10
    No Suffering              Extreme Suffering

How much are you suffering due to your fear of the future?

    0  1  2  3  4  5  6  7  8  9  10
    No Suffering              Extreme Suffering

Figure 6.4 Sample Questions from "Comfort Assessment." Reprinted with permission of Health Partners, Minneapolis, MN.

Figure 6.5 Highest Level of Suffering Reported by Patients for any Category of Suffering, at Baseline. Reprinted with permission of Health Partners, Minneapolis, MN.

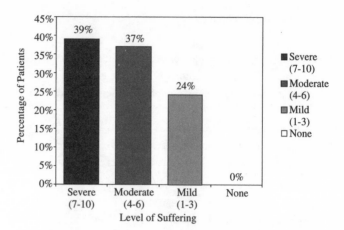

Patients found relief from suffering primarily through contact with family, friends, and hospice staff, including knowledge and comfort given by a nurse; prayer and the Bible; and medical treatments. To cope with suffering, patients turned to others, including spouses and children and hospice staff, as well as coworkers; prayer; and "my outlook on life." Patients generally reported that their ability to cope was medium (29 percent) or high (64 percent); 7 percent rated it as low.

The team measured results in part through self-reports by nurses, social workers, and clergy on the value of the comfort assessment in improving patient care. The project reported several findings:

- All patients surveyed reported some degree of suffering in at least one of the categories.
- There was no significant correlation between pain level and any category of suffering.

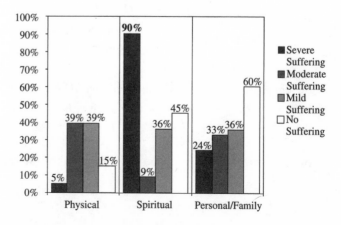

Figure 6.6 Patient Suffering Levels (by Category). Reprinted with permission of Health Partners, Minneapolis, MN.

- Patients experienced the highest rates of severe suffering (24 percent) in the personal/family category.
- Many patients (45 percent) reported no spiritual suffering.

Staff reported that the suffering assessment tools added value to patient care. For instance, the assessment "helped identify the 'real' worries, i.e., client concerned about his elderly mother and the effect his dying would have on her."

## ★Help Patients Address Issues of Meaningfulness and Spirituality

Because life's emotional and spiritual issues can become even more important to so many people as they approach death—and to the people who love them—organizations need to honor and respect this aspect of a patient's experience. Doing so requires creativity and sensitivity and an awareness that supporting patients' spiritual needs can bolster support for their physical and emotional needs.

### Take a Spiritual History

Dr. Christina Puchalski of the George Washington University and the National Institute for Healthcare Research has developed a questionnaire she uses to teach doctors, nurses, social workers, and medical students how to take a spiritual history. The acronym for the assessment is FICA—Faith or Beliefs/ Importance or Influence/Community/Addressing Issues.
  Specific questions to ask include:

| | |
|---|---|
| **F**(aith): | What is your faith or belief? Do you consider yourself spiritual or religious? What things do you believe in that give meaning to your life? |
| **I**(mportance) | Is faith important in your life? What influence does it have on how you take care of yourself? How have your beliefs influenced your behavior during your illness? What role do your beliefs play in regaining your health? |
| **C**(ommunity) | Are you part of a spiritual or religious community? |

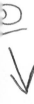

---

### Ways to Provide Care in the Hospital or Nursing Home

- Provide bedside journals for patients, with some explanation that patients and families can write (or sketch) their thoughts, stories, concerns, hopes, and fears.
- Encourage clinicians (when appropriate and if they have enjoyed a long-term and friendly relationship with the patient) to write a few notes to the family about the patient.
- Assemble "comfort packs" to keep at nurses stations. These packs include tape players, meditative or religious music tapes, and spiritual or religious readings.
- When appropriate, send sympathy cards or "thinking of you" notes. Most families appreciate the gesture.
- Develop protocols to refer families to bereavement support groups. Some people benefit from sharing their experiences with others.

---

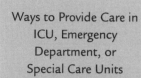

Is this of support to you and how? Is there a person or group of people you really love or who are really important to you?

A(ddress)    How would you like me, your health care provider, to address these issues in your care? (Referrals to chaplains, other spiritual resources, further discussion)

| Ways to Provide Care in ICU, Emergency Department, or Special Care Units |
|---|
| • Give pagers to families, especially those caring for patients in the home and those keeping vigil for critically ill loved ones in hospitals. Pagers give families "permission" to leave the patient's bedside. |
| • Set up a comfort room where families can rest, shower, sleep, and find solitude or gather in privacy. |
| • Provide bereavement support and follow-up to families whose loved ones die unexpectedly—in the ER, for example, after worsening of a long-term illness, or after a sudden illness. |
| • Develop responses for families that are in crisis, overwhelmed, depressed, or exhausted. |

Taking a spiritual history is basically listening to a patient's stories, to their beliefs, their fears, and their hopes. Discussing beliefs is a good way to introduce other issues about end-of-life care. FICA is meant to be used as a guide to introduce the conversation about spirituality. A complete spiritual history takes less than two minutes, so it can be used in any setting. Of course, if deeper issues arise, the conversation may take longer. Asking patients about their spirituality is a way to help them tap into their own sense of hopefulness. This method seems to be acceptable to physicians while promoting a conversation patients find helpful. To date, more than 60 medical schools are teaching the method, and many physicians have begun to use it.

### ★Provide Institutional Resources for Activities on Meaningfulness and Spirituality

All institutions can integrate chaplains into the health care team. Everyone in the organization—doctors, nurses, social workers, chaplains, administrative and housekeeping staff, and nurses aides—can play a role in supporting patients at the end of life. Spiritual services to consider providing include:

- Quiet and private rooms, as well as chapels or meditation rooms, where patients and loved ones can participate in prayer or sacred ritual, including listening to music
- Staff who have the time to listen to patients and loved ones express their concerns and needs
- Opportunities for quiet reflection and time to touch and hold patients who seem to want physical contact
- Opportunities for staff to participate in sacred rituals, such as prayer, when patients and loved ones invite them to do so

- Time and space for families to practice religious rituals (prayers need not be interrupted to deliver meals or take vital signs)
- Opportunities for staff to process their own grief and reactions as they care for dying patients
- Staff training in spiritual issues and how to address those issues with patients, families, and loved ones
- Resource rooms for patients and families that offer literature, sacred reading, tapes, etc.

Organizations that offer chaplaincy programs need to explain to patients and loved ones what the program can offer them. Many patients are reluctant to call on hospital chaplains for fear of being preached at; let patients know that chaplains receive special training, have no desire to "convert" patients, and can offer comfort, guidance, and practical resources to patients of any religious background as well as patients who are not religious at all.

### ★★★Offer Bereavement Counseling and Services in All Settings

People faced with life-limiting illnesses grieve many losses in the course of their illness—the loss of the future, the loss of independence, the loss of privacy. Patients may benefit in talking about these losses with bereavement counselors. At the same time, families and loved ones grapple with both anticipatory grief and the grief that comes when a loved one dies.

Although hospices offer bereavement counseling and support programs, many other care programs do not—even though patients often die in ICUs and ERs. Several Breakthrough Series teams developed new bereavement programs or revamped existing programs to offer more services to more people.

#### ★★★Coney Island Hospital: Bereavement Services in an Acute Care Facility

Coney Island Hospital, a 434-bed acute care facility, serves a community of 750,000 and has the largest proportion of elderly among the hospitals in Brooklyn. Many patients who die in the hospital arrive there as the result of some crisis, not always at the end of a chronic illness. The group planned ways to create bereavement services tailored to their population, aiming to support the grieving process of families in need. Among the many changes tested were:

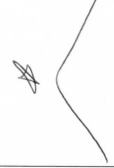

- Open (to all interested participants) and closed (ongoing, with constant membership) bereavement groups
- Mobile team to visit families
- Follow-up calls to families
- Individual counseling, on site or by referrals
- Staff training on assessing bereavement and intervening appropriately
- Baseline established for future studies to match individuals with the appropriate level, intensity, and type of service

The interventions were successful. Of the 50 families initially assessed, 40 remained in the study. Of these:

- 6 attended bereavement groups.
- 7 received visits from the mobile unit; 6 received counseling while on the hospital's medical units.
- 10 were referred for mental health therapy.
- 15 reported that a follow-up call and card were all that was needed, while 2 refused the phone call and services.

Following the bereavement intervention, families reported feeling that they had some control over their grief. All staff who participated in the bereavement counseling reported that it helped them to understand better the grief process and to incorporate their awareness into their practice.

### ★★★University of Utah Hospital

The Breakthrough Series team at the University of Utah Hospital in Salt Lake City aimed to improve supportive care to families whose loved ones had died in the hospital; the specific goal was to provide follow-up supportive care to at least one family member of all patients who had died within the four hospital units involved in the Breakthrough Series.

Changes tested included establishing end-of-life teams on these units, including the ICU and the neuro-critical care unit. Each unit tailored its involvement based on the patients in its care. All agreed to try three targeted interventions that could be measured:

1. Within one to two weeks of death, a unit nurse would send a family member a "thinking of you" card.
2. Within one month, a nurse or doctor on the unit would

call a family member and tell them that an information
packet about grief and grief support resources would be
mailed.

3. Within six weeks, a follow-up packet, including a letter
from the unit staff, a list of common grief responses, and
a list of bereavement services in Utah, would be mailed.

Nurses found that the telephone calls were difficult to make:
The additional time and effort required by the calls sometimes
forced them to extend their work hours or come in on days
off. Nurses were anxious about what to do should the family
seem to need help, so nurses were given a list of crisis center
phone numbers in each Utah county. A script was drafted for
nurses. When families were reached, they seemed to appreciate
the contact.

The cards and packets, although slightly more time-consum-
ing, were completed more frequently. This was accomplished,
in part, by a committed volunteer, who donated many hours
of service to the project. To the group's surprise, not all patients
had a home address—for instance, those who had arrived from
nursing homes and prisons or who were homeless had no
address or next-of-kin to contact.

By the end of the Breakthrough Series, most units were
sending cards to all families, some of whom sent notes of
appreciation. During the study period, 91 patients died in the
four units.

Nurses' follow-up efforts were an important intervention,
and both patients and staff expressed appreciation for the interaction. Families appreciated the extra effort, and nurses felt a
sense of completion in the care they had provided. In the
past, staff had wanted to follow up with families but had no
organized method for doing so.

The University of Utah Hospital is building on work accomplished by the Breakthrough Series team, appointing a Bereavement Coordinator who is working with the hospital to develop
grief and bereavement services.

## Conclusion

See what your organization can do to achieve some of the
targets originally proposed to the Breakthrough Series quality
improvement teams, such as:

- Having more than 90 percent of families report that their
loved one received tender care, that their emotional needs

were addressed, and that professional caregivers said or did something meaningful

- Having more than 90 percent of families say that they would want to receive similar care should they become seriously ill
- Asking doctors or nurses to make at least one follow-up call to each bereaved family, offering families an opportunity to ask any remaining "medical" questions, and screening for the need for grief counseling
- Having more than 90 percent of families report that they cannot recall a time when they were kept "in the dark," heard cruel or uncaring remarks from health care professionals, or felt their beliefs or practices were disregarded
- Doubling the rate at which patients and families agree that the "last few weeks or months were especially meaningful"
- Having patients' spiritual beliefs assessed on a routine basis by all members of the health care team

A popular expression describes people as "spiritual beings having a human experience" rather than human beings having a spiritual experience. At life's crossroads—births, deaths, marriages—we are often reminded of just how spiritual life is and of how important it is to attend to relationships, families, and our own sense of meaning. Perhaps at no time is the sense stronger than it is during the dying process. By honoring the spiritual in each person, health care providers honor our humanity. Programs that encourage and promote such attention promote a sense of worth, dignity, and respect for patients and loved ones.

### Innovators Need to Know

- Dying patients need medical and nursing care—but they also need emotional and spiritual support and opportunities to address important relationships and to be with loved ones.
- Families and loved ones need care and support during the difficult period of caring for a dying person.
- The end of life can be a time for growth and meaningfulness.
- Spirituality can encompass any of the ways in which people seek greater meaning to their lives—and institutional practices can respect individual spirituality and offer pa-

tients time and privacy for comfort, peace, prayer, and
ritual.
- Bereavement support for families is a crucial element of
  good end-of-life care.


## Resources

American Association of Pastoral Counselors
  9504-A Lee Highway
  Fairfax, VA 22031-2303
  Phone: 703-385-6967
  http://www.aapc.org

American Hospice Foundation
  1130 Connecticut Avenue NW, Suite 700
  Washington, DC 20036
  Phone: 202-223-0204
  Fax: 202-223-0208
  http://www.americanhospice.org
  Offers an excellent series of pamphlets on how to deal with
grief and serious illness in the workplace

Hospice Foundation of America
  2001 S Street NW, Suite 300
  Washington, DC 20009
  Phone: 202-638-5419
  http://www.hospicefoundation.org
  Has an entire audiotape series, "Clergy to Clergy: Helping
You Minister to Those Confronting Illness, Death and Grief,"
along with several helpful books

National Association of Catholic Chaplains
  P.O. Box 070473
  Milwaukee, WI 53207-0473
  Phone: 414-483-4898
  Fax: 414-483-6712
  http://www.nacc.org

National Institute for Healthcare Research
  6110 Executive Boulevard, Suite 908
  Rockville, MD 20852
  Phone: 301-984-7162
  Fax: 301-984-8143
  http://www.nihr.org

National Hospice and Palliative Care Organization (NHPCO)
The NHPCO Store
200 State Road
South Deerfield, MA 01373-0200
Phone: 800-646-6460
http://www.nho.org

# Continuity of Care

## Improving Patient Confidence in the Health Care System

What is the health care system? A local physician's office or HMO in which a patient may see one of several providers, including advanced practice nurses, physician assistants, and physicians? A community-wide network of providers, encompassing many providers and services, from durable medical equipment suppliers to radiology offices, from doctors' offices to long-term care facilities?

Or does it include the range of community-based services that serve the seriously ill and dying, such as Meals-on-Wheels, various forms of visiting volunteer services, worship communities, and senior centers? Perhaps units within one system, such as different hospital wards, really function as a system.

It is, of course, all of these elements and more. With so many large and complex organizations delivering, organizing, and paying for care, it is little wonder that the "system," which is actually many subsystems, is often fragmented.

From a patient's perspective, the system can be impersonal, uncommunicative, and disorganized. Because our health care system seems so reliable in treating infections or dealing with medical crises, patients expect it to perform well for them when they are dying. Patients rely on the system and its providers to do the right thing for them—but problems occur at many points on the care continuum, from a failure to transfer patient records to a lack of plain talk about dying, from being seen by strangers to dying in hospitals rather than homes.

Health care providers and organizations struggle to balance competing demands for their time and attention—the sheer volume of record keeping, for instance—that remembering or trying to collaborate with others may receive low priority. Organizations and providers may not communicate with one

In the last nine months of Mrs. H's life, she never really knew which health care professional was leading her care. There was the orthopedist, who read her X rays and recommended that she talk to an internist. There was her primary care doctor of 45 years, who retired and left no referrals to other physicians. There was the internist, who was younger than her grandchildren and seemed too inexperienced to empathize with what she was going through. And there were the oncologist, the urologist, another orthopedist, a rheumatologist, a physical therapist . . . When she was referred to hospice, it came with a new team of strangers—licensed practical nurses, a nurse for the morphine pump, a chaplain, a few social workers, and an ever-changing cast of health aides. They sometimes mentioned another doctor, a hospice doctor, but Mrs. H. never met him. Once, the internist showed up at her home to check on her. A private woman, she was irritated by this constantly changing cast of characters, whom she viewed as strangers intruding on her life. Repeating her medical ➡

another quickly enough. Patients may be bounced from one setting to another without much notice or explanation. When patients and families navigate this expanse, they may often feel that they've set out without compass, map, or guide, only to find themselves in a strange and frightening place. In such cases, quality of care is diminished.

Mrs. H., her family, and her family caregivers realized too late—and her professional providers never seemed to realize—just what such fragmented care means for dying people. As more groups begin to at least think about providing comprehensive, integrated care for the dying, perhaps the current situation will improve. Continuity of care has to be at the core of reliable and trustworthy systems of care for dying patients and their families. Continuity can ensure that patients and families know who their care team is, who is in charge, and where to turn for help and guidance.

Creating continuity within your organization and throughout your community may be a daunting task. In the IHI series, groups rarely tackled the problem, and even then, they rarely achieved much. The status quo—which does not object to "dumping" patients from one facility to another, which has any number of professional caregivers coming in and out of patients' lives, which does not always know patients' wishes and preferences—is an embarrassment to us all. Recognizing this, however, should not paralyze us. Instead, our poor track record for continuity of care should motivate us to improve things now. Through the Plan-Do-Study-Act model for change, even this enormous task can be broken down into manageable components, problems for which solutions seem evident. Even minor changes, such as guaranteeing that a patient will always know who is leading his or her care team, can lead your organization to improved continuity of care.

Each day, most of us encounter some form of technological wizardry that tracks one or another aspect of our lives, from the kind of toilet paper we usually buy to the location of our express mail packages. The proliferation of such technology has not yet enabled much improvement in the health care industry. Privacy issues notwithstanding, it seems reasonable to consider using bar codes, for example, to track where patients are in a health care system, which providers they have seen, and which medications they are on. Some managed care organizations rely on technology to track patient care and costs and can report on which provider saw which patient when and for what, and what treatment was recommended. Perhaps health care organizations can develop similar systems to communicate with and about patients and their needs and can extend that tracking process across provider organizations. Probably, though, nothing quite fully takes the place of a doctor or nurse who has known the patient and family for some time.

## In This Chapter

Some organizations have begun to demonstrate just how coordinated health care improves care of seriously ill and dying patients. This chapter features the work of several programs and describes what can be done to create coordinated care in other organizations. Suggestions include:

- Setting goals that promote coordinated care
- Making and keeping specific promises to patients
- Reducing patient transfers, especially when patients are near death
- Coordinating care within and across treatment settings
- Giving patients and families one or two points of contact
- Creating a process through which health care providers can communicate with one another about patient care
- Making patient preferences known and accessible to all health care providers

Comprehensive, coordinated care reflects the complexity of human life, with its rich array of physical, emotional, social, and spiritual needs, and allows the health care system to better meet patient needs.

### ★★★On Lok Senior Health Services

Begun 25 years ago, San Francisco's On Lok Senior Health Services offers integrated, community-based care to frail elderly participants in their own homes and communities. In 1997, the federal government moved its Programs for All-Inclusive Care of the Elderly (PACE) from its demonstration status to that of a permanent provider. PACE sites rely on integrated financing—from Medicare, Medicaid, and private sources—to offer clients a range of health care services, transportation, food, and social activities, as well as physical, recreational, and occupational therapy. At the same time, PACE operates within a capitated payment system, putting each program at financial risk for all patient care.

A TROUBLED SYSTEM

history over and over to different people exhausted and saddened Mrs. H. and her family.

Along the way, Mrs. H. lost her privacy, along with any faith that the system would do well in caring for her. In her final days, a different nurse came to the house every day to cover for the regular hospice nurse, who was on vacation. Their failure to coordinate care was evidenced by their differing approaches to relieving the pain of Mrs. H's pressure sores. One told the family to ignore the sores, another told the family to change the dressing, another told the family to turn Mrs. H. every few hours, and still another told the family not to move her, since she did not have long to live.

The last 72 hours of her life were spent on the inpatient hospice ward, where a new group of doctors and nurses came in and out and where her family unraveled, confused and afraid, while she lay confused, though sometimes asleep.

A multidisciplinary team serves as a case manager for each patient; the team includes physicians, nurse practitioners, nurses, social workers, recreation/occupation therapists, home health aides, dieticians, and drivers. PACE transports some clients to adult day care daily.

To be eligible to enroll, a patient must be over 55 years old, must be Medicaid-certifiable for nursing home care, and must live in the program's defined geographic area. Patients must be eligible for Medicare; those eligible only for Medicare must pay the Medicaid portion of the fee out of pocket. The program is designed especially to meet the needs of low-income elderly people.

When a patient enrolls, the entire team assesses his or her clinical and social situation, helps develop a care plan, delivers appropriate services, and allocates necessary resources. At enrollment, the team also discusses advance directives with patients and families; directives are then reviewed periodically.

PACE participants usually have several diagnoses—for example, heart disease, Alzheimer's, and stroke. Every member of the PACE team plays a role in providing preventive health care services, such as medication monitoring, nutritional assessment, evaluation of home safety, and respite care. The average PACE participant is in the program for about three years, until death. Because PACE team members come to know each person and family rather well, the team can detect subtle changes in health status, mobility, nutrition, and so on. The care plan is adjusted accordingly.

PACE seems to generate cost savings: In a 1993 study, savings to Medicare were estimated to be 14 percent to 39 percent when compared to fee-for-service. PACE also has a lower average number of hospital days than does the general Medicare population. This rate is notable primarily because the general Medicare population includes people who are well and those who are sick—unlike PACE, which includes only the very ill and frail, and a majority of patients who have many serious illnesses.

PACE programs exemplify a coordinated care system. For instance, in one San Francisco site, clients participate in adult day programs, which include meals, activities, companionship, and health care; others live at the site. Clients and staff enjoy a rapport based on months and years of daily interaction—a far cry from the alienation that occurs when nursing home patients who are dying are transferred to hospitals for each complication and back again. Because PACE staff are expected to observe changes in client behavior, moods, or physical status, the team can adapt to meet changes in a patient's needs.

## ★Set Goals That Promote Continuity

For patients and family caregivers—and the staff who work with them—the lack of continuity in care is disruptive and stressful. The people working in the system (not just the system itself) start to feel like inhumane automatons—even if the reality is that most people who care for the dying are deeply caring and committed to their patients. When care is continuous, patients can generally expect a certain standard of care, and they sense that an integrated team is providing trustworthy, continuous care.

Going from provider to provider and place to place creates a sense that one's care is fractured, disorganized, or substandard. Frequent transfers, changes in staff, or a general lack of knowledge about the patient erode patient and caregiver confidence that the health care system is working for them, rather than working on its own agenda.

Quite simply, without long-term relationships, providers cannot make promises to patients. Furthermore, in such circumstances, only understandings that have been made explicit (and, so, are quite rigid) can be counted on. Without a shared history, valuing the person becomes a hollow exercise, and unstated, intimate understandings are impossible or unreliable.

Developing systems of care that focus on a standard of continuity is critical. Systems need to be committed to standards of pain and symptom relief, of advance care planning, and of patient and family inclusion. As described in chapter 2, systems and teams need to be willing to make promises to patients: promises that patients will know who their treatment team is, that they will know who to call in the middle of the night (and that someone will be there to take the call), that

A Whole-Community Model for Care at the End of Life (*Continued*)

charitable organizations, support groups, and government agencies
- Interdisciplinary palliative care teams which recognize that patients and families are members of the team

*Source*: Institute of Medicine, 1997

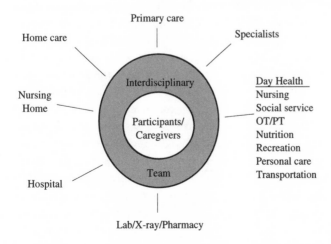

Primary care

Home care

Specialists

Interdisciplinary

Nursing Home

Day Health
Nursing
Social service
OT/PT
Nutrition
Recreation
Personal care
Transportation

Participants/
Caregivers

Team

Hospital

Lab/X-ray/Pharmacy

Figure 7.1 Coordinated Care Model, PACE. Reprinted with permission of the National PACE Association, San Francisco, CA.

responsive and reliable individuals are dedicated to working with the patient for a safe, dignified period at the end of life, and that their preferences and values will be honored.

Organizations can set very specific aims that will promote continuity, enabling patients to feel that the system does, in fact, care about them. One example is to limit patient transfers between units or health care settings to create the confidence and familiarity that allow patients and families to trust the health care team. Organizations should strive for specific goals. Some that can be readily achieved are described below:

- People living at home generally remain at home, where services come to them. Those in medical emergencies or unable to remain at home receive care tailored to medical and emotional needs.
- People near death are never transferred from one unit or facility to another just to save money or satisfy utilization review criteria.
- People die under the care of key personnel who are always available to them—and plans are made to address possible disruptions in care.
- Families keeping vigil for dying patients have access to supportive services, such as a sleeping room and bereavement support.

### ★Set Standards for Continuity Based on Promises to Patients

Setting institutional standards for continuity is a basic step in bringing the issue to health care providers' attention. Standards may be very basic, such as ensuring that no more than two or three nurses ever visit one hospice patient at home, or guaranteeing that all patients will know who their primary health care providers are and how to contact them.

Another route to setting standards is to make promises to patients and families. Chapter 2 describes the promises some organizations are committed to making to patients and families. Early in the course of caring for dying patients, health care providers should aim to make promises to patients about the overall system of care: promises about a level of performance that all providers agree to maintain. Patients and families should feel confident that they will encounter few crises or emergencies which are not quickly resolved through the health care team and that when emergencies occur, those who attend to the patient will know and respect the patient's preferences.

What can you promise patients? Try some specifics. Can your organization make any of these promises to a seriously ill patient?

- If your pain is above a level 3, we will revise your treatments within an hour.
- If you need help at any time, even in the middle of the night, someone you have met before will respond to your call within 30 minutes.
- If you are transferred to the hospital from your home, we will make sure that the hospital staff are aware of your treatment plan and preferences and that your medical records are available.
- Wherever you receive care, you will know who the leader of your health care team is.
- If you experience nausea, shortness of breath, or any other troubling symptoms, we will work around the clock to bring them under control.

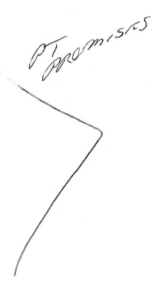

*PT promises*

Making and keeping promises is a way to start making care more reliable for patients and their caregivers.

## Make Only Essential Transfers of Dying Patients

Transfers and staff changes create very real problems for patients and providers. The average hospital patient may see as many as a dozen different physicians and a dozen different nursing personnel in one day! Home care patients, too, may see a number of different health care providers—nurses, health aides, physical therapists, counselors, and volunteers. The personnel parade can take an emotional toll on patients and their caregivers. Repeated transfers or changes among health care providers contributes to a loss of empathy, intimacy, trust, and promise keeping—the very factors so critical to good care at the end of life.

Being transferred from one unit to another—from the ICU, for instance, to a general medical ward, when the patient has only 48 hours to live—can be very disruptive to patients and families.

Transfers create the following kinds of problems for patients, families, and health care providers:

- Relationships built over time and based on trust cannot be developed or sustained.
- Settled care plans are lost.

- Treatment schedules are disrupted.
- Explicit and implicit understandings between patient and provider are lost or misunderstood.
- Specific prescriptions may not be provided in a timely manner.
- Discordant opinions or treatment plans may create anxiety and confusion.

For systems, transferring patients from one setting to another—from the nursing home, for instance, to the emergency room—permits a critical lack of accountability. Everyone involved with the patient's care can fall back on not knowing enough about the patient, his or her preferences, or his or her treatment plan. It is easy to claim that something is not one's problem, duty, or responsibility.

In many systems, various units do not even view themselves as being integrated or interdependent. The emergency medical system may not view itself as having some accountability to the intensive care system, which in turn does not see itself as part of the medical/surgical system. Each operating unit views itself in isolation from the others; it is as if a quarterback just decided to pass without even looking for a receiver.

What can organizations do to prevent unnecessary transfers? They can develop the capacity to meet patient needs, regardless of which unit they are in, along with policies of "compassionate nondischarge." These policies, which are already in place at several Catholic hospitals, require that hospitals keep patients, rather than discharge them, when death is likely to occur within 48 hours, even if a hospital level of care is unnecessary. This would mean not discharging those who are very near death from the ICU to a medical floor, or not discharging to homes those who would do better to remain in hospitals.

★★Coordinate Patient Care across and within
   All Operating Units

Continuity of care requires an integrated approach to care. Professionals and health care institutions accept the ongoing responsibility of caring for dying patients. The health care aide who visits a patient on Monday also visits the patient on Wednesday. The treatment plan used at home is followed in the hospital. A patient being cared for in an integrated system does not have to explain to ER staff that she is enrolled in hospice. No one has to search for a DNAR order—and one order is honored everywhere. The system operates cohesively and coherently, and patients and families trust providers—and the health care system—depending on it for care best suited to their disease and circumstance. In this system, all members share a commitment to key elements of care, such as pain relief or bereavement support.

★★*EverCare Program,*
*United HealthCare Corporation*

EverCare is a demonstration program operated since 1986 by a national managed care organization, Minneapolis-based United HealthCare Corporation (UHC). UHC serves nearly 20 million people in all states and manages 19 health plans, with a total of 1.6 million enrollees. It has been a Medicare risk contractor for almost 15 years.

EverCare is a five-year demonstration project sponsored by the U.S. Health Care Financing Administration at nine sites nationwide. Its primary goals are to improve management of specialized acute care and to restructure service delivery and financing for the frail elderly in nursing homes. Like PACE, the program emphasizes preventive medicine and early intervention and limits unnecessary care. And, like PACE, EverCare receives comprehensive capitated payments, putting it at risk for virtually all Medicare-covered costs.

EverCare is available to Medicare-certified nursing home residents on Medicare (Parts A and B or Part B only) but not enrolled in hospice or an end-stage renal disease program. Once enrolled, members must continue to pay Part B premiums. Capitated, risk-based financing of all acute medical services provides flexible use of funds.

The EverCare team includes a physician and a nurse practitioner trained in geriatric medicine; while the nurse conducts the initial assessment, the nurse and doctor together develop the care plan. The nurse practitioner serves as the case manager and communicates with the patient's family. By using a provider team to monitor patients, the program promotes continuity. Because the team has several patients at one site, visits are more frequent, and the team develops a stronger relationship with patients and with nursing home staff. The nurse visits each patient at least monthly and is available during working hours; on-call backup is available after regular hours.

The nurse practitioner can also pre-authorize hospitalization and appointments at other medical facilities. If the nursing home staff are concerned about the need for acute care, the nurse practitioner examines measures to be taken and, if hospi-

## Some Elements of Coordinated Care

- There are defined procedures for patient transfers.
- Follow-up mechanisms are used regularly.
- There are designated primary care providers.
- There are integrated patient information systems.
- Medications travel with patients.
- Follow-up calls and contacts are made.
- When transfers are expected, anticipatory planning meetings are held.
- Relationships among different health care systems are standardized.

*Source*: Institute of Medicine, 1997

talization is required, consults with hospital staff to discuss the patient's care.

To date, the program's results indicate a 30 percent decrease in costs compared to fee-for-service equivalents and a one-third reduction in hospital admissions. However, it has been difficult to expand the program because HMOs are reluctant to target the frail elderly, whose care they have little experience managing; physician networks are reluctant to take on the financial risks of a large geriatric population, because a special understanding of the nursing home environment is essential—and some groups are unable to develop this relationship.

### ★★★Give Patients and Families One Point of Contact

Staffing issues and needs—vacations or holidays—can make it hard to assign any given staff person to any given patient. And yet patients and families need to have as small as possible a group of reliable clinicians on whom they can rely virtually around the clock to answer questions, address changes in treatment plans, or respond to crises. In the Detroit Receiving Hospital, for instance, all families with loved ones dying in the ICU can page the palliative care nurse, who then responds immediately to their concerns, fears, or problems. Patients and families know that when they need help, someone they have met and trust will respond.

Hospice has earned a reputation for providing comprehensive care by offering patients access to physicians, nurses, social workers, pastoral care, and community volunteers. The "24/7" (24 hours a day/7 days a week) availability of a good nurse is essential to hospice patients and families. Other health care organizations can emulate this by encouraging an interdisciplinary approach to care of the dying.

Patients and families can also get to know a few key people on the care team. Obstetrical practices offer a model for this approach. Pregnant women routinely meet each obstetrician in a practice, so that they will at least have met the physician who is on call when they go into labor.

### ★★Hope Hospice

As a quality review tool, Hope Hospice in Fort Myers, Florida, measured the number of visits by different nurses. The group uses its database to track which health care providers have visited a patient and what services were provided. Hope Hospice then uses the reports to review continuity of care. The hospice teams also review data about unscheduled visits, which may indicate uncontrolled symptoms, a fall, or some other crisis. If three or more nurses see a patient in any week, the quality review team looks into why this happened: Was there a set of special services that required a different nurse at morning, noon, and night? Or did staffing problems mean that the three nurses were chosen willy-nilly?

The team found that once it kept the number of different professionals visiting a patient to a minimum, continuity was more easily maintained. The group found that continuity influenced patient satisfaction. For example, one care team had many nurses and health aides seeing patients; and, at the same time, morale was low and complaints were high. After the Breakthrough Series team coached its colleagues on how to plan staffing needs, the caregivers reported feeling better about their work, and patient complaints subsided.

## ★★Franciscan Healthcare Systems

Franciscan Health Systems of Tacoma, Washington, includes community hospitals, care centers, home care and hospice programs, and a physician health system network. The Breakthrough Series team aimed to improve patient access to supportive services as a way to increase patient and family satisfaction and reduce hospitalizations and emergency room visits. This team is credited with first using the "surprise" question, which it used to encourage doctors to refer patients to supportive care. The team asked doctors, "Would you be surprised if this patient died within the year?" Using this approach, referrals increased from one each month to six. The enhanced referrals and the improved services ended up yielding better care and a 400 percent increase in hospice revenues. (This increased revenue has helped to extend the program to other facilities throughout the Franciscan system).

Community volunteers were a key element in helping patients find and use supportive services. The eight volunteers were mostly women who had recently retired from positions that had made them very involved in the community. Each month, sometimes more often, the volunteers called patients and caregivers to discuss their needs and recommend appropriate services. These conversations also gave patients a chance to express their concerns, fears, and worries. Volunteers let program staff know how patients responded and whether additional services or help was needed. The program also ensured that patients had opportunities to make plans for future care.

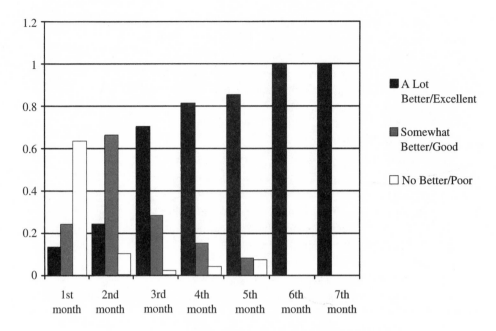

Figure 7.2 Patient Satisfaction per Month in EOL Program. Reprinted with permission of Franciscan Health Systems, Tacoma, WA.

The team found that once supportive services were in place, patient satisfaction with end-of-life care improved dramatically. The following chart shows just how much improvement the team managed in seven months. In the first month of enrollment, more than 60 percent said that their satisfaction was no better than before Supportive Services started or was poor; seven months later, 100 percent reported that their satisfaction was a lot better or excellent. Remember, these were patients who were, at the same time, becoming sicker.

### ★★Set Up Communication Systems for Health Care Providers Who Share Care for a Group of Patients

Providers need the opportunity to talk to one another about patients for whom they share care. For many Breakthrough Series teams, the project was the first time that professionals from different hospital units—such as oncology and hospice or primary care—worked together to improve a system, in part just by communicating with one another.

*** Kaiser Permanente, San Diego*

San Diego's Kaiser Permanente team developed a collaborative planning process between hospice and oncology units, primarily to reduce patient pain and the need for urgent admissions. The process encouraged a consistent approach to pain management for hospice and oncology units and offered patients a full continuum of care as they moved from oncology to hospice care. (For details, see chapter 3 on pain and symptom management.)

### ★★★Make Patient Preferences Accessible and Known to All Health Care Providers

For health care organizations with sophisticated patient information systems, the issue of transferring records may seem obvious. However, as the Breakthrough Series teams found, many organizations need to improve record transfers to ensure that DNR orders, advance care plans, and other vital information is transferred from one setting to another.

Some states have developed quick ways to make sure patients' wishes are known by all health care providers who are treating them, or who may treat them, such as EMS crews. Among the strategies being used are:

- DNR orders printed on brightly colored paper, posted on medical records and in prominent places in the home
- Wrist bracelets indicating a patient's DNR wishes
- Prescription medicine vials containing emergency information, to be carried in glove compartments and stored in freezers, where EMS personnel have been instructed to look for them

*** Oregon's POLST—Physician Orders for Life-Sustaining Treatment*

Oregon uses the one-page Physician Orders for Life-Sustaining Treatment (POLST) Document to help health care providers honor patients' treatment wishes. Printed on unmistakable bright pink card stock, the form is attached to the front of medical records in hospitals and nursing homes. The document is a physician order form that records patient preferences and treatment intentions and is meant to enhance the appropriateness and quality of care. The form contains specific orders on whether a patient wants to be resuscitated and lists any limits on medical interventions to be used—specifically, antibiotic use and feeding procedures. Physicians review the document with patients and families, but patients do not actually complete it; the POLST is not a substitute for a living will or durable power of attorney.

According to a 1998 study by the Center for Ethics in Health Care at Oregon Health Sciences University, POLST is effective at limiting unwanted treatments. Of 180 nursing home patients who had indicated DNR on their POLST, not one received CPR, was admitted to the ICU, or received ventilator support. Only 2 percent were hospitalized to extend life. Of the 38 people who died during the year of the study, 63 percent had an order for narcotics, and only 2 died in an acute care hospital.

Dr. Susan Tolle, director of the Center, says the study shows that "the POLST form focuses efforts on the patient's comfort, creating a positive plan that serves the patient." Tolle believes that several features of the form make it effective:

- It is standardized statewide, improving the likelihood that it will be recognized and respected.
- Because of its shocking pink color, it cannot be ignored and is easy to find.
- The orders to limit life-sustaining treatment are clearly printed on the front, making them easily located.
- The form is written in plain English, making it easy for staffs of nursing homes, home hospices, home health agencies, as well as covering physicians, to understand it.
- The specific language requiring comfort measures encourages attention to pain and suffering—and relieving both.

Tolle notes that another reason POLST is so effective is a five-year, statewide education initiative, as well as Oregon's commitment to providing resources to support patients dying at home.

The POLST was developed in response to concerns about problems in respecting DNR orders when patients were transferred from nursing homes to hospitals. The document is meant to reduce unwanted transfers and, for most patients, limit intensive medical interventions. To date, 175,000 forms have been distributed statewide, and hundreds more have been distributed around the country.

Oregon has made another important improvement by redefining the scope of practice for EMTs and first responders and for their supervising doctors. EMTs and others are now directed to respect patient wishes to life-sustaining treatments and to comply with physician orders, such as those in the POLST document.

## A Story of Continuity: Sister Antonine's Final—Great—Adventure

Angoon is a village of 600 residents on Admiralty Island in Alaska; there are more bears than humans on the island, which also boasts more than 9 million acres of a national wildlife preserve. Angoon was the vacation destination chosen by Sister Antonine, OSF, a 76-year-old Roman Catholic nun of the Franciscan Sisters of Baltimore, in July 1996. She had been a nun for almost 60 years and had spent most of her life teaching in poor urban communities on the East Coast. Recent years had been difficult for her—the Mother Superior of her convent was brutally murdered in 1992, her brother died in 1991, and her two sisters died soon after, one in 1993 and one in 1994. Sister Antonine had been with her sister Anna, who suffered a massive heart attack at home, was resuscitated by a rescue squad, and endured invasive hospital procedures before dying a few hours later.

Subsequent years continued to be a struggle: in 1995 and 1996, she suffered a series of strokes and had been hospitalized with a broken hip and fractured arm. In the 1950s, she had undergone open-heart surgery, and in the late 1980s, she underwent surgery to replace a heart valve. She was a tiny, frail woman. She was determined, however, that she would visit Alaska, and when a distant young cousin who taught in Angoon invited her to visit, she immediately accepted. At first, her Mother Superior did not believe Sister Antonine was well enough to travel; however, Sister Antonine enlisted Sister Mary Margaret, a "young" nun of 74, to accompany her. Despite her doctor's advice and warnings of blood clots, the two nuns took off for Angoon in July 1996.

They enjoyed three days of fantastic nature, travel adventures, bear sightings, halibut fishing, and dinners with the Tlingit Indians who live in Angoon. Then, on July 24, as they returned to a small apartment after dinner, Sister Antonine suffered another stroke, this one massive (she said to Mary Margaret, "I just don't feel well"). It was almost midnight, in the midst of a storm. Sister Mary called Sister Antonine's cousin, who contacted the local nurse, who radioed to Juno for help in evacuating Sister from the island. Eventually, a Coast Guard helicopter arrived to medevac her to a hospital. At first, the medics were reluctant to allow Sister Mary to come with them. When she insisted, they relented, gave her a helmet, and raced through the storm to the chopper, which took them to Sitka, a larger city on a nearby island.

There, she was hospitalized in a former naval station hospital, Mt. Edgecumbe. As the pilot left, he gave Sister Mary Margaret his phone number and told her to call if she needed help. That night, Sister Antonine was placed on a ventilator, for a brief trial to evaluate whether her condition was likely to improve. A nurse made up a bed for Mary Margaret, brought her a warm drink, and comforted her.

By the following morning, Sitka's Catholics had mobilized to help the two nuns—people visited the hospital, brought food, prayed with Sister Mary Margaret, and took her into the town. The local priest gave her his car to use and offered her the rectory.

Throughout the ordeal, people remained with Sister Mary Margaret, who was often at Antonine's side, praying. The two women had been friends for more than 40 years. When studies showed the extensive brain damage caused by the stroke, the hospital doctor consulted the Mother Superior, who agreed that Sister Antonine's ventilator should be removed and that she should be allowed to die peacefully and naturally. Less than 12 hours later, she died. The Mother Superior flew to Juno, where Sister Antonine's body was taken and cremated.

Sister Mary Margaret recalls the generosity of the town, the hospital and its staff, and the Coast Guard pilots—and she laughs when she says, "I promised to bring her home, and I did." Incredibly, this remote Alaskan community had created a care system that showed remarkable continuity, comprehensiveness, and competence.

### Innovators Need to Know

- Organizations can begin to create continuity by making and keeping promises to patients.
- Tracking the number of different health care providers a patient sees in a short period is a good way to measure continuity of care.
- Patients and families need to meet the health care team and become familiar and comfortable with several members, while having a single point of contact.
- Reducing transfers, especially of dying ICU patients, can reduce family distress.

## Resources

EverCare
  9900 Bren Road East
  Minnetonka, MN 55343
  Phone: 612-936-6833
  http://www.uhc.com/about/specos/evercare.html

For more information on PACE, contact:
  National PACE Association
  1255 Post Street, Suite 1027
  San Francisco, CA 94109
  Phone: 415-749-2680
  Fax: 415-749-2687
  E-mail: npace@pacbell.net
  http://www.natlpaceassn.org

For more information on POLST:
  OHSU Center for Ethics in Health Care L101
  3181 SW Sam Jackson Park Road
  Portland, OR 97201
  http://www.ohsu.edu/ethics
  To order a sample form, write to ethics@ohsu.edu.

# PART III

---

# ARRANGEMENTS TO PROMOTE REFORM

While rapid-cycle changes described in previous chapters offer a model for improving patient care, organizations can promote systemwide change through administrative improvements and reform. The chapters in this section describe current arrangements or practices in four specific areas and then look at ways to improve or change those practices for everyone's benefit, not only patients and families but staff as well.

Chapter 8 describes models for hospital-based palliative care units and consultations, which extend hospice principles to patients who are ineligible for hospice, either because of their prognosis or because they desire to continue aggressive treatment although they realize that their diseases are eventually fatal. (For instance, new treatment regimes allow HIV/AIDS patients to live much longer, but issues of advance care planning and palliation of symptoms are still critical to these patients and their loved ones.)

Chapter 9 discusses how Medicare now reimburses end-of-life medical expenses and suggests what managers need to consider in structuring and financing any new program to care for patients at the end of life. The chapter describes how programs can bill Medicare appropriately and discusses the likely income that such billing will generate.

Chapter 10 offers ideas on how groups can use their management information systems—whether they are very basic or cutting-edge technology—to measure quality improvement endeavors.

Chapter 11 looks at some of the issues and concerns surrounding personnel who work in end-of-life care, such as offering bereavement counseling to staff and creating career paths for paraprofessional workers.

Previous chapters included many examples of how groups have applied quality improvement methods to create change. The following chapters describe the exemplary efforts some groups are trying: Although their progress and accomplishments have not all been rigorously tested or measured, their ideas seem to be good ones, and worth consideration by others.

# Hospital-Based Palliative Care Consults and Units

Many organizations, eager to do something about end-of-life care, decide that what's needed is a palliative care unit or consult service. There are many advantages to this course, but it does entail risks and difficulties. Before choosing this course, consider the current patient census, existing services that might benefit dying patients and their loved ones, and how a palliative care unit or program would work with other programs, such as hospice and home care.

Palliative care units and services are an excellent approach to care for seriously ill and dying patients—including those who live for years with their illnesses. With their focus on pain and symptom management and psychosocial support, such programs are now underway or have been developed in many communities nationwide. However, not every community can support a program, and every community has different needs or expectations for their services.

The best way to get a good idea is to get a lot of ideas.
—Linus Pauling

## In This Chapter

Groups that plan to establish palliative care services or consults must consider many elements, ranging from how to select the patient population to how to bill for services. This chapter describes issues that tend to emerge when organizations begin to consider their need for palliative care services and the goals for such a program; the types of programs that can be established; how programs or consults fit within an institution; and the staff and resources needed to create a palliative care service.

Addressing these issues requires managers and clinicians to reflect on their institution's organizational structure and its goals for improving end-of-life care.

> The World Health Organization defines palliative care as "the active total care of patients whose disease is not responsive to curative treatment . . . [when] control of pain, of other symptoms, and of psychological, social and spiritual problems is paramount."

## What Is Palliative Care?

Palliative care, sometimes described as supportive care, means different things to different people. Even among health care professionals, there is not always consensus on what palliative care is or should be. Some clinicians question whether and how palliative care differs from hospice care; others wonder what distinguishes palliative care, with its focus on relieving symptoms and comforting patients, from basic, good medical practice.

Most often, palliative care is described as a way to meet the physical, mental, and spiritual needs of chronically ill and dying patients. The philosophy underlying palliative care, however, is not unique to any disease or illness. In fact, some claim that palliative care describes the kind of relief from suffering all patients need. But with its attention to relieving symptoms and meeting patient goals, palliative care is certainly an approach from which those near the end of life most benefit.

Clinicians tend to associate palliative care with oncology and believe that palliative care is what is given when aggressive, curative treatment no longer works. Many clinicians believe there is a demarcation line between when cure-oriented care ends and palliative care begins; others believe the transition is far more gradual and less clear-cut. Clinicians may believe that palliative care requires patients to forgo other treatments, such as radiation or chemotherapy. Although this is indeed the case with some traditional hospice programs, palliative care need have no such requirement.

Andrew Billings, MD (1998), director of the Palliative Care Service at Massachusetts General, describes palliative care as "comprehensive care, provided by an interdisciplinary team, for patients and families living with a life-threatening or terminal illness, particularly where care is focused on alleviating suffering and promoting quality of life." He adds, "Major concerns are pain and symptom management, information sharing and advance care planning, psychosocial and spiritual support, and coordination of care, including arranging for excellent services in the community."

The Last Acts Palliative Care Task Force has released a booklet called "Precepts of Palliative Care," which can be integrated into end-of-life programs and services. The precepts (included in the Resources section on page 327 at the back of this book) focus on respecting patient goals, preferences, and choices; providing comprehensive care; using interdisciplinary resources; addressing the concerns of family and caregivers;

### Goals of Palliative Care Services

- Assure that patients and families receive excellent pain control and other comfort measures
- Give patients the information needed to participate in decisions about care
- Offer emotional and spiritual support and practical assistance
- Obtain expert help in planning care outside the hospital
- Continue to received good services in the community

*Source*: Billings, 1998

and building systems and mechanisms that support palliative care programs, as well as research and evaluation of them.

## Building a Model That Works

Several models exist for palliative care programs in hospitals: dedicated inpatient units, palliative care experts, consultative services, or some combination of the three. Some programs rely on a nurse practitioner to coordinate care throughout medical-surgical wards; others rely on a team of physicians to make consults. Some programs have a very structured mechanism to receive referrals; others use physician outreach and networking for referrals.

### ★★★Northwestern Memorial Hospital

Organizations that set up palliative care consults expand the opportunity to educate many health care providers about the goals and practices of palliative care. Charles von Gunten, MD, former director of the palliative care consult service at Chicago's Northwestern Memorial Hospital (and now medical director of the Hospice of San Diego) describes it this way: "Besides yielding direct benefits to the health of patients and their families, consultation serves a second important purpose. Physicians learn about developments and approaches to patient care through consultation. The consultation represents an example of learner-centered learning. The referring physician (the learner) has identified the problem(s) that need solving, and the new material is clearly relevant to the problem at hand" (von Gunten et al., 1998). Its educational focus is on improving provider ability to assess and manage pain and other symptoms; improving clinicians' ability to communicate with patients and their loved ones; and improving knowledge and awareness of palliative medicine as a resource that can help physicians.

In a survey of providers who had referred patients to the palliative care consult team, Northwestern found that attending physicians, physician house staff, medical students, and ward nurses all learned from the experience. During the four years in which the service has been operated, requests for direct training through it have gone from none to more than 200 medical students, as well as 30 residents for direct clinical experience (von Gunten et al., 1998). Trainees have indicated many other goals for their experience, such as improving their

## What's in a Name?

If defining palliative care itself is a difficult task, naming a program can seem almost impossible. One children's cancer program tried to deal with a charged turf issue by calling its palliative care program the "advanced cancer support program." The hospital's oncologists objected, asking if their work was "just basic cancer support." The group then tried to describe it as a comfort unit—and met with more objections. Finally, the group settled on "palliative care," although most patients and families were not familiar with the term. Other groups have used the concept of "extensive" or "advanced" illness in describing their patient population. A few groups are calling their programs "MediCaring."

Regardless of what they are called, such programs offer patients and families the kind of comprehensive, supportive care so essential to people facing serious and complex diseases.

own level of comfort in dealing with death and dying, and developing ways to apply palliative care approaches to other fields of adult medicine.

Many programs, like the one at Northwestern, involve provider training and outreach. The task may include educating colleagues about palliative care, facilitating communication among the many providers who work with a patient, and teaching students, interns, and residents about pain management.

### ★★★*Memorial Sloan-Kettering*

For almost two decades, Memorial Sloan-Kettering in New York City has offered supportive care services to its patients. Today, the Pain and Palliative Care Center is patient- and family-oriented and operates based on a collaborative approach between a clinical nurse specialist, a doctor, and a social worker. The clinical nurse specialist coordinates care. Consultation team members cover areas including psychiatry, rehabilitation, nutrition, and spirituality. Although the team is based at Sloan-Kettering, its focus is on patients living in the community. Each of the two clinical nurse specialists on the team serves from 12 to 15 patients and families.

The clinical nurse specialist performs many roles:

• Handles day-to-day management and relief of patients' pain and other symptoms
• Provides liaison between the primary treating physician, the patient, and the community's resources
• Understands each patient's disease process, effective symptom control, and the specifics of psychosocial dynamics, and coordinates all who are involved in caring for the patient
• Follows patients through telephone calls, as well as home and clinic visits (for example, before discharging a patient, the clinical nurse specialist contacts the local doctor and discusses pain management and other symptom-control techniques that have been effective)
• Contacts community nurses and makes appropriate referrals
• Contacts the patient's local pharmacy to make sure the prescribed analgesics are available and, if not, locates another pharmacy

### ★★*Detroit Receiving Hospital*

In 1986, Detroit Receiving Hospital, a Level 1 Trauma Hospital, established the Comprehensive Supportive Care Team, designed as a nurse-directed collaborative practice between a physician and an advanced practice nurse to provide comprehensive, comfort-focused care to dying patients and their families. Services are offered after a transfer of service from the admitting physician/resident team, or in consultation with the primary team. The supportive care team provides clinical ethics consultation related to end-of-life issues, teaches staff and students, and conducts clinical research.

The primary medical or surgical physician/resident team refers patients who are not expected to survive hospitalization. The team evaluates each patient and independently determines whether or not they can be of help to the patient. If so, the team accepts the patient and develops a comprehensive therapeutic plan that addresses patient and family wishes regarding life-sustaining measures, comfort, and psychological and spiritual needs.

The advanced practice nurse and physician round together daily and evaluate and revise the therapeutic plan as needed. The advanced practice nurse has institutional prescriptive privileges that permit her to serve as the primary provider responsible for each patient.

Patients referred to Supportive Care from the ICU are moved to a special area of dedicated beds where the therapeutic plan is implemented. This process provides a triage option for the ICU and privacy and unrestricted visiting for the dying patient and his or her loved ones. The patient remains with the Comprehensive Supportive Care Team until death or discharge, unless a change in condition warrants a return to the referring service for more vigorous treatment.

Figures 8.1, 8.2, and 8.3 reflect a few facts about the service, including trends in referrals and in the average length of stay, which has gone from 13 days in 1986 to 4 days in 1997. Hospital charges are reduced dramatically when patients are cared for by the Supportive Care Team. Traditional care for 31 anoxic encephalopathy patients averaged about $35,000; Supportive Services provided care for 31 similar patients at a cost of about $12,000.

## Selecting a Model: Service or Unit or Both?

Despite the example of the Detroit Receiving Hospital, for the most part, the costs and benefits of palliative care programs are not clear-cut; as with much in this field, few studies have been done, although many promising programs are under way. Here are some questions to consider:

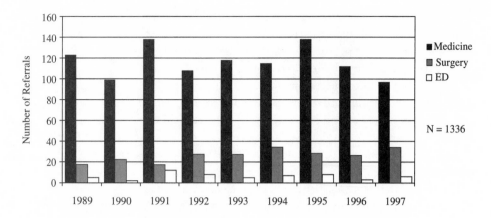

Figure 8.1 Referral Sources for the Supportive Care Team. Reprinted with permission of Detroit Receiving Hospital, Detroit, MI.

- What problems will palliative care address?
- Is a palliative care unit or consultation service part of the solution?
- If so, how would the group measure its progress?
- What other elements are needed to solve the problem(s) identified?
- Can the program be sustained financially? How will it be funded? (See chapter 9 for a detailed discussion of financing end-of-life care.)
- How will providers bill for care?
- What effect will the unit have on overall costs? Will engaging more patients sooner and providing them with increased levels of care increase costs? Or will costs be reduced, as patients and families get the support and treatment they need to prevent symptoms or costly—and avoidable—hospitalizations?

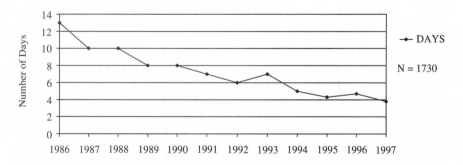

Figure 8.2 Average Length of Stay for Supportive Care Team Patients. Reprinted with permission of Detroit Receiving Hospital, Detroit, MI.

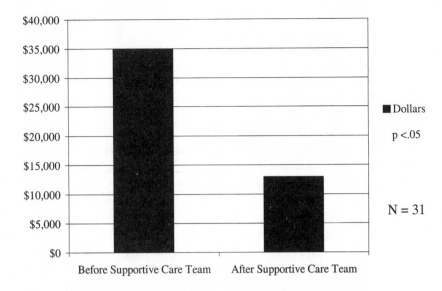

Figure 8.3 Hospital Charges for Encephalopathy Patients, Supportive Care or Usual Care. Reprinted with permission of Detroit Receiving Hospital, Detroit, MI.

- Which staff are available? Will new staff be hired or necessary? How much and what kind of training will be needed?

Strategies for gathering this kind of information include:

- Retrospective chart reviews, both qualitative and quantitative
- Inpatient questionnaires and interviews
- Family questionnaires and interviews, by phone or in focus groups
- Focus groups with physicians, nurses, medical students, and others
- Roundtable discussions with house staff
- Management information system (MIS) data collection on hospital deaths
- Monitoring and assessment of a select group of current end-of-life patients

*Source*: Zuckerman, 1998

Once this study has been completed, organizations must next consider how to present the proposed project to health care staff and how to anticipate and respond to their concerns. When organizations finally select an approach, they must develop a way to manage the program and provide day-to-day administrative support for tasks such as grant writing, funding, research and analysis, and outreach. Some programs are managed within geriatrics or pain service. Still others hire new staff for their units or consults.

## Responding to the Concerns of Health Care Providers

Many clinicians will likely welcome the palliative care unit for its increased support and guidance in dealing with end-of-life problems. Some providers may be reluctant to "give up" patients to palliative care teams, or to lose contact with longtime patients.

Others may feel that teams are an intrusion. Indeed, in one New York City hospital, doctors said they would view a palliative care team as a "death squad."

Successful palliative care programs are generally viewed as an adjunct to care, not as a replacement. Some new palliative care programs report that within a few months of start-up, providers have begun to refer patients regularly or call for advice and help. Many colleagues take the advice or recommendations of the palliative care teams. Northwestern Memorial Hospital Hospice/Palliative Medicine reports that in one fiscal year, its palliative consultative service received 524 total requests for consultation. Since the program's inception, the number of consultations per year has increased by approximately 10 percent each year; by 1997, the program was receiving an average of 60 consultations each month.

One leading medical center operates a palliative care consult service and an inpatient unit with a few beds scattered throughout the facility. When it first began, physicians were sometimes reluctant to refer patients. One even had to be persuaded to accept a palliative care consult for a young woman for whom a cure was impossible—and who continued to seek treatment, unaware that her prognosis was fatal. Still hoping for a cure, the woman, a single parent, had not made plans for guardianship of her daughter. When the palliative care team heard about the case, the team decided it was critical to encourage and support the oncologist in discussing the patient's prognosis with her. While the oncologist spoke to his patient, the team remained nearby, ready to help. The following day, the woman met with a team member to begin developing plans for her child, who was also present and talked about her concerns and fears.

## Enrolling Patients and Measuring Satisfaction

Unlike hospice, which is limited by Medicare reimbursement policies in the kinds of patients it can admit by virtue of their prognosis, palliative care programs often see patients for whom prognosis is uncertain. Some programs take patients in the early stages of congestive heart failure, helping them live with their disease by controlling symptoms. Many see patients who may have more than a year to live.

*CHF*

Within this broad framework, palliative care programs are able to serve patients with cancer, HIV/AIDS, congestive heart failure, emphysema, stroke, sickle-cell anemia, Alzheimer's, and dementia. In general, referrals can come from within the hospital itself, from other community organizations, from chart reviews, and from patient and family requests for service.

To determine their referral base, organizations need to gather and analyze information about deaths in the community, collecting data such as:

- Location and cause of death
- Timing, frequency, and length of hospitalizations
- Cost of patient care
- Community-based resources

### ★★★Good Samaritan Regional Medical Center

During its year-long project for the Breakthrough Series, the team from the Good Samaritan Regional Medical Center in Phoenix, Arizona, established a palliative medicine program. A nurse practitioner who reports to the medical director leads the program, which operates as a separate unit within the hospital. The multidisciplinary team includes social services and pastoral care.

Good Samaritan uses several methods to track performance, such as referral sources, patient disposition, and money saved

Table 8.1 Referral Sources

| Referral sources | Total | Discharge | | | | |
| | | Died | SNF* | Home | Hospital | Hospice |
| --- | --- | --- | --- | --- | --- | --- |
| Academic medical service | 13 | 1 | 5 | 3 | 4 | 1 |
| Palliative medicine director from geriatrics practice | 65 | 6 | 36 | 22 | 1 | 10 |
| Other geriatric practice | 2 | 1 | 2 | — | — | 1 |
| Misc. hospital referral | 4 | 1 | 1 | 2 | — | 1 |
| Consults only | 16 | 4 | 2 | 2 | 8 | 1 |
| Total | 100 | 13 | 46 | 29 | 13 | 14 |

*SNF—skilled nursing facility

Reprinted with permission of Good Samaritan Regional Medical Center, Phoenix, AZ.

Table 8.2 Financial Effect of Palliative Medicine Service

| Patient | Age | Diagnosis | Hospital LOS* | Palliative LOS | Cost | Cost Avoid+ |
|---------|-----|-----------|---------------|----------------|------|-------------|
| A | 91 | CHF, renal failure, pneumonia | 3 | 11 | $4,060 | $1,000 |
| B | 86 | Dementia, Atrial fibrillation | 0 | 2 | $850 | $1,000 |
| C | 77 | Intracerebral bleed | 10 | 7 | $11,574 | $15,000 |
| D | 87 | Dementia, hip fx, pneumonia | 0 | 3 | $1,487 | $3,000 |
| E | 93 | Dementia | 0 | 1 | $649 | $1,000 |
| | | | | Total | $18,620 | $21,000 |

*LOS: length of stay, after referral

+Cost avoid: estimates based on ICU days avoided by consultation or transfer to Palliative Medicine Service

Reprinted with permission of Good Samaritan Palliative Care Unit, Phoenix, AZ.

or costs avoided. Tables 8.1 and 8.2 chart the data Good Samaritan collected on these variables.

The team from Good Samaritan also surveyed families for satisfaction with the health care service, both before and after the palliative care service was established. Before it was created, only 30 percent of families said that doctors or nurses had talked to them or to the patient in ways they could understand about end-of-life issues. Little more than nine months later, 100 percent of those surveyed said such conversations had occurred.

★★★*Parkland Health & Hospital System*

Chapter 2 highlighted the accomplishments of Parkland Health & Hospital System, a public hospital serving Dallas County, Texas. The Parkland Breakthrough Series team focused on improving patient access to palliative care services. Specifically, the team aimed to increase by half the number of medical oncology patients who received palliative care services before the last month of life. Palliative services were defined to include pain management, hospice referral, social and spiritual referrals, and primary care. This service was integrated into an existing team—another model for teams and organizations to consider.

To evaluate the program's success, Parkland measured:

- Percentage of patients receiving palliative services before the last month of life
- Length of time from palliative care referral to death

- Percentage of patients who achieved pain management goals
- Percentage of patients referred to social services, pastoral care, and hospice
- Patient and family satisfaction

The charts that show Parkland's success are given in chapter 2. For instance, the average number of days in which a patient received palliative care services went from 11 to 60, and the percentage of patients receiving services rose from 40 to 80. The Parkland team attributes its success to careful case management and weekly multidisciplinary team meetings. (See the appendix, page 299, for Parkland's referral flowcharts.)

The next step in Parkland's cycle will include a focus on improved patient understanding of hospice care, increased advance care planning, and better pain management. The service will also be expanded beyond the oncology unit.

## Marketing the Program to Clinicians and Others

Many programs "market" their services to providers and organizations, usually through outreach and education activities, such as newsletters, stickers, brochures, and telephone cards. For instance, the palliative care service at New York's Mount Sinai Hospital prints and distributes a quarterly palliative care newsletter to 8,000 individuals associated with end-of-life care. Another New York hospital, Saint Vincent's, has distributed a brochure about its palliative care service to almost 800 doctors who have hospital admitting privileges, and it also distributes other promotional items, such as phone stickers for medical-surgical units and Rolodex cards for doctors. The program hosts a lecture series featuring talks by national experts on palliative care.

### ★★★Franciscan Health Systems

Franciscan Health Systems, based in Tacoma, Washington, aimed to improve access to and increase patient satisfaction with supportive services. Franciscan's team took several approaches to increasing access to care, primarily by increasing provider referrals to hospice and supportive care. The group tested several approaches to encourage doctors to refer patients whose diagnosis of heart disease or cancer gave them a prognosis of less than 12 months to live.

The group found that the most effective way to get referrals was to show doctors a list of patients with serious diagnoses and ask, "Would you be surprised if this patient died in the next year?" Tactics that didn't work included a self-referral brochure for patients and a resource list in each exam room. Doctors and other staff who viewed the video "Supportive Care of the Dying," which describes the needs of dying patients, were more likely to increase referrals. Increased referrals had a significant effect on Franciscan's hospice:

- Referrals increased from one per month to six per month
- Length of stay increased by half
- Hospice revenues increased by 400 percent

Supportive Care program staff are based in the system's clinics, where their presence serves to remind clinicians that the program is available. Physicians can also continue to follow their patients.

### Set Standards and Procedures

Like all medical services, palliative care units require standards and procedures. Many organizations use standing orders in

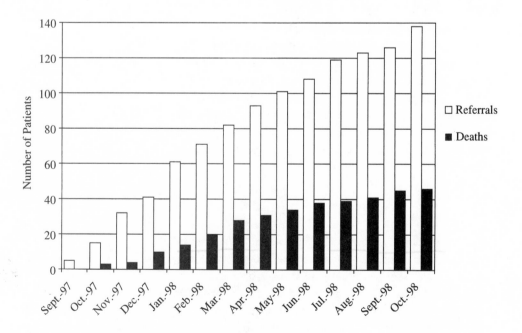

Figure 8.4 Patient Referrals and Deaths. Reprinted with permission of Franciscan Health Services, Tacoma, WA.

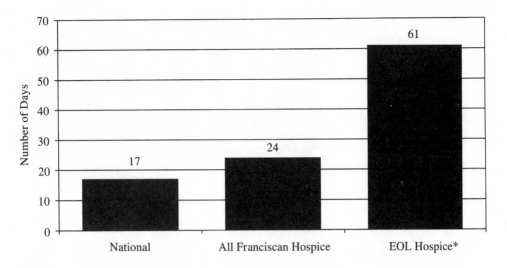

*End of Life care recipients use of hospice

Figure 8.5 Median Length of Hospice Service. Reprinted with permission of Franciscan Health Services, Tacoma, WA.

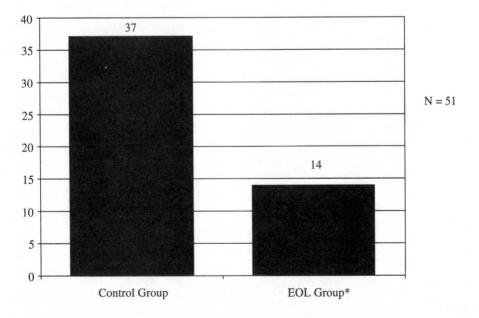

*End of Life care recipients

Figure 8.6 Number of Hospitalizations, Last Year of Life. Reprinted with permission of Franciscan Health Services, Tacoma, WA.

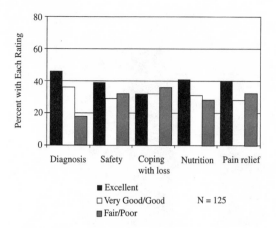

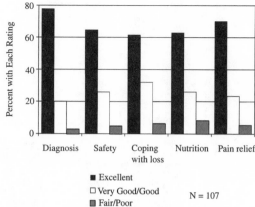

Figure 8.7a Satisfaction before Supportive Service. Reprinted with permission of Franciscan Health Services, Tacoma, WA.

Figure 8.7b Satisfaction after Supportive Service. Reprinted with permission of Franciscan Health Services, Tacoma, WA.

their palliative care programs to help ensure that patients receive prompt attention and treatment for a range of problems.

★★*Community Memorial Hospital*

Community Memorial Hospital of Menomonee Falls, Wisconsin, is a suburban, nonprofit hospital with 208 beds. In 1997, it had 6,700 discharges, 200 patient deaths from all causes, and 575 newly diagnosed cancer patients.

With the goal of establishing a palliative care program, the improvement team submitted a proposal to its administrative group and its medical staff executive committee. The group aimed to reduce by half the physical symptoms, emotional impact, and resource utilization of dying patients through palliative care initiatives. The group focused on five key dimensions for improvement, setting specific goals within each domain:

- Case finding (e.g., 90 percent of patients report they are well informed of medical situation)
- Pain management
- Support and meaningfulness for patient and family
- Advance care planning
- Continuity of care

Based on its extensive list of standards for patient care, Community Memorial Hospital clearly establishes what patients and providers can expect from the program; these are

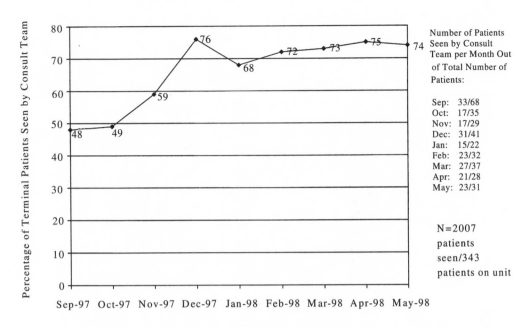

Figure 8.8 Patients Seen by Consult Team. Medical/Oncology Inpatient Unit-Terminally Ill Patients. Reprinted by permission of Community Memorial Hospital, Menomonee Falls, WI.

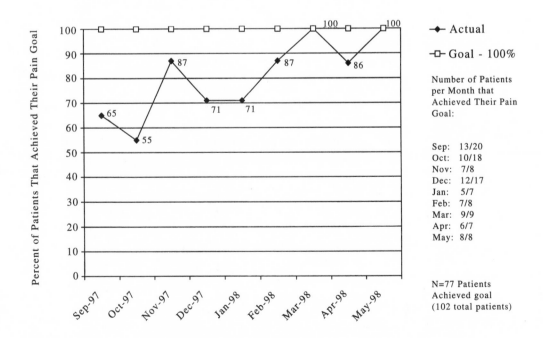

Figure 8.9 Patient's Pain Goal Achieved. Medical/Oncology Terminal Inpatients (with pain). Reprinted by permission of Community Memorial Hospital, Menomonee Falls, WI.

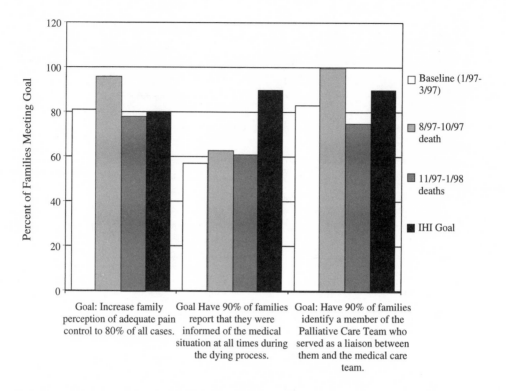

Figure 8.10 Family Satisfaction Questionnaire Results. Questionnaire mailed 2–3 months after patient's death. Reprinted with permission of Community Memorial Hospital, Menomonee Falls, WI.

highlighted in the group's instrument "Standards of Palliative Care," which is provided in the appendix.

The programs have been successful. The number of patients seen each month went from about half of terminally ill patients in September to about three-quarters by May. When the program began, 65 percent of patients reported that their pain goals were achieved; eight months later, that figure had increased to 100 percent.

The communication plan set out by the Community Memorial Hospital Palliative Care Program is an excellent outline of how programs can work with other providers and can give patients and families information. It is included in the appendix.

### Innovators Need to Know

The ways in which most people die—and will die in the future—will not fit into any particular "box" or program. Services that adapt to patient and family needs, offering support and help for end-of-life concerns even when patients are receiving aggressive treatments, will best meet the needs of many dying patients. Whether groups develop palliative care units or consults, they will improve the end-of-life experience of patients and their loved ones.

- Organizations can tailor palliative care services to meet patient needs and institutional missions.
- Palliative care programs offer "teachable moments" for all staff involved in caring for seriously ill patients.
- Palliative care programs expand hospice-like service to an array of patients with diseases that will prove fatal over the course of many months or several years.
- Careful analysis of existing services and programs, and of ways to integrate these with a palliative care program, is essential.
- Programs can be led by different practitioners, from physicians with expertise in palliative care to certified nurse specialists with similar expertise.

## Resources

American Academy of Hospice and Palliative Medicine
4700 W. Lake Avenue
Glenview, IL 60025-1485
Phone: 847-375-4712
Fax: 847-375-6312
E-mail: aahpm@aahpm.org
http://aahpm.org/

"Guide to Hospice/Palliative Care," covering such topics as pain management, dyspnea control, and psychological, social, and spiritual distress.
http://www.aahpm.org/Primer.htm

*Journal of Palliative Medicine*
David E. Weissman, MD
Palliative Care Program Director
Medical College of Wisconsin
Froedtert Hospital East
9200 W. Wisconsin Avenue
Milwaukee, WI 53226-3596
E-mail: dweissmn@hemonc.mcw.edu

# Medicare Reimbursement

Most of the model programs that have demonstrated good care for patients at the end of life are sustained by cross-subsidies within their organizations or by grants awarded by private foundations. Foundations, other private organizations, and some government programs have supported advances in the end-of-life field and in quality improvement programs. However, programs that rely on such funds can rarely be sustained indefinitely—much less replicated widely.

No current reimbursement strategy regularly matches financial incentives with desirable care. As a result, health care managers interested in developing new programs for end-of-life patients need to consider not only cash flow but also the effects of various funding strategies on the tendency to create—or to sustain—patterns of inadequate care for dying patients.

Each funding method in Medicare has different incentives for and barriers to providing quality care to patients at the end of life. In the current framework, most providers cannot afford to earn a reputation for providing excellent care in difficult cases—that is, care that is complex and expensive but also includes continuity, medications, counseling, and nursing.

Why focus only on Medicare? Because most other reimbursement systems are similar, and because three-quarters of deaths occur while the patient is in the Medicare system. Since the 1980s, more than a quarter of annual Medicare expenditures have been accounted for by the 5 to 6 percent of beneficiaries who died that year (Lubitz and Riley, 1993). Because most elderly people are sick for a few years with the illness that eventually claims their lives, one may reasonably estimate that nearly half of Medicare expenditures go for the care of

> Modern society must learn how to assure that dependent and disabled persons can live well, despite living for a long time with eventually fatal illnesses.
>
> —American Geriatrics Society

eventually fatal illnesses, and care for serious and eventually fatal illnesses represents a substantial proportion of the services most health care organizations provide.

Any one patient, at any one time, can be in only one of the three Medicare payment systems: fee-for-service, full risk capitation, or hospice. In most circumstances, the patient is presumed to be in Medicare fee-for-service unless the patient has chosen to enroll in a capitated system or in hospice. These are summarized below and are explained at length in later sections.

### Capitated, Risk-Bearing Payments

In this model, Medicare reimbursement essentially equals the local per capita rate (the "AAPCC") times the number of enrollees. The minor adjustments for age and gender do not usually add up to a substantial effect; the more substantial adjustment for nursing home residence affects few beneficiaries (unless that is the target population).

Currently, only a few managed care plans provide care for large numbers of seriously ill Medicare patients. For a few years, Medicare capitation saw dramatic growth; but since July 1998 the proportion of Medicare beneficiaries enrolled in managed care plans has been holding at about 15 percent, or 5 million beneficiaries (HCFA Medicare Managed Care Cost Report, http://www.hcfa.gov). Plans have no incentive to enroll or retain patients with substantial care needs. Since Medicare does not yet have any adjustment for severity of illness, managed care plans cannot afford a reputation for excellence in caring for the seriously ill, because that would attract patients whose expenses are predictably higher than reimbursements.

Seriously ill patients could actually benefit from the continuity, comprehensiveness, and flexibility in service array that capitated risk-bearing managed care plans usually provide. However, the costs of enrolling or retaining unusually sick patients have prevented such innovation. The Balanced Budget Act of 1997 aims to correct this distortion by requiring a system of risk adjustment (for expected utilization for sick patients), starting in the year 2000. The form of these risk adjusters is still quite uncertain, and it is likely to be delayed and also implemented in phases.

In capitated managed care, the cash flow, the locus of risk, and the organization of the physician providers are all quite variable. In traditional HMOs, the physicians were a closed panel, the provider group owned the hospitals, and providers were responsible for clinics and the risk for costs. Now many managed care contractors collect the capitation but pass both the money and the risk through to provider groups who serve many such contractors. Accountability can be difficult to locate.

If a manager in such a system aims to assess the merits of a special service for the seriously ill at the end of life, that manager will be able to estimate the cash inflow for existing patients fairly directly (at least until risk adjustment is initiated). However, what matters most are two elements that can be much more difficult to estimate. The first is to estimate the effects on case mix of having such a service: Will it attract high-cost patients disproportionately? If substantial, adverse risk selection would obviously prevent establishing the new service. The second is to estimate the effects on recent costs of having such a service. If current costs are running five times the AAPCC (not an unusual figure) and the new service promises to cut costs to twice the AAPCC, then encouraging the new service might well be wise, so long as it does not attract more high-cost beneficiaries.

Some well-controlled systems will be able to predict the utilization of a new service. However, another variable to consider is the degree to which eligible beneficiaries are likely to use the service. Such data may not be readily available but can be estimated with some accuracy as a program begins. Parameters for continuation or revisions can then be built into the development plan.

## Hospice

Medicare reimbursement for hospice is based on a per diem, all-inclusive rate, so its core funding is predicted by multiplying the home care hospice rate by the number of patients and days on service. This reimbursement approach means that hospice incentives are more like those in capitated managed care than in fee-for-service. However, hospice's comprehensive service array (it even includes most prescription drug costs), its enrollment limitations (only people with "prognoses of less than six months" are eligible), and its avoidance of hospitalization and high-tech interventions make it quite different from the other reimbursement models. (More about hospice is included later in this chapter.)

## Fee-for-Service

Most of Medicare is in the fee-for-service sector, and most payments are linked to the setting and the service. Incentives for providers in fee-for-service care generally encourage patterns of care that expand services, rather than prevent future exacerbations or provide coordinated care with many different kinds of services. To estimate reimbursements in fee-for-service, one has to estimate numbers of patients, the duration of services in each setting, services per patient per unit time in each setting, reimbursement rates, and denial and appeal effects. These are spelled out in the following section, which describes fee-for-service payments according to setting (e.g., home health, skilled nursing facility, hospital).

### In This Chapter

This chapter, which is generally organized by treatment setting, provides information about how Medicare could reimburse providers for services to the seriously ill. This chapter:

- Shows how a comprehensive program for end-of-life can bill Medicare appropriately for services rendered
- Helps managers assess alternative strategies, limit financial risks, and anticipate shortfalls even when they are not reasonably avoidable
- Helps estimate the income likely to be generated through such billing

This chapter cannot, of course, construct a business plan for any single organization. Instead, the information and tables here enable readers to explore ways to tailor a plan that provides services to patients with advanced illness. It focuses only on the background considerations regarding how Medicare can be billed, in various settings, for specially tailored programs that serve dying patients. To generate a financial plan in this rapidly changing environment, a manager will need to estimate costs and revenues for various strategies. Organizations can estimate their own costs for each specific type of service, based on the type and number of patients to be served over a period of time. Managers must also assess the match of services with their patients. The service array for patients who are poor, who use home care or nursing care, or who have no family support will be quite different from the service array designed for patients who have extensive financial and family support.

Some unusual Medicare payments are not discussed here: PACE (Program of All-Inclusive Care of the Elderly), Evercare, and Social HMOs. These effectively provide capitation rates for special populations: nursing home dual eligibles (Medicare and Medicaid) for PACE, nursing home residents for Evercare, and a deliberate population mix with expanded benefits for Social HMOs. They all offer real opportunities for excellent palliative care, but they are not available everywhere and may take quite some time and effort to establish.

## Medicare Payments for Fee-for-Service Programs

Most fee-for-service payments to health care programs are based on the nature of the program; most people with serious illness at the end of life will use a combination of home health care, hospital care, and nursing home care. Here we review major considerations surrounding reimbursement in the three major programs by which fee-for-service care is organized.

### Home Health Care

Medicare will cover home health care for beneficiaries who meet four criteria. The beneficiary must:

- Need intermittent skilled nursing care or physical therapy or speech language pathology
- Be homebound
- Be under a physician's care plan
- Receive services from a Medicare participating home health agency (HHA)

Once a beneficiary qualifies, Medicare will pay for the following services, if medically reasonable and necessary:

- Part-time or intermittent skilled nursing care
- Part-time or intermittent home health aide services
- Part-time or intermittent physical therapy or speech language pathology
- Continued occupational therapy services
- Medical social services
- Durable medical equipment (subject to 20 percent coinsurance)

Medicare does not cover prescription drugs or personal care provided by home health aides (custodial care) if this is the only care that the patient needs. The Social Security Act contains blanket exclusions of coverage for custodial care (personal care unrelated to skilled treatment of a specific illness or injury) and personal comfort items.

Home health care had been growing dramatically under a fee-for-service reimbursement, limited mainly by eligibility requiring skilled services. The Balanced Budget Act of 1997 (BBA) instituted major changes in payments to home health agencies, initially under the Interim Payment System (IPS) for fiscal years 1998 and 1999. A home care Prospective Payment System (PPS) is to begin on October 1, 2000. The IPS and the PPS have dramatically increased financial risks to programs and diminished potential returns from home care, and many have left the field. The combined effect of the new regulations will require many agencies to reduce their average cost per visit and average cost per patient, which usually means limiting enrollment and the number of visits and aiming to have patients whose costs are lower and whose need for services is shorter.

Many home health providers who have traditionally cared for patients with serious and complex illness now need to balance patients whose care is expensive with those whose care is cheaper because their stays are shorter. The new aggregate cost limit per beneficiary will be different for every agency. Each agency's own case mix will determine its ability to care for seriously ill patients. Projecting the patient mix requires a large and stable patient mix. This, in turn, requires avoiding adverse bias in referrals—in other words, avoiding a reputation as the place to go for good care for serious illness.

From the perspective of many managers, the IPS translates into an annual flat fee per patient (who qualifies). This reimbursement strategy creates a serious problem for patients who most need end-of-life care: those with substantial disability, complex illnesses, and unpredictable timing of serious need. Most agencies will have no problem caring for short-term, low-maintenance clients within the reimbursement cap. Patients who need wound dressings changed a few times, or who need supervision of glucose monitoring for their first few weeks at home with diabetes, will be "winners" for home care programs.

Patients who need more intense or prolonged care, and those who come to the agency late in the course of their disease, will far exceed the reimbursement cap. To prevent significant financial losses, the agency needs to recruit low-cost patients while limiting services to high-cost patients. Administrators must carefully manage the case mix.

Many patients whose costs are expected to be quite high have either been denied admission or been preemptively discharged because managers believed such action was essential in order to stay under the reimbursement cap. Whether or not this is the case, this mindset is making it much more difficult for very sick patients to get the care they need.

## Reimbursement for Home Health Agencies

Under the new payment method, home health agencies will be reimbursed the lowest of:

1. Their actual allowable costs
2. The aggregate per visit costs, limited to 105 percent of the national median
3. A new aggregate per beneficiary limit*

* The per beneficiary limit is usually based on payments per patient at that agency, including nonroutine medical supplies, during federal fiscal year 1994.

At the same time, major efforts continue to move these patients out of hospitals quickly and to keep them from using nursing homes. The denial of home health services could effectively mean that they have no Medicare-paid services. Having the cap rate set by reimbursement levels of five years ago exacerbates the scarcity of services for the seriously ill.

Home health agencies have come under scrutiny for fraud; investigations seem to have focused on the merit of visits, on billing for visits not made, and on abuse of the provision of durable medical equipment. Providing medically certified skilled services to people with serious and eventually fatal conditions has not been a particular locus for allegations of fraud.

Most agencies have already calculated their new per beneficiary limit and will have made some decisions about their increased risks. The accompanying chart will help to determine what the service reimbursement will be for each service to each patient. To estimate financial returns, a manager needs to multiply the cap by the number of patients, then modify that based on the likely service array actually provided.

### Skilled Nursing Facilities

The BBA also instituted a new Prospective Payment System (PPS) for Medicare in skilled nursing facilities (SNFs). Under the PPS, SNFs receive per diem payments. There will be a three-year, phased transition from facility-specific rates (reflecting the individual facility's historical cost experience) to standardized federal rates. Medicare's changes here are aimed to affirm that the Medicare SNF benefit is *only* a postacute, short-term benefit, meant to decrease hospital use.

The per diem payments that the new PPS makes are case-mix adjusted to reflect the actual resource intensity a resident needs. To make the case-mix adjustment, the SNF PPS clinically groups SNF residents by using the Resource Utilization Groups, version III (RUG-III), a classification system that groups residents according to average daily care needs. Under the new PPS, the Minimum Data Set (MDS) will determine rates for each SNF resident by placing patients in one of the 44 RUG-III groups. Although the MDS was developed for clinical evaluation and guidance for the care plan, it will now be the foundation for determining each SNF resident's Medicare payment.

Because Medicare SNF reimbursement depends on a "skilled need," only the most acute first 26 RUG-III categories are sure to be reimbursed. The higher payments are connected to intensive rehabilitation services, such as physical therapy

---

**Average Reimbursement per Home Care Visit, 1997\***

| | |
|---|---|
| Average cost of home visit (by anyone) | $77 |
| Nurse | $98 |
| Therapist (physical, occupational) | $90 |
| Home care aide | $54 |
| Homemaker | $52 |
| Other (social workers, other professionals, etc.) | $89 |

\* Updated by the average annual rate of increase of Medicare per visit charges, which was 4.7 percent between 1987 and 1995 (HCFA, Office of Information Service, 1999).

following orthopedic surgery. The increment for unstable medical conditions is small, and most patients with serious and complex but stable illness will not qualify for any Medicare payment. For example, if a family caregiver can be trained to provide an ongoing service, it is generally difficult to claim that the service continues to be a skilled one (even if the SNF requires a nurse to provide it). Each RUG corresponds with a set per diem payment rate: The higher the ranking, the higher the payment.

Residents receive a single RUG-III ADL (Activities of Daily Living) score that measures their ability to perform these activities (on a scale of 4 to 18; higher scores represent greater functional dependence and a need for more assistance). The major categories include (in hierarchical order) rehabilitation; extensive services; special care; clinically complex; impaired cognition; behavior problems; and reduced physical function. The first 26 RUG-III categories always qualify for Medicare Part A coverage. Other categories require individual coverage determination.

The chart categorizes patients by rehabilitation needs: The ADL score (second column) coupled with the category-specific score (third column) correspond to the RUG code (fourth column).

Stays that follow unusually brief hospital stays (early discharges), and vice versa (bounce-backs), come under complex rules that make the facilities financially responsible for some of one another's actions. One net effect of these billing changes is to force SNFs to take a lead in integrating services. It is not clear yet what results that will yield.

Other than hospice investigations, the care that SNFs provide to dying patients has not come under scrutiny for fraud or abuse. Of course, dying residents will usually retain Medicare coverage for their SNF stay for just a short time, perhaps two weeks after a hospital discharge. They usually do not qualify for rehabilitation, and their conditions, while complex and hazardous, are often stable for long periods. Thus, these patients may not qualify for substantial periods of Medicare coverage in a skilled nursing facility.

Managers addressing SNF coverage for residents who are sick enough to die face perplexing financing issues in considering whether to field a special or enhanced set of services. They will have to understand both the option of using hospice services and the potential for reimbursement under Medicaid and from private sources. Certainly, the experience in Oregon and elsewhere shows that very frail and very sick persons living in SNFs

Table 9.1 Average Daily Rate for Highest RUG Code, by Category

| Category | ADL score required | RUG code | Average daily rate for highest RUG code in each category (nursing, rehab, and nontherapy case mix) |
|---|---|---|---|
| Ultrahigh rehab | 16–18 | RUC | $424.97 urban<br>$359.28 rural |
| Very high rehab | 16–18 | RVC | $327.57 urban<br>$272.97 rural |
| High rehab | 15–18 | RHC | $300.33 urban<br>$245.46 rural |
| Medium rehab | 15–18 | RMC | $295.70 urban<br>$239.48 rural |
| Low rehab | 4–13 | RLA | $198.00 urban<br>$160.13 rural |
| Extensive services *CI | Greater than 7 | SE2 | $242.20 urban<br>$188.70 rural |
| Special care | 17–18 | SSC | $210.71 urban<br>$164.70 rural |
| Clinically complex **DI | 17–18 | CC2 | $209.71 urban<br>$163.78 rural |
| Clinically complex **DI | 4–11 | CA2 | $157.66 urban<br>$155.66 rural |

*CI is the abbreviation for clinical indicators.

**DI is the abbreviation for depression indicators.

can receive good care until death without being moved to hospitals. However, the Medicare SNF benefit is not a prominent factor in financing that care.

### Hospitals

Hospital stays for Medicare patients are usually covered by a flat fee, based on the Diagnosis-Related Group (DRG). The DRG system was designed to group patients with similar resource consumption and length of stay patterns into categories with a set rate for reimbursement. For example, a Medicare patient who enters the hospital with bronchitis and asthma and experiences complications will be assigned to DRG 96, and the hospital will receive an average payment of about $3,280.

Hospitals are at special risk when initiating end-of-life care services. There are some striking examples of inpatient services with designated beds that have published information about good outcomes and sustainable finances (von Gunten, et al.

1998). When organized as inpatient hospital services, however, these programs risk eventual investigation of whether some of the patients served really had to have been in the hospital. The question of who should be in the hospital is obviously central to the question of whether Medicare should pay a DRG for the hospital stay, but there is no settled answer. Essentially, a fiscal intermediary can make a patient-by-patient judgment, and the hospital has to take on the burden of appeal. Formally, the fiscal intermediary can allege that the patient was in the hospital but not receiving services that required hospitalization (sometimes proposing that the person could have been served in a skilled nursing facility, sometimes simply that the person could have been served somewhere else). In either case, reimbursement for the stay is denied. Usually, the hospital cannot collect from the patient, so this situation presents the possibility for substantial bad debt. A patient who is in the hospital and receives opioids for pain management, along with family support and chaplain services (and no surgery, consultations, diagnostic procedures, etc.), seems to be a person at risk of such "downgrading" from hospital-level reimbursement.

Creating a service or unit that might concentrate such patients might well be risky. It seems that everyone knows of a case like this happening somewhere, sometime, but no one knows the rate or the degree of risk. Financial risks will be lower for units that have lots of "doctor-requiring" interventions on the usual patient (e.g., intrathecal anesthesia, radiation treatments, intravenous vasodilators, or inotropic drugs). In units with very short stays (such as ventilator withdrawal cases), the risks of adverse financial decisions (under fraud and abuse investigations) are reduced. However, a unit that really caters to the many patients who need close monitoring for symptoms and peaceable deaths is likely to have to organize such services as a licensed nursing facility or inpatient hospice rather than as a hospital.

In addition, hospital management might well have to consider the financial effect of strategies for caring for end-of-life patients—especially since these strategies can reduce hospitalizations. Some disease management approaches in congestive heart failure have cut hospitalization by more than half (Rich, 1999). The variation in practice patterns for treatment of dementia and frailty of old age is quite substantial. If a hospital is in a setting in which most dementia patients are hospitalized for every fever and most die with gastrostomy tubes, the management would do well to consider the financial consequences of a potential shift toward more care at home and less intensive medical interventions.

## Medicare Payments for Physician Services

Medicare usually pays physicians for procedures and for what it calls "evaluation and management" services (E&M), a category under which payment for most patients with advanced, long-term illness is likely to come. Each E&M bill requires two codes: one for diagnosis and one for how extensive the service was. The diagnosis codes extend to every patient setting, but the coding for how extensive the services were varies by the setting and by whether the service is an ongoing one for an established patient or a first assessment of a patient. Medicare puts many limitations on the frequency of billing possible, but none of these is peculiar to seriously ill patients. (For more basic billing information, go to http://www.ahima.org or http://www.mgma.org.)

Documentation in the medical record about the work involved for a patient—the systems affected, time spent, and complexity—determines coding for how extensive the service provided was. This process has been a flash point for fraud and abuse investigations. As a result, fiscal intermediaries, the Health Care Financing Administration (HCFA), and medical groups are working out guidelines for review. Managers and planners will have to stay current on the issue as it evolves.

Most patients with advanced illness will have several diagnoses that require many medications; many will be relying on family caregivers, who must bear the stress of caregiving and of loss; and patients themselves must face with their own emotional and spiritual concerns as they approach the end of life. It is likely that the billing profiles of physicians who specialize in serving this population will be quite different from their colleagues whose patients do not have serious and complex illness. For example, an oncologist whose patients have an array of cancer diagnoses will have many short checkup visits that balance the longer visits very sick patients require. An oncologist whose practice focuses solely on patients with advanced illness will bill primarily for longer visits. Because such disparity tends to invite scrutiny, physicians in this area must attend to the need for careful documentation and billing. Without it, a review by the fiscal intermediary might well precipitate billing denials and fraud allegations.

Physician claims are sometimes denied because two physicians practicing in the same specialty cannot bill for ongoing services to the same patient at the same time. Because physicians who focus on treating seriously ill and dying patients have no specialty recognition, this claim restriction is a particular problem. In the previous example, the general oncologist and the oncologist who specializes in advanced illness are both oncologists. If the general oncologist wants his colleague to see the patient as well, that claim might be denied unless the bill uses appropriate E&M codes that differentiate between the services.

This restriction is especially problematic for the general internists and family physicians who typically serve hospices. Despite their substantial expertise in working with patients at the end of life, they cannot advise their physician colleagues who have the same "specialty" training. Often, billing for the symptom by the palliative care physician and for the underlying illness by the primary physician is sufficient.

This problematic billing restriction means that physicians or managers interested in developing palliative care services should first contact their Medicare intermediary. Some intermediaries will allow exceptions and approve concurrent care by two physicians in some circumstances if the service can be proved (sometimes on a special documentation form) to be fundamentally different.

### Northwestern Memorial Hospital and Mt. Sinai Hospital

Chicago's Northwestern Memorial Hospital offers a palliative care consultation service in its acute care facility. The palliative care team comprises a nurse, attending physicians, rotating fellows, medical residents, and medical students. The full consultation—for example, talking with the patient's family members or other loved ones—could take several visits. Comprehensive results of the consultation are recorded in the patient's medical record; the team makes its recommendations surrounding a treatment plan directly to the attending physician.

To avoid the suggestion that the patient did not need hospital services, consultants do not discuss hospice services in the chart notes, unless hospice will clearly be part of a discharge plan. If there is need to clarify or justify the acuity needs of the patient, the consultant makes this explicit in the note. For example, intensive nursing care and frequent physician assessments often require an inpatient hospital setting.

For organizations making their first attempt at offering a palliative care service, the consult model may be a good place to start. It provides a basis for educating patients, other physicians, and family members about the purpose of palliative care. This model has very few overhead costs. A dedicated multidisciplinary palliative care team and an organizational structure within which it can operate are all that is needed.

---

Billing Patterns for
Palliative Care
at Northwestern

- Northwestern Memorial Hospital reports that during one fiscal year, the four attending physicians on the team billed initial consults almost entirely with the code 99254, which is a level 4 visit consisting of a complete history, a comprehensive exam, and moderate level of medical decision making (a total of 275 times).
- Forty-nine percent of the billed charges were collected.
- Repeated visits were billed as subsequent care codes, not as follow-up consultation codes, since the consult team is usually managing symptoms or providing direct care.

Often the effects on improving services are well worth the risks of denials or of simply not being able to bill enough to fund the program, at least for a while.

The palliative care team at New York's Mt. Sinai Medical Center provides only consults and works in conjunction with other attending physicians. The team uses the standard CPT (Current Procedural Terminology) billing codes for the first three inpatient palliative care consults, billing all as initial consults; if the physician is the patient's primary attending, the code for initial visits is used. The Mt. Sinai team once estimated that the average cost of a consult was $300, although the mean Medicare payment for such consults, in their experience, was $150.

Physician services to very sick patients in an office, home, or nursing facility follow the same pattern, with a set of E&M codes for each setting, graded by intensity of services and (for some) whether it is an initial evaluation. In the examples given in Table 9.2, "intermediate" is defined as an E&M visit that requires at least two of the following three components which include coordination of care with other providers or agencies:

- Detailed interval history
- Detailed examination
- Medical decision making of moderate complexity

Usually, the presenting problems are of moderate to high severity and require physicians to spend 40 minutes with the patient and the family. The "values" (payments) for the mid-range of an intermediate visit (which will be the low end for services to these complex patients) for new and established patients are shown in Table 9.2.

## Know the Codes

Palliative care billing codes are those used for initial hospital care: 99221, 99222, or 99223 (along with the patient's ICD-9 diagnosis). As with other services, the intensity of the visit escalates the coding. A palliative care doctor would bill a moderately complex inpatient visit for a patient with congestive heart failure as 99222 (with an ICD-9 of 428.0).

Any subsequent palliative care consults are billed as subsequent hospital inpatient services: 99231, 99232, or 99233.

Table 9.2 Midrange Payments for Intermediate Visit, New and Established Patients

| Level of service | New patient code | Established patient code | Pay |
|---|---|---|---|
| Office visit | 99204 | | $121.06 |
| | | 99214 | $69.52 |
| Nursing facility visit | 99302 | 99302 | $79.99 |
| Subsequent nursing facility visit | N/A | | — |
| | | 99313 | $71.55 |
| Home care visit | 99343 | | $115.73 |
| | | 99349 | $99.61 |

A physician can bill Medicare for the oversight of a care plan if the time that the physician spent organizing care for that patient exceeds 30 minutes (CPT 99375) or 60 minutes (CPT 99376) of their own direct time during one month. The average reimbursement for these services is about $65 for the first 30 minutes.

Fiscal intermediaries have their own "triggers" for reviewing physician records for patterns of overbilling. Intermediaries might look at physicians who often see patients in nursing facilities more than once a week or who usually bill at the "top end" of E&M services. With adequate documentation, the claim should be paid. Physician services to hospice patients (provided that the physician is not an employee of the hospice) are billed exactly the same as they would be for a nonhospice patient. One exception is that the fiscal intermediary must determine whether inpatient hospice care should be billed as a home visit or as a hospital visit, because the two require different E&M codes. Since the HCFA 1500 form does not designate "hospice" as a site of care, it is up to the intermediaries to determine how an inpatient hospice visit should be billed. There is no established practice.

### Medicare Payments for Hospice Services

The Medicare hospice financing structure is very different from its other reimbursement programs. Most hospice payments are based on an all-inclusive per diem rate, except for physician services, which are mostly paid in the conventional manner (Part B physician billing). The Medicare hospice benefit is available only to individuals who are eligible for Medicare Part A, whose physicians certify that the prognosis is "less than six months," who understand the nature and purpose of palliative care, and who understand that by selecting hospice, they waive their right to certain other Medicare services. For qualified patients, the benefit includes most costs for prescription drugs, durable medical equipment, and care provided through an interdisciplinary team that assesses the needs of each patient and family and develops and implements an appropriate care plan. Hospice patients are distinctly less likely to have surgery, hospitalization, resuscitation, or other "high-tech" interventions (though these services are not explicitly precluded by the Medicare regulations).

When they were first established, the hospice rates covered virtually every service required, with the possible exception of long-term assistance by an aide. The BBA defines a covered hospice service as "any other item or service which is covered by Medicare and is indicated as necessary for the treatment of the terminal illness and related conditions." Medicare Part A will reimburse a hospice for two 90-day periods and then repeated 60-day periods during a patient's lifetime (so long as the patient remains eligible) and for services that the interdisciplinary team identifies as necessary for the palliation and management of their terminal illness. These services include:

- Physician services (if that physician is part of the hospice team)
- Nursing care
- Medical appliances and supplies
- Drugs related to the terminal illness
- Short respite care
- Home health aide and homemaker services
- Physical therapy, occupational therapy, and speech/language pathology services
- Social services, including bereavement
- Nutrition and dietary counseling

The Medicare hospice benefit is paid at one of four rates:

- Routine home care
- Continuous attendance at home
- Inpatient respite care
- General inpatient care (or inpatient symptom management care)

For any one hospice program in one year, the aggregate number of inpatient days, both general and respite, may not exceed 20 percent of the aggregate total number of days of hospice care provided. This requirement makes it difficult for people to receive hospice services if they do not have a suitable home environment or a family caregiver. All payments to all providers for hospice patients are through the hospice program, except for non-employee physicians who submit conventional bills under Medicare Part B, and also except for a few billings for services for illnesses other than the terminal illness, such as an acute injury. Table 9.3 shows the average daily Medicare reimbursement rate.

Hospices have generally competed on amenities and visibility, not on measures of quality or efficiency. The standards of hospice service are incomplete and not well studied. However, it seems likely that there are substantial variations in practice and in quality among hospices.

Table 9.3 Daily Medicare Reimbursement Rate, 1999 (by Service Type)

| Type of service | Daily Medicare reimbursement rate, 1999* |
|---|---|
| Routine home day care<br>  Individuals receiving hospice at home | $97.11 per day |
| Continuous home care<br>  Individuals in a crisis with skilled care for at least 8 hours within<br>  a 24-hour period, only for brief periods of crisis and only as neces-<br>  sary to maintain the individual at home | $566.82/day or $23.62/hour |
| Inpatient respite care<br>  May be provided for no more than five days at a time | $100.46 per day |
| Inpatient symptom management care<br>  Care may be provided in a hospital, skilled nursing facility, or<br>  freestanding inpatient hospice facility | $432.01 per day |

*Varies a little by area wage index.

As hospice has evolved, so too has palliative care for patients at the end of life—including the development of several costly strategies. Palliative chemotherapies for cancer and pain medications can now cost more than the daily hospice rate, for example. Thus, hospices now need to evaluate ways to maintain financial viability while providing the necessary range of health care services.

In general, patients who are dying of a serious nonmalignant disease, such as congestive heart failure (CHF), do not qualify for the hospice benefit because they do not meet the prognosis requirement. Hospice benefits were designed around the disease trajectory for cancer, in which patients follow a fairly predictable course.

The National Hospice Organization wrote *Medical Guidelines for Determining Prognosis in Selected Non-Cancer Diseases* (Stuart, 1994) for enrolling people with nonmalignant disease into hospice; most intermediaries use something similar. However, data from the SUPPORT study imply that these criteria will dramatically limit hospice availability without substantially helping to ensure that hospices do not enroll many patients who live much beyond six months (Fox et al., 1999). Under current rules, hospices can probably serve only about one-quarter of the patients who will die with CHF and obstructive lung disease. Because diseases such as heart failure are so common, and because many of these patients will live in hospice for more than a month, this seems to be a good opportunity for hospices to gain experience (with little financial risk) in meeting the needs of these patients. If good services can be designed, perhaps a modified benefit (or substitution of a different benefit) will eventually enable more access.

Hospice payment for nursing home residents is a thorny subject, primarily because Medicare will not reimburse both the hospice and the nursing facility for care provided to a nursing home resident. Facilities receive better payments from Medicare than from their next best alternative (usually Medicaid), so they are not eager to have patients or families consider hospice enrollment when the patient might qualify for Medicare skilled nursing facility benefits. However, Medicare does not pay for the core services of most nursing home residents, so this problem affects a limited number of patients, usually during their first few weeks in the nursing facility.

Since the beneficiary "holds" the hospice benefit, it would seem that hospice services should be available wherever a person lives. For many years, that was the case. A person living in a nursing home (and having that bill paid for privately or by Medicaid) was eligible for hospice services. Since the hospice per diem rate is almost the same as the usual nursing home daily rate, this could be a substantial infusion of money. However, the hospice payment requires that the hospice team control the plan of care, while nursing home licensure requirements insist that the nursing home team be in control of the plan. This obviously leads to a complex interaction. Now most Medicaid payments for nursing home stays for Medicare hospice patients are reduced to about 95 percent and are given to the hospice program. The hospice program and the nursing home must have a contract that spells out their relationship. Obviously, such arrangements vary by states and institutions.

This issue is controversial. Some people contend that nursing facilities should be able to provide hospice services and that the rates they receive should reflect their services. Others contend that nursing facilities are not now and are not likely to be good at end-of-life care and that a Medicare beneficiary who is a nursing facility resident should not be denied hospice care. For now, both funding streams are available and the attenuation, if combined, is not substantial.

Innovators Need to Know

- Medicare does pay for services to those with serious and eventually fatal illnesses.
- Billing Medicare can be very complex and requires focused attention.

- Because of geographic differences in fiscal intermediary practices, institutions must get to know their own fiscal intermediaries.
- Programs that want to develop and offer palliative care and hospice services might first focus on a small set of services in a specific setting, such as a palliative care consult in a hospital unit.

### Resources

The best resources on this subject come from HCFA itself, and they include:

- 1997 E&M documentation guidelines: http://www.hcfa. gov/audience/planprov.htm
- Physician fee schedule: http://www.hcfa.gov/medicare/ pfsmain.htm
- RUG categories: Federal Register, May 12, 1998

For more basic billing information go to http://www.ahima.org or http://www.mgma.org.

Material for this chapter also forms the basis of: Fowler, N. M., Lynn, J. Potential Medicare reimbursements for services to patients with chronic fatal illnesses. *Journal of Palliative Medicine* 2000; 3:165–180.

# Beyond Number Crunching

*Ways to Use Information Systems
in Quality Improvement*

## 10

Information management is critical to good patient care: Tracking clinical data, along with the administrative data for billing and staffing, is a key element for resource management. Groups aiming for breakthrough change should view the information system as a tool that can be quite efficient in measuring patient care and the effects of change on that care.

Measuring change is essential, but it must not overwhelm the team's work or become its central task. Groups do not want to devise elegant measures for a lack of improvement!

One way to be more efficient in improvement work is to use the management information systems (MIS) developed for service delivery, either patient care or program management, as a quality improvement tool. For example, an automated medical record can have a "pop-up" query asking if an ICU patient has an advance directive. This prompt is likely to get questions asked and responses documented. By having this query in every medical record, the system can put in place an automated record to tally advance care plans.

Hospital record-keeping systems routinely collect data that can be used to measure quality improvement. For example, staffing data can become a measure of continuity of care: How many nurses visited a hospice patient in one week? How many hospice patients saw more than three different home health aides in any given week? How many families called the after-hours answering services? (For more details, read chapter 7 to learn how Hope Hospice used this approach to improve continuity of care.) How many late-stage heart failure patients were admitted to the hospital emergency room? Financial data can show when cases are opened or closed (and, as a result, how long a patient was in a system) and the services billed for

> If you don't know where you're going, you'll probably get lost.
>
> —Yogi Berra

the patient (e.g., home infusion therapy, skilled nursing care, and so on).

Looking at administrative data from a different perspective can reveal much about where change is needed—and the effect of such change.

## In This Chapter

Health care programs require systems to gather information to manage services and billings. In some organizations, these systems are also designed to monitor and support quality improvement. This chapter gives ideas for how to use the MIS for improvement and introduces some rather extraordinary systems developed specifically to support quality monitoring and improvement. The major ways teams have used MIS to improve end-of-life care include:

- Creating a list of patients, or a registry
- Promoting change with record system innovation
- Monitoring improvement with periodic tallies in existing systems
- Monitoring improvement with customized outcomes information

## Review the Management Information System

The clear starting point in using the MIS for quality improvement is to review the system to understand what it collects, how it works, and how teams can cull (or contribute) information using it. Here are some basic questions to consider:

- What are the components of the information system?
- Who uses each component?
- What information is available?
- What information is not available?
- How reliable is the information?
- How readily, and how quickly, is it available?
- How hard is it to modify data?

Remember to consider all of the ways the organization regularly collects information or data. One improvement team developed a bereavement questionnaire, only to have the first respondent point out that she had answered similar questions from the hospital chaplain's office just a few days earlier! In nursing homes required to use the extensive Minimum Data

Set (MDS) tool, a great deal of information will already have been gathered. Sometimes marketing, nursing, or billing departments have data that would be useful—and that would not require additional patient surveys.

A quick review enables an improvement team to find what its members know—or don't know—about the organization's record-keeping and information management processes. What can the MIS do? Can it track the outcomes relevant to the team's improvement projects? What kinds of information can be used to enrich quality improvement efforts? Are there ways to use information from the financial system—for example, tallying diagnostic tests or procedures used on patients with certain diagnoses—to track quality improvement measures? The process itself can generate quality improvement endeavors.

## Make the MIS Do Double Duty

Although there are probably many ways an MIS can be used to make improvement activities more effective and efficient, here are four that come up frequently and that have proven useful in rapid-cycle change projects.

### ★Create a List of Patients, or a Registry

Groups often want to start projects by creating a list of "all patients with _____ (a particular condition)." Usually, one way to accomplish this is to review medical records. If a team wants to track the rate of severe pain on the hospital's third floor, the denominator has to be the patients on that floor over a specified time. If a team wants to track and improve continuity of care by making opioid drugs available after hospital discharge among patients who have trouble paying for medication, the registry might be a list of all patients who are receiving opioids in their last two days of hospitalization. That list might be readily made from pharmacy or billing records, even if the hospital does not have an automated clinical record.

Sometimes the MIS-generated list needs to be reviewed and revised. For example, one team uses its MIS to generate a monthly list of all patients (and their diagnoses) seen by each particular physician in a primary care clinic. The physician then reviews the list for people who are "sick enough that death in the next few months would not be a surprise." The team uses the resulting patient list to target counseling, symptom management, advance planning, and family support.

One institution aimed to improve decisions about resuscitation. One very efficient monitor was the simple rate of CPRs at death divided by total deaths.

In short, information systems are useful in creating lists of patients with whom to target interventions or monitor events.

## ★★Promote Change with Medical Record System Innovation

Depending on a team's aims and its information system, changes to the system itself can be worth trying. Some teams have created important changes just by modifying their usual forms. And since health care providers are used to keeping and seeing many records, they expect to contribute to them. One move that teams can try for a wide variety of aims is to change something about the information being recorded. If a standard history and physical form has space for "pain and symptoms," "preferred decision makers," or "spiritual issues," those things are much more likely to be recorded—and to be brought up with patients and loved ones.

One very popular change is to alter the bedside chart for hospital patients so that pain is recorded every time vital signs are taken (see chapter 3 on ways to improve pain management). One nursing home made a similar and effective change by using the last line of the "problem list" for a synopsis of advance care plans. Having a space to be completed made quick reference easy and ensured that the issues were addressed.

The record system itself can be the basis for innovation. Statewide, Oregon uses a hot-pink form called the POLST, Physician's Orders for Life-Sustaining Treatment, to communicate plans about resuscitation and other important aspects of rescue treatment. The form is valid in every treatment setting in the state—home, ambulance, nursing home, and hospital (see chapter 7 for more details).

The possibilities for using automated patient record systems as quality improvement tools are numerous. Automated systems can provide prompts or follow-up inquiries. One team is trying a query that pops up whenever an ICU patient is discharged. The query asks, "Do we know what this patient would want if he/she were ever so sick again?"

## ★★Monitor Improvement with Periodic Tallies

Sometimes, the existing MIS contains the numerator and the denominator for a study. A team that aims to reduce exacerbations of heart failure can tally emergency room visits and/or hospitalizations for a patient population defined as ever having been hospitalized for heart failure. If the team knows that virtually all exacerbations will be treated in its facility, it can track improvement entirely from billing data. In general, existing administrative data can be used to track most aims that center on utilization rates.

Other items commonly found in administrative data are prescription drugs, orders against resuscitation, and treatments for specific problems, such as skin breakdown. Since there is virtually no justified use for meperidine in chronic pain, a simple declining rate of its use helps to document improvement in prescribing practices.

Even if a team needs to measure some other aspects of care to be sure of improvement, having some core measure that is so easy to obtain (and thus never has missing values) is a real boost to enthusiasm. Most team members love clinical care and evidence of improvement—but they only tolerate data collection. It is easier to stay involved if data collection and measurement are easy.

### Track Improvement with Customized Outcomes Information

Something very special happens when the patient or family outcomes that the improvement team aims for are a prominent part of routine data collection. In the VITAS hospice system, patients are routinely asked about comfort, spiritual peace, and family relationships. This makes it possible to compare programs in different cities or to track the performance of one clinical team over time. Since the questions are appropriate to clinical issues, staff do not see recording them as requiring additional effort.

The Minimum Data Set now required by federal regulation of nursing facilities has similar features. Every few months, function and comfort are routinely recorded for every nursing home resident. In aggregate, facility performance over time on these measures is readily tracked.

### Systems That Help Manage Improvement

Not every organization needs its own custom-made computer system. Most can use off-the-shelf programs to generate spreadsheets, tabulate and graph data from chart reviews, and present information to others. Smaller organizations can build ties with similar organizations in their state or region, pooling resources to develop a computerized MIS. A simpler approach is to find a similar organization, ask about its MIS, and ask if the software can be purchased and customized.

Three large organizations that focus on end-of-life care have developed computerized systems that streamline administrative functions and improve continuity of patient care for chronically ill or dying patients. In general, these systems provide the tools to improve case management, which in turn can improve patient care. Smaller organizations cannot invest the resources required to develop new systems—but they can use these models for ideas about how to work the MIS to create breakthrough improvement.

### ★★Franklin Health

Franklin Health, Inc., of Upper Saddle River, New Jersey, describes its mission as caring for the "sickest 1 percent" of society. The organization relies on nurse care managers to work directly with patients and families, health care providers, and insurers to develop treatment plans, coordinate care, and facilitate information flow. Franklin uses a Web-based information system, Patient Management System '98, to track patient care and quickly update medical records during late-stage disease management.

Case managers enter information when patients are admitted to the Franklin Health System and then use the system to track patient goals, patient and family issues or concerns, treatment plans and actions, and outcomes.

The system aims to promote information sharing between the patient and treating physician—and to improve communication among the field case manager, the health plan, and the nurse and physician case supervisors. Team managers can access patient data at any time. To safeguard patient privacy, only employees with the appropriate Web browser and passcode have access to patient information, and only for patients who are in their care. Approximately 60 care managers use the software to track visits to patient homes, as well as hospital and nursing home stays.

Eventually, Franklin will make the system available on-line at a secured site that other organizations could access to track patient care. Such Web-based computing would permit widely dispersed organizations to enter data for their own tracking purposes. In a sense, such a system would be like a grocery store card, which marketers use to follow individual purchases to tailor marketing and which managers use to change orders and track inventory. Using aggregate data, managers and care-givers can assess the entire care system to identify areas needing improvement and can monitor progress as changes to the system are made.

### ★★*Hospice of the Florida Suncoast*

Hospice of the Florida Suncoast, based in Largo, has developed software tailored specifically to track end-of-life care by monitoring clinical and administrative tasks. The Suncoast is currently establishing direct on-line connections for some 850 clinicians—doctors, nurses, social workers, and physical, recreational, and occupational therapists. The system links clinical staff with billing staff, enabling the group to code and submit bills electronically. Employees use the system to submit time records and patient visits.

Three years in the making, the system was built around the ideas and recommendations of senior-level managers, clinicians, field and administrative staff, and end users. Fifteen care teams, each responsible for as many as 100 patients, now use the system to record services provided.

When admitting patients, a team member uses a laptop to key information. Teams report that the presence of the computer does not seem to intimidate or bother patients, especially when staff members explain how the system works and how it can tailor and improve care. Whenever staff members make home visits and enter data, they sit beside the patient or family, who can then see what is being written and ordered. The system is less labor-intensive for clinicians, who can update care plans in approximately seven minutes, far less than the time once required to return to the office and manually update records.

Flexibility is built into the computerized system. For example, its forms can be modified and tailored to each patient's particular needs or case. Clinicians rely on the system to get a patient "snapshot," taking a quick look at key issues such as pain scores and medications. This "snapshot" is especially useful for on-call staff who may not be familiar with specific issues for a patient.

When problems occur, the system prompts the clinician with solutions and flags the record. Clinicians use the system's prompts to define goals, interventions, and outcomes. This information is analyzed to assess how well different interventions work, with which patients, and under which circumstances. This information is then entered into the system so that clinicians can learn from experiences with other patients and can seek "best practices" for particular problems, symptoms, and diseases. The University of Central Florida is in the process of using these data for benchmarking studies.

### ★★VITAS Healthcare

Patients in the hospice system operated by VITAS Healthcare of Miami self-report pain in an automated record-keeping system that clocks visits to patients by physicians, nurses, home health aides, and social workers. Although the computerized system does not replace paper medical records, it does serve as a real-time tool for tracking and changing patient care.

Teams use the Missoula-VITAS Quality of Life Index to track patient-reported information on five dimensions of experience: symptoms, functional status, interpersonal relationships, emotional well-being, and transcendence. A patient might categorize pain at a level 2 or 3; however, the team might notice during the chart review that after the patient is bathed, pain scores jump to a 6. The team would then work with the patient to take additional medication an hour before the visit.

Using the system, staff can respond quickly to patient and family needs. Each team, which includes about 12 employees assigned to 40 to 60 patients, has almost instant access to patient records. Using electronic links to local vendors, staff can quickly order medications, durable medical equipment, and so on. Similarly, when a patient dies, the system faxes vendors to pick up equipment from the patient's home, a process that saves families the burden of making such arrangements.

The computerized system now contains approximately 100,000 records and, at any given time, is tracking almost 5,000 active records. VITAS uses the data to examine severity of illness, admissions and deaths, patient demographics, staff turn-

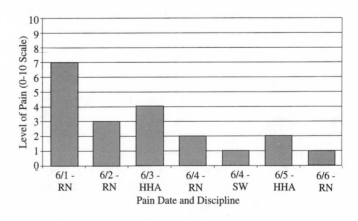

Figure 10.1 Last Pain Reading, John Doe 12345. Reprinted with permission of VITAS Healthcare Corp., Miami, FL.

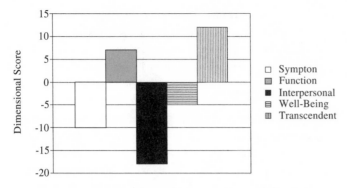

Figure 10.2 Missoula-VITAS Quality of Life Index, One Day Reading, John Doe. Reprinted with permission of VITAS Healthcare Corp., Miami, FL.

over rates, staffing ratios, length of visits and stay, the diagnostic mix of patients in a team, and continuity of care.

The information is reported in easy-to-read charts, shown in Figures 10.1, 10.2, and 10.3, that display patient status and progress.

Employees who visit a patient can either phone in data about the visit (including information for their own time sheets) or enter it via keyboard. Phone-in reports are usually done the day of the visit and can track clinical data such as pain severity. Other reports, such as bereavement visits, are usually entered into the computer within a week of the visit.

### Innovators Need to Know

• Tracking changes through data collection is essential to know whether a change is an improvement.

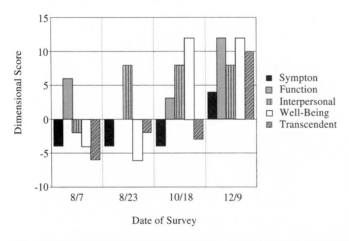

Figure 10.3 Quality of Life Survey, John Doe #012345. Reprinted with permission of VITAS Healthcare Corp., Miami, FL.

- Go beyond information collected for clinical records and use other information systems to track quality improvement: Billings can track emergency room admissions for heart failure patients, for instance, and human resources can determine how many different providers visited a patient in any given month.
- Paper medical records provide a starting point for finding patients to include in interventions and for periodically tallying specific changes.
- Changing the information on existing forms to include new questions—e.g., "Do you have an advance directive in your medical record?"—can be its own innovation.

## Resources

Franklin Health, Inc.
   10 Mountain View Road
   Upper Saddle River, NJ 07458
   Phone: 201-512-7067
   http://www.franklinhealth.com

Hospice Institute of the Florida Suncoast
   300 East Bay Drive
   Largo, FL 33770-3770
   Phone: 727–586-4432
   http://www.hospiceweb.com/states/florida/institut/
   institut.htm

VITAS Healthcare Corp.
   100 South Biscayne Boulevard, Suite 1500
   Miami, FL 33131
   Phone: 305-350-5923
   http://www.vitas.com

# 11

# Caring for Caregivers
## *Helping Staff to Provide Good Care*

Service industries thrive on customer satisfaction. In health care, staff can bring compassion and warmth to each patient encounter—or, through inattention or lack of concern, can compound a patient's stress. In end-of-life care, staffing issues are even more critical than in most other business and health interactions. Whether staff meet a customer's needs ultimately influences how customers—dying patients and their loved ones—experience one of life's most profound transitions.

Good end-of-life care depends on the ability of staff to routinely provide what is, in fact, an intense degree of care.

The needs of dying patients can range from the dramatic to the mundane. Patients may need expert interventions to treat complex symptoms, or families may ask a volunteer to help with grocery shopping. In each instance, and at every point in between, clinicians and administrative and support staff must be able to anticipate patient needs, when possible, and to respond confidently, quickly, and effectively.

Because gravely ill patients have an array of emotions, symptoms, and needs, caregivers must be deeply committed to patient care. Regardless of their professionalism, those who work in end of life encounter emotional challenges—the unpredictability of death, the repeated losses, the interaction with grieving and overwhelmed family members and loved ones. Although their potential for burnout is high, those who work in this field generally first speak of their satisfaction in caring for patients and families.

Never be afraid to try something new. Remember, amateurs built the Ark. Professionals built the Titanic.

—Anonymous

179

## In This Chapter

Resources on personnel abound, so this chapter focuses on a narrow slice of human resources: the special issues faced by organizations whose workers care for the dying. This chapter describes:

- Building and strengthening interdisciplinary teams
- Providing opportunities for career advancement, including cross-training
- Offering bereavement and counseling services for staff

People who work for end-of-life programs, from receptionists to oncologists, are often drawn to the field because of their own experiences with dying friends and family, and are often committed to improving end-of-life care. Most people who work with the dying do so out of a deep love for humanity and a passion for what they do. Their hearts often lead them to the field, and their personalities keep them at it. It is this heartfelt conviction and dedication to improving the status quo that often distinguish people who work with the dying from those who work in other realms of health care.

## Building Interdisciplinary Teams

By its very nature, health care demands that people from different disciplines collaborate on patient care. Good end-of-life care, however, requires more than multidisciplinary care—it requires an interdisciplinary approach in which, while each team member has a defined role, each often takes on other roles too. Team members need to understand their roles within the context of the team and to understand and appreciate colleagues' roles as well.

All team members—professionals, paraprofessionals, and volunteers—need to feel that they are equals and that each can offer ideas and recommendations about how to improve care and routine operations. On Lok Senior Health Services exemplifies this approach in the way it relies on its drivers to observe how patients are doing—if they seem to be stiff or sluggish or if they have trouble moving. Drivers report their observations to the care team, who can then act on the information.

Good teams do not just happen; they happen by design. Members are recruited, screened, reviewed, and observed as they interact with others. Team members need to communicate with each other, review their work together, work out problems and barriers, and share successes and failures. Analogies for teamwork abound in American culture, from professional to intramural sports, from large corporations to community activism. No matter where they perform, teams represent a complex array of relationships, which take energy and time to develop and sustain. Today's environment of rapid change challenges the best of teams to keep up.

End-of-life care relies on several levels of teamwork. Not only must members of the care team work together; so, too, must clinical, administrative, and financial teams. When teams work well, patients benefit because their care plan considers the clinical situation and the use of financial and community resources. As in family systems, when any member of the team is overwhelmed, exhausted, or tuned out, others in the team live with the consequences and may find themselves compensating for one another.

It is important to note, however, that not every patient requires the service of every team member. Some patients may primarily need physician or professional nursing services; others will only want to interact with social workers or chaplains at a particular time. Some families may require extensive support and come to rely on volunteers to help with routine activities such as transportation to medical appointments or grocery shopping; still others will cope with transportation but will look to home health aides for help with laundry and cooking. Health care managers must balance the diversity of needs by having an array of staff—often both paid and volunteer—to meet an array of patient and family needs.

Here are goals to consider when fostering interdisciplinary teams:

- Annual reviews include an evaluation of each team member's professional objectives and obligations.
- Retention rates and employee surveys indicate high levels of job satisfaction.
- Each team member participates in planning for the operating unit or division.
- The majority of team members attend most team meetings.
- Each team meets its quality indicators at least 95 percent of the time.
- Patients and families express satisfaction with the care provided by the team.

### Team-Building Strategies

A team-building focus can pay off in several ways. As individuals become more effective in working with other team members, the team becomes more effective. The team can learn how to examine its own work and progress and identify areas for improvement.

Breakthrough Series faculty member Connie Jastremski recommends that organizations recognize the following trigger points that indicate a need for team building:

- Decreased productivity or effectiveness
- Increased number of complaints about staff or quality of care
- Conflicts among staff members
- Confusion about assignments or unclear roles
- Decisions that are misunderstood or are not carried through properly
- Apathy or lack of interest and involvement among staff members
- Ineffective staff meetings; low participation in group decisions
- Start-up of a new group that needs to develop quickly into a team
- High dependency on or negative reactions to the manager

If a team decides to engage in a team-building process, it should be sure to establish objectives for it, such as:

- Write a mission and purpose statement for the team.
- Establish roles and responsibilities for team members.
- Develop a conflict-management procedure.
- Examine and improve the team's problem-solving strategies.
- Improve the group's communication skills.
- Develop respect, if not actual friendship, among team members.

### Effective Team Meetings

Interdisciplinary team meetings are designed primarily to coordinate the patient's plan of care. They also offer team members an opportunity to talk about particular experiences with patients and families, review ideas and problems, and grieve loses. Team meetings are a primary opportunity to deal with issues of change and growth and to encourage all members to attend and participate.

Many programs encourage all employees involved in a patient's care, including health aides and nursing assistants, to attend team meetings. The structure of each meeting should be consistent and should include enough time to address the status of each patient being reviewed, including ways to meet his or her needs and staff recommendations and responses. Tips for successful team meetings include:

- Getting feedback about what is—or is not—working
- Asking questions such as, "What single thing could we do this week to improve (for example, our communication with the admissions staff)?"
- Listening to ideas and recommendations
- Providing opportunities for leadership
- Acknowledging changes and adaptations the team has made
- Anticipating and projecting next steps
- Whenever possible, laughing and enjoying one another and the opportunities to make a real difference in the lives of patients and families

### Building Morale

In 1997 the Ohio Hospice Organization and Fortman & Associates surveyed 84 member hospices on several topics, including factors that hospice administrators believed contributed most to staff morale. Beyond employee benefits, the most frequently cited factors included:

- Open communication, including "open-door" management
- Highly functioning and cohesive teams of competent and capable staff
- Good communication skills
- High levels of autonomy and self-direction
- Clear definitions of roles and accountability
- Mission focus

The survey also asked, "What has your organization done that has been most helpful in improving or maintaining a high level of morale?" Here are their responses:

- *Recognition*—A focus on recognizing, appreciating, and celebrating individuals and teams. Examples included sending personal notes, celebrating special days (e.g., days or weeks designated for specific disciplines or professions), peer recognition at staff meetings, and celebrations for success (and, at times, just for the sake of celebrating).
- *Support*—Opportunities to share stories. Examples included support groups, birthday luncheons, staff retreats, staff picnic, casual dress days.
- *Communication*—Tracking, displaying, and communicating important statistical and operational data in a snapshot, graphic format. Examples included: town hall meetings, small group task forces, and transition teams.
- *Team building*—A commitment to team participation in goal setting, as well as team-building opportunities and exercises and cross-training.
- *Staff involvement*—Self-directed teams; staff decision-making authority.

### Interdisciplinary Team Training

Clinical and administrative teams need to share a common sense of purpose, framed by their organization's mission and driven by best practices and patient needs. At the same time, a committee cannot provide clinical care. Instead, all team members must have authority to act within the team framework and within professional and regulatory guidelines. Whenever necessary, team members must be able to respond to needs or questions that are not really "in the job description." A social worker may visit a patient and find that he or she is in severe pain. Although the social worker cannot administer medications or increase dosages, he or she can work with the patient and family to contact clinicians, make the patient comfortable, and stay until the crisis has been resolved. Just knowing what is likely to be done puts the social worker in a good position to increase the family's confidence and to get problems solved effectively. Similarly, physicians may need to know the basics about community services, such as Meals-on-Wheels, and be able to give families this information when necessary. When physicians demonstrate real understanding of a community, patients and families tend to feel that professional caregivers are truly concerned for their well-being and comfort, beyond what basic medicine requires.

Groups can take many approaches to cross-training. For instance, during orientation periods, new staff can be introduced to key personnel who can explain their work and its significance to the patient's care. Staff may "shadow" one another for half a day to learn more about hands-on work. Key personnel can hold occasional brown-bag lunches during which they discuss advances in the field, emerging trends in patient care, or systemwide improvements in information systems. By attending team meetings, all staff have an opportunity to learn about each other's work, to ask questions, and to gather information.

The Breakthrough Series has revealed several effective orientation and training programs. Among them, the Palliative Care Center of the North Shore focuses on training members of its interdisciplinary teams on how to provide patient- and family-centered care. All team members are required to understand key elements of end-of-life care, such as pain and symptom assessment and management, family dynamics, pastoral care, and psychosocial concerns. Once new employees have completed orientation and are ready to be in the field, they accompany more experienced staff members on patient visits. This process usually begins during the first week of work.

In Massachusetts, Fallon Healthcare System, the University of Massachusetts, and the Harvard Geriatric Education Center have developed a program to train residents and nurses to provide interdisciplinary care of the elderly in community settings. The month-long program includes day-long sessions in which residents and nurses spend mornings attending team meetings, participating in quality improvement activities, evaluating resource utilization, and participating in ethics committee meetings. Afternoon sessions are spent participating in long-

Table 11.1 Staff Training Modules

| Module 1 | Module 2 | Module 3 |
|---|---|---|
| Introduction | Communication and collaborative problem solving | The PACE model of care |
| Why teams? | Group process and team facilitation | Roles of team members |
| Team definitions | Conflicts and resolution | Individual discipline vs. team problems/goals |
| Factors affecting team development and function | Styles of dealing with conflict | Resource allocation and risk management |
| Development phases of interdisciplinary teams | Avoidance | |
| Types of leadership roles | | |

Reprinted with permission of On Lok Senior Health Services, San Francisco, CA.

term care and rehabilitation medicine, either during home visits or at the day health centers. Through this process, students learn about administrative aspects of care, participate in patient care in a variety of settings, observe social worker and physical therapist assessments, and make home visits.

In California, On Lok Senior Health Services provides a half-day orientation to all new employees on the role of interdisciplinary teams. Physicians, nurse practitioners, home care and clinic nurses, physical therapists, social workers, occupational therapists, recreation therapists, dietitians, and intake staff participate. The On Lok program features three modules, each lasting approximately 90 minutes.

## Career Advancement and Continuing Education

Professionals interested in advancing their careers can usually pursue specific steps or procedures to do so. But for others involved in health care, progress may not be so clear. To some employees, it may seem that their positions offer no room for advancement or improvement.

In an age of nursing shortages and high turnover rates for paraprofessional staff, administrators must come up with ways to help employees to find satisfaction with their current positions while pursuing opportunities for advancement. One way to do this is to offer employees ongoing training and education programs. Some organizations have improved retention of certified nursing assistants (CNAs) by offering classes and programs to enhance professional caregiving skills. Skilled and competent CNAs are encouraged to return to school to further their education and reach their own potential. With support and encouragement, paraprofessionals can also advance in allied health professions, such as administration, grief counseling, emergency medical services, and chaplaincy.

### ★Calvary Hospital

At New York City's Calvary Hospital, a 38-year-old program trains and certifies individuals to become Cancer Care Technicians (CCT), paraprofessionals who assist nurses in meeting the needs of cancer patients and their families. After one year in the hospital, nurse's aides are eligible to participate in the CCT training program, which includes studying the physiological, psychosocial, environmental, and spiritual needs of cancer patients. In addition to being competent in these areas, CCTs must be able to work well with others, have sound judgment, demonstrate initiative, and use good communication skills. There are four levels of CCT paraprofessionals, which creates room for advancement. The program encourages participants to pursue professional nursing education.

According to the program's director, the CCTs help relieve patient and family suffering while affording nurses more time to perform tasks only they can provide. In their work, CCTs follow nursing guidelines to manage problems such as skin breakdown, malnutrition, impaired coping, safety risks, and bleeding precautions. CCTs participate in ongoing training through lectures and skill-building workshops sponsored by nurses, physicians, and others from the interdisciplinary team, including pastoral care.

For those interested in developing similar programs, Calvary offers a "Train the Trainer" program for other hospital educators. (For information on contacting Calvary, see the Resources section on page 327 at the end of this chapter.)

## Offer Employee Counseling and Education about Death and Dying

People who work in end-of-life care face experiences most other workers do not: Answering services receive late-night calls from families in crisis; nursing home receptionists answer calls from people who may not yet know that a loved one has died; data entry clerks key information about a patient's death. In each instance, the staff person faces, however briefly, a sense of loss.

Organizations whose staff work with seriously ill and dying patients must attend to the bereavement needs of staff, from direct care workers to medical records clerks. Teams can help staff by providing opportunities for them to reflect on their own beliefs and feelings about death and dying. Shared memorial services and sharing family expressions of gratitude also help.

As part of its new employee orientation program, the Palliative Care Center of the North Shore offers a session titled "Personal Death Awareness." After completing a written exercise (an adapted version of which appears below), staff members meet in small groups to exchange thoughts and ideas. The program is designed to help employees understand and clarify their own ideas about the meaning of death and dying. Such awareness can promote empathy for patients and families and enable employees to be more effective in their work with dying patients.

### Personal Death Awareness Exercises

The following exercises are intended to help you learn more about yourself and your feelings and beliefs about death and dying. The notes you make on these pages are for you alone, and you need not share them with others.

Set aside a quiet time and place to reflect on these exercises. Allow yourself to be reflective. You may need two or three hours to complete these exercises.

**Exercise 1:** Draw a straight line of any length with a beginning and an end. Consider this line to be your total life span. Place a slash mark at any point along the line where you think you are today in your life's chronology.

Complete the following fill-in-the-blanks statements:

I expect to live until age _____.

I am now _____.

When you compare your present age to the age at which you expect to die, how much of your life do you find you have already lived? Half? Two-thirds? One-quarter? Now look at the line you drew. How does your estimate of the time you have left to live on the life-span line compare to your numerical estimate? ➡

Personal Death
Awareness Exercises
(*Continued*)

How did it feel to commit
yourself to a definite life
span? Some people worry
that they may "jinx"
themselves by doing this. Old
superstitions rise up and
haunt them. Does this
concern you? Were you
uncomfortable? If not, why
do you think you felt
comfortable doing this? Take
a minute and answer these
two questions.

**Exercise 2:** The first death
that I experienced was the
death of:

I was _____ years old.
At that time, I felt:
I was most curious about:
The things that frightened
me most were:
The feelings that I have
now as I remember that
death are:
The most intriguing thing
about the funeral was:
I was most scared at the
funeral by:

➡

Some programs hold occasional memorial services during
which staff members can remember and acknowledge the lives
of patients who have been in their care. In some communities,
staff use this time to remember and honor their own loved
ones who have died.

Other organizations offer grief and bereavement counseling
to staff members; larger organizations may have half- or full-
time staff dedicated to this position. In some cases, staff are
referred to counselors and mental health professionals to work
through personal issues.

Administrators need to be tuned in to how staff are doing
and how they are coping with patient deaths or family needs.
In some cases, administrators may notice a "red flag" that a
problem is developing. One administrator explained that if a
troubled family repeatedly calls on only one clinician to respond
to its questions, or if a staff member becomes extremely
attached to a patient, administrators will ask that the staff social
worker speak to the employee. Professional boundaries offer
some protection from exhaustion and burnout. Boundaries are
often hard to maintain, and they still offer only partial protection. People working with very sick patients and families usually
need some counseling from time to time.

Professionals and staff working in end of life need time and
opportunity to recognize their own humanity, to consider their
own mortality, and to integrate—and separate—their personal
and professional lives.

### Innovators Need to Know

Observing and experiencing an interdisciplinary team as it cares
for a dying patient and supports a grieving family is like watch-
ing an orchestra prepare for and then perform a symphony.
The conductor knows how each bar of music should be played
and how it should sound, but the individual musicians only
focus on their own section, with the conductor's direction.
They rehearse intensely and persist toward perfection. In the
end, the audience enjoys a beautifully played symphony. The
audience is not aware of, and probably doesn't care about, the
chaos, exhaustion, and frustration experienced by musicians
working under deadlines and striving for perfection.

Like musicians, members of the interdisciplinary team must
focus on their role in caring for individual patients. At the same
time, however, they must have a conductor's sense of how the
final piece should sound. Unlike in an orchestra, however, in

palliative care, members may be asked to "change instruments" at any time—even in the midst of a performance.

- Interdisciplinary teams provide the framework for excellent end-of-life care.
- Good teams do not just happen—they happen through time, training, and commitment.
- Team meetings provide a forum for staff to discuss patient issues and to address concerns about the organization or team itself.
- Team-building strategies are a way to reinforce the team's mission and goals.
- Paraprofessional staff benefit from ongoing training and opportunities to participate in in-service training programs.
- All staff members face issues of grief, bereavement, and loss and need time to reflect or grieve when patients die.

## Resources

Calvary Hospital
  Patricia Terrell, RN, MPH
  1740 Eastchester Road
  Bronx, NY 10461
  Phone: 718-518-2244
  http://www.calvaryhospital.org

*A Kick in the Seat of the Pants*, by Roger von Oech. New York: Harper & Row, 1986.

*Managing Transitions: Making the Most of Change*, by William Bridges. Reading, MA: Addison-Wesley, 1991.

*Personal Coaching for Results: How to Mentor and Inspire Others to Amazing Growth*, by Lou Tice. Nashville: Thomas Nelson, 1997.

*Playing Along: 37 Group Learning Activities Borrowed from Improvisational Theater*, by Izzy Gessell. Duluth, MN: Whole Person Associates, 1997.

*The Team Handbook: How to Use Teams to Improve Quality*, by Joiner Associates, Inc., Madison, WI. To order call 800-669-8326.

---

Personal Death
Awareness Exercises
(*Continued*)

---

The first personal acquaintance of my own age who died was:

---

I remember thinking:
The death of _____
has been the most significant for me. It was significant because:
The most recent death I experienced was
when _____
died _____ years ago.
The most traumatic death I ever experienced was:
At age _____, I personally came close to death when:

**Exercise 3:** Do you view death as a beginning or an end? Do you mourn or celebrate death or do both? Do you have tradition and ritual to serve you in the dying process? Are feelings about death universal or are they unique to individuals and cultures?

Adapted with permission of the Palliative Care Center of the North Shore, Evanston, Illinois

# Using Law and Policy to Improve End-of-Life Care

**12**

Dr. S is the coroner and family practitioner in Sleepy Town, USA. In most years, one dead body is pulled out of the river that flows past town; Dr. S has to declare death and do an autopsy. This year things are different: So far, 14 dead bodies have been hauled out of the river. Dr. S finally decides to look into what's happening, even though it's not really his job. At some point, he realizes, he has to redefine his job. He has to go upriver and figure out what is going on.

> Any change is resisted because bureaucrats have a vested interest in the chaos in which they exist.
>
> —Richard M. Nixon

Like Dr. S, innovators aiming to improve their systems may need to go upriver. It is not always enough to focus on improving existing systems, since internal change alone cannot change external forces, such as Medicare reimbursement schemes or public policy. Even though it may not be part of the usual job description for health care workers, they may want to step back and think about the laws, regulations, financing mechanisms, and cultural barriers that block excellent care at the end of life. This chapter aims to direct these advocates to "go upriver" and define and address barriers to good care.

Health care is frequently the subject of federal and state legislation, which govern aspects of prenatal care, abortion rights, emergency services, and experimental treatments. End-of-life health care, however, has rarely been the direct focus of any federal or state regulations, other than laws governing patients' decision-making authority. There are no standards, for instance, governing how end-of-life care is provided to Medicaid and Medicare beneficiaries. There are no laws requiring that health care organizations collect and submit data about the circumstances in which patients die—even though most of those deaths are paid for with federal funds. There are not even national outcome standards surrounding Medicare-certified

## Important Legal Actions on End-of-Life Care

- 1976: *Quinlan v. New Jersey*: The U.S. Supreme Court allowed the parents of young woman in a persistent vegetative state to remove her from a life-sustaining ventilator. The Court authorized removal on the basis of a right to privacy.

- 1983: Medicare Hospice Benefit: Medicare began providing reimbursement for hospice programs caring for the terminally ill.

- 1986: *Bouvia v. Superior Court*: The California Court of Appeals found that a 27-year-old competent woman with severe cerebral palsy had the right to forgo life-sustaining treatment.

- 1990: *Cruzan v. Director, Missouri Department of Health*: The U.S. Supreme Court decided that states are free to adopt evidentiary standards to indicate when a family member can make end-of-life decisions for one unable to do so. Five justices recognized a constitutional right of competent people to refuse life-sustaining treatment.

➡

hospice care, although some efforts toward this end are now under way.

Influencing policy and legislation at all levels of government can be part of quality improvement in end-of-life care. Laws often arise in response to increased public scrutiny or demand, as has been the case with physician-assisted suicide. Unfortunately, this issue has detracted from the attention that should be focused on other equally compelling and difficult end-of-life issues, such as adequate pain relief or changes in federal laws that regulate how opioids are prescribed.

Teams that work to push these and other issues into the public arena and onto the political agenda can create improvement through changes in our social and cultural views of death and dying.

### In This Chapter

Innovators face challenges created by current law and policy. This chapter provides a brief history of legal actions in end-of-life care, then offers specific advice on areas for change, along with examples of successful programs and initiatives. Topics include:

- Changing misconceptions about how people with severe and chronic live and eventually die
- Eliminating legal barriers to prescribing pain medications
- Advocating for public investment in health services and basic research on end-of-life issues
- Pushing for a more appropriate health care service mix to correct patterns of resource availability

### Change Assumptions and Boost Expectations about the End of Life

Despite the advances in increased life expectancy, we have not paid much attention to aging, living with serious illness, or dying. Just talking about dying remains a social and medical taboo. The emphasis on medical prowess has created an expectation that medicine can prolong life almost indefinitely. Patients and health care providers alike expect the end of life, when it comes, to be a predictable period, one that brings increasing disability, misery, and suffering and little redeeming merit.

Cultural expectations that the dying must suffer mean that few families threaten to take legal action when terrible suffering does occur; physicians have little fear of sanctions; and few groups lobby for change.

## Some Suggestions for Changing the Current Situation

1. Advocate for regional and federal health care report cards that include end-of-life issues.

Many public and private organizations are setting standards for health care provided in managed care settings so that employers and the elderly can select the best plans. The National Committee for Quality Assurance (NCQA), the voluntary association for quality in managed care plans, has a set of quality measures it calls HEDIS (Health Plan Employer Data Information Set). In the most recent version, HEDIS 3.0, NCQA was interested in including quality measures focused on the end of life. However, none were found to have been used enough to ensure a definite link between health care providers' behaviors and better quality.

The Foundation for Accountability (FACCT), which aims to help large purchasers of health care, including Medicare, to purchase high-quality care, has named end-of-life care as one of its priority areas for development. FACCT gathers data to communicate a wide range of information about quality to consumers and to create condition-specific quality reports.

Some state and federal agencies have developed consumer report cards for different kinds of medical care, such as mental health care; others have created consumer report cards to rate managed care firms operating in their states. Benefits managers, employers, and health care consumers can push to add end-of-life issues, such as pain and symptom management, to these report cards.

2. Push for laws that address genuine choice at the end of life, rather than the appearance of choice.

The focus on physician-assisted suicide, which could offer patients only the "choice" of either suffering terribly until they die or causing their own death, has stifled debate around real

---

Important Legal Actions
on End-of-Life Care
(*Continued*)

- 1991: Patient Self-Determination Act (PSDA): This federal measure mandated that health care institutions receiving Medicare or Medicaid funding give patients written information about their right to participate in medical decision making and write advance directives.

- 1997: *Washington v. Glucksberg, Vacco v. Quill*: The U.S. Supreme Court found, in two unanimous decisions, that there is no constitutional right to assisted suicide. The Court indicated that the issue is one that state legislatures should determine. Several justices' opinions can be read as having established that Americans have a right to palliative care.

- 1997: Physician-assisted suicide: Oregonians reaffirmed legalization of assisted suicide through a second voter referendum, making Oregon the first state in the country where the practice is legal.

---

choices—such as where to die, which medications to receive, and how to access appropriate services.

**3.** Expand content of advance directives.

Many state advance directive forms are limited to clear-cut decisions, with no room for the uncertain times that accompany the end of life. Most forms do not, for instance, include blanks for people to say that they would be willing to undergo a trial on a ventilator for a week before having it removed. Directives can be expanded to include more information and more choices that reflect the continuum of serious and eventually fatal illness. (Chapter 5 details ways to improve advance care planning.)

**4.** Fund public forums, newsletters, and hearings about end-of-life issues.

Your organization can organize public forums—town meetings—where individuals can gather to talk about end-of-life issues. Approach local chapters of disease organizations, such as the American Cancer Society or the American Heart Association, and ask to be included on the agenda for their next meeting. Talk to local business organizations, such as chambers of commerce or voluntary groups, and get on their agendas. Team members or representatives can approach their state legislature to request a public hearing on the state of end-of-life care in the community. The possibilities are there—and increased public interest in the subject is likely to generate some turnout.

**5.** Work with state end-of-life commissions.

By early 1998, at least 30 states had established commissions or task forces to examine end-of-life care issues. Attorneys general, governors, private organizations, the medical community, and individuals spurred the formation of many of these panels. In at least six states—California, Colorado, Illinois, New Jersey, Tennessee, and Virginia—law or legislative resolutions mandated that panels be created. These groups are charged with assessing historical and current practices, educating health care professionals and consumers, examining the effect of law on end-of-life care, providing resources, and piloting new programs, among other activities. A list of sites that have received grants from the Community-State Partnerships to Improve End-of-Life to establish such bodies can be found at the Web address http://www.mid.bio.org/npo-map2.htm.

6. Talk to the media about improvement
   efforts under way—or problems in end-of-
   life care in the community.

The media is receptive to stories about organizations that have improved care of the dying, especially when stories include ways that patients' lives were changed. Doing a good job of caring for society's most vulnerable people makes for good press and publicity. Members of the community—many of whom fear dying in pain—will be relieved to hear that a local organization is doing more to care well for the dying and to make good care the norm.

## ★★U.S. Department of Veterans Affairs

The VA is the largest integrated health care system in America. In recent years, the VA has focused on the needs of aging and seriously ill veterans and has implemented a networkwide performance standard that targets two high-priority areas for improving end-of-life care: advance care planning and pain management. Patients who have severe diseases, such as congestive heart failure and chronic obstructive pulmonary disease (COPD), are included. Hospitals can meet the standards in two ways: by referring patients to hospice care and by documenting specific services for patients, ranging from advance care planning to pain management. Performance evaluation looks at a center's progress toward the standard.

With its national advance care planning project, the VA is aiming to have advance care plans in place for 95 percent of its seriously ill patients. When the project began, about half of these patients had such plans. After three months of an intensive effort to increase patient-provider communication about pain management, advance directives, and other end-of-life issues, almost 70 percent of the most severely ill patients had made advance care plans.

The VA is also turning its attention to improving pain management with a project called "Pain as a Fifth Vital Sign" to ensure that all of its health care sites make pain assessment as routine as taking a patient's blood pressure or temperature. Coordinated by a multidisciplinary team representing various health care fields, the program features increased education for patients and providers, along with better documentation of pain assessment and treatment. Clinicians will learn how to interpret and respond to patient reports of severe pain; patients and families will learn the importance of talking to providers about pain; and the health care system will track pain scores in patients' medical records. The VA has earmarked more than $3 million for staff training and pain management research.

The VA has been a leader in improving care of the dying: In 1991, it issued an official policy that all veterans needing and choosing hospice care would be provided with such care, either through the VA or through referrals to community hospice resources. In the years since, the VA has mandated that each of its medical centers establish a hospice program according to its needs and resources.

### ★Minnesota's Revised Advance Care Planning Forms

Minnesota's Health Care Directive law streamlines and strengthens the use and application of health care directives statewide. The new law replaced legislation guiding the use of living wills and durable power of attorney for health care forms. It clarifies all presumptions: that the health care directive is presumed to reflect the patient's wishes, that it is properly executed, that the patient was competent when the directive was written, and that the directive is legally sufficient unless there is clear evidence to the contrary.

### ★Illinois Coalition for Improving End-of-Life Care

Beth Walston, RN, PhD, began a campaign to empower lay-people in Illinois to have the ability to make informed choices about their dying and to educate and inform the public about the choices available to dying patients and their families. In February 1997, she submitted draft legislation to Illinois state senators; in May 1997, Senate Resolution No. 76 was passed, creating a task force to study end-of-life issues. In December, a group of health care professionals and interested citizens formed the Illinois Coalition for Improving End-of-Life Care to promote awareness. The coalition has sought and received community and foundation support. By 1998, the group had grown to include interest groups from around the state and had begun to network with others around the country.

### Eliminate Legal Barriers to Prescribing Pain Medications

Legal and ethical concerns persist about providing adequate doses of opioids for pain and other symptom relief. Myths about the potential to create addicts among terminally ill patients or about the risk of hastening or causing death with overdoses of opioids are hard to overcome.

Doctors who practice state-of-the-art pain management, including prescribing relatively large doses of opioids for dying patients, too often feel threatened by investigation, trial, loss of license, and even criminal penalties if state medical examiners boards or the Drug Enforcement Administration (DEA) claim inappropriate or excessive use and prescription of opioids. Prescribing laws that require strict tracking and reporting of controlled substance use compound these problems.

In fact, research shows that the incidence of addiction in cancer patients treated with opioids is extremely small. Although physical dependency occurs with opioid treatment, it does not lead to any adverse behaviors.

Drugs such as morphine and other opioids used in pain relief are often thought to hasten death, despite a lack of evidence to support that assumption. Because of this fear, some doctors are concerned that use of effective drugs will be seen as having engaged in active euthanasia (i.e., actively killing a patient via lethal injection). (More on this topic is found in chapters 3 and 4.)

Since 1998, Congress has been considering legislation that would have allowed the DEA to determine whether high doses of controlled substances had been used with the intent to hasten death, rather than just an intent to relieve pain. Adding such a threat to physician practice would have hindered effective pain management even further.

The discussion of this proposed law indicated shortcomings in what many policymakers know about pain management and relief: Like many people, they misunderstood the role of opioid analgesics in pain relief. In 1999, new legislation designed to focus on improving pain management was introduced, along with legislation to promote more research into end-of-life issues, increased public access to information, and greater federal attention to the issue.

Legislative efforts are few and have largely focused on pain, ignoring other symptoms that cause the dying to suffer needlessly. Although pain is often cited in surveys about fears of dying, other symptoms can also be quite distressing. Many people may suffer from other symptoms, such as dyspnea, weakness and fatigue, nausea, mouth and skin problems, and depression and anxiety, for long periods during the course of their illness. These symptoms can go on for months or years, not only in the final days or weeks of life. Like pain, these symptoms may be ignored, and they have not been subject to legislative or policy efforts at improving care. And, like pain, many of these symptoms can be relieved, especially if health care providers understand how common—and treatable—they are.

### Some Ideas Innovators Can Try

1. Push for medical school and continuing medical education classes that concentrate on pain and other symptom relief as a distinct and important part of end-of-life care.

A 1993 study by the Eastern Cooperative Oncology Group assessed physicians' attitudes and knowledge about pain control and found that pain assessments were rare in clinic visits and that education on pain management was substandard. Only when new and practicing doctors know that symptom relief is an essential part of practice will patients benefit from current knowledge.

The American Medical Association developed the Education for Physicians on End-of-Life Care (EPEC) project to ensure that practicing physicians have the knowledge and skills to provide the best possible care to dying patients. The curriculum covers key competencies for all doctors, including fundamental skills for palliative care, ethical decision making, symptom management, communication, and psychosocial aspects of care at the end of life. Each meeting lasts for two and a half days and features didactic and interactive learning opportunities. The project aims to educate 250 physician-educators who can then go on to train others and adapt the curriculum to their specific needs.

2. Advocate for federal research that focuses on the aggressive treatment of pain and other symptoms commonly experienced by dying patients.

Many agencies within the Department of Health and Human Services conduct basic and health services research on serious and life-limiting diseases, yet almost none conduct research on how these diseases affect the end of life and how pain and suffering can be relieved.

3. Track and educate physicians who underprescribe pain medication.

Physicians who routinely care for dying patients—such as on-cologists, geriatricians, and internists—can be expected to prescribe some level of opioids. Those who prescribe insufficient amounts, based on the number of dying patients treated, or prescribe inappropriate drugs or dosages could be sent reeducation materials by state medical boards.

4. Eliminate duplicate and triplicate
   prescription forms.

States with duplicate or triplicate prescribing forms for controlled substances should eliminate these forms. Some states, including New York, have recently done so. Studies have shown that when such prescription systems are instituted, the prescribing of Schedule II opioids decreases, while the use of less heavily regulated (and less effective) analgesics increases.

In 1998, New York's governor signed a bill eliminating the requirement for triplicate prescription forms for narcotic pain relievers. Sponsors of the measure expressed hope that the new bill would prompt New York doctors to prescribe pain medication more often for seriously ill patients. The law also changed definitions of "addict" and "habitual user" so that doctors will no longer have to report patients who are legitimately taking controlled substances to the State Department of Health.

5. Develop electronic monitoring forms for
   opioid prescriptions.

Some states now use electronic systems to monitor controlled substance prescriptions. With this monitoring, states can readily detect when high volumes of prescriptions have been given for extended periods. The Wisconsin legislature, for instance, created an "interagency diversion prevention and control program" to coordinate the work of state and federal agencies in using existing information and resources to address and identify the sources of drug diversion. More recently, several states, including Massachusetts, Oklahoma, and Nevada, have developed electronic prescription monitoring programs, known as electronic data transfer (EDT) programs. California is testing such a program as a possible replacement for its triplicate prescription program, the oldest of its type in the country. States are studying the effect of EDT programs on drug diversion and on legitimate prescribing for pain and other symptoms.

6. Reduce malpractice premiums for physicians
   who take additional courses.

This was a step taken by Copic, a medical liability company that covers 75 percent of Colorado's physicians: Throughout the state, Copic offers one-and-a-half-hour courses on pain management. Doctors who complete the course earn one of five points needed to receive a discount in their malpractice premiums. The course was developed in response to legislative activity surrounding physician-assisted suicide, which led to many reports of untreated pain among dying patients. Among the course's goals are to reduce suffering and to increase health care professionals' ability to recognize and refer patients to pain specialists and to increase their knowledge of pain assessment, pain medications, and auxiliary pain management methods.

## ★Advocate for Health Services and Basic Research on End-of-Life Issues

Many federal agencies, primarily the National Institutes of Health (NIH), the Agency for Healthcare Research and Quality (AHRQ), and the Health Care Financing Administration (HCFA), influence health care delivery, either by directing state-of-the-art treatment and research or by funding services. These organizations can be pushed to use resources to fund new research on relieving symptoms at the end of life, developing guidelines, and monitoring effectiveness. Health care services research can provide educational resources and revised approaches to health care delivery. Studies that determine how differences in costs and outcomes are related to problems in clinical care can point to directions for improving care.

The Institute of Medicine report *Approaching Death* suggests many avenues for study. Its recommendations can serve as a guide to those interested in conducting research or in advocating for increased research funding:

1. People with advanced, potentially fatal illnesses and those close to them should be able to expect and receive reliable, skillful, and supportive care.

2. Physicians, nurses, social workers, and other health professionals must commit themselves to improving care for dying patients and to using existing knowledge effectively to prevent and relieve pain and other symptoms.

3. Because many problems in care stem from system problems, policymakers, consumer groups, and purchasers of health care should work with health care practitioners, organizations, and researchers to:

a. Strengthen methods for measuring the quality of life and other outcomes of care for dying patients and those close to them

b. Develop better tools and strategies for improving the quality of care and holding health care organizations accountable for care at the end of life

c. Revise mechanisms for financing care so that they encourage rather than impede good end-of-life care and sustain rather than frustrate coordinated systems of excellent care

d. Reform drug prescription laws, burdensome regulations, and state medical board policies and practices that impede effective use of opioids to relieve pain and suffering

4. Educators and other health care professionals should initiate changes in undergraduate, graduate, and continuing education to ensure that practitioners have the appropriate attitudes, knowledge, and skills to care well for dying patients.

5. Palliative care should become, if not a medical specialty, at least a defined area of expertise, education, and research.

6. The nation's research establishment should define and implement priorities for strengthening the knowledge base for end-of-life care.

7. A continuing public discussion is essential to develop a better understanding of the modern experience of dying, the options available to patients and families, and the obligations of communities to those approaching death.

## ★Create a More Appropriate Service Mix to Correct Patterns of Resource Availability

Various factors affect the availability of good end-of-life care. Even basic demographic issues can have a drastic effect on how and where people die. According to the *Dartmouth Atlas of Health Care* (1998), produced by researchers at Dartmouth Medical School and the American Hospital Association, people in some areas of the country tend to die mostly in hospitals, while in other areas they are more likely to die at home. In some regions, half of all Medicare beneficiaries who died were in hospitals, while in other regions that rate was only 20 percent.

What makes this statistic so important? In a local health care system that has a relative oversupply of hospital beds, there will not be much of a system—or incentive—to get doctors to visit nursing homes or private residences; the community will expect that people die in the hospital. On the other hand, circumstances will force a system in which there are few hospital beds to develop more efficient home care, more ways to support very sick patients and their families at home, and strategies that often lower health care costs—while risking underservice at home.

Further, neither managed care nor fee-for-service structures include appropriate financial incentives to parallel the services that most people facing the end of life need. The Institute of Medicine report describes the problems people with chronic or progressive illnesses face in managed care. For instance, the composition of provider networks and other practitioners reflects the needs of the entire enrolled population and is not likely to reflect the diverse health care needs of people with chronic illnesses. Current capitated payment systems encourage enrolling low-risk people—plans do not want to enroll high-cost, chronically ill people. Fee-for-service plans are not a real match for this patient population, either, given the variety of needs—and the need for comprehensive, coordinated care—over extended periods.

### Initiatives That Would Support Suggestions for Improvement

1. Reform the structure of current reimbursement rates, thus appropriating funds to improve health care for those who need multiple services in their final weeks.

It is not uncommon for people to die with multiple diseases and costly health care needs. Reimbursement mechanisms need to be altered to allow for this scope of services at the end of life and allow providers to tailor care to the needs of each patient.

2. Promote structures that value continuity and reduce incentives to treat episodically.

This change needs to come not only from individual providers but from the entire health care system. Our focus needs to change quite dramatically. Physicians who treat a patient from the onset of chronic illness should follow up and continue to be involved even after the patient has been referred to hospice, for example. Instead of bouncing patients from hospital to nursing home to home care—with a different health care provider in each setting—patients should be attended by a team that understands the patient's overall needs. Such continuous care requires a different approach and changes in medical education, physician practice, and consumer demand and expectation.

**3.** Pay for continuity.

To accomplish continuity of care, the health care financing system must also change direction. Insurers need to create incentives to promote continuous, flexible end-of-life care. For instance, Medicaid could give providers incentives based on avoiding disruptive transfers to and from nursing homes.

**4.** Revise the hospice benefit.

The way the Medicare hospice benefit is written and interpreted allows for too much variation based on facility and geographic region. The various fiscal intermediaries that enact eligibility guidelines vary in their flexibility and allowance for provider subjectivity. No matter how rates are set, it is advantageous for the hospice to choose the lower-cost patients. The narrowly interpreted language of the Medicare hospice benefit, "six months or fewer to live," has resulted in median lengths of stay of less than 30 days in many programs. Various strategies could expand and regularize eligibility and service mix.

**5.** Provide palliative care services
   in many settings.

End-of-life care is most prominently available through and funded for in hospice programs. Hospice includes a range of medical and social services with some emphasis on palliative care. Hospice programs may operate or contract for inpatient services and may even run their own freestanding inpatient facilities.

However, most hospice care is provided in the patient's home. Indeed, most hospices require that patients have a home and a caregiver available to provide assistance. These restrictions limit hospice availability for many people, including those who have no family and those who do not have a home in which hospice services can be provided.

Many hospitals now offer palliative care services, aimed at treating symptoms and reducing suffering. These programs do not have the kinds of restrictions posed by hospice services and are able to meet the needs of more diverse populations, including those whose diseases are not swift killers, those who do not have caregivers, and those whose prognosis goes beyond the six-month hospice rule.

**6.** Establish standards for end-of-life care in
   nursing homes.

Nursing homes and other long-term care facilities need to assure that plans are in place for most expectable emergencies.

Further, nursing homes should have in place both transfer practices and review processes to determine whether such moves cause patients and/or families unnecessary distress. All staff should be trained to communicate with patients and families about change in status or preferences for "do not resuscitate" orders. Patient dignity should be emphasized as well.

7. Promote grassroots and
   community-based programs.

Many organizations become involved in state- and community-wide programs to increase awareness of end-of-life issues, encourage communication among various health care organizations, and achieve some economies of scale.

•Albemarle Home Health and Hospice, which spans 12 counties in rural North Carolina, is establishing a statewide demonstration through the state's office of rural health. The program would create a single point of entry for patients with life-limiting diseases. Albemarle presented information about end-of-life issues to the annual meeting of North Carolina's public health association, trying to expand the base of organizations that see a role for themselves in this field. Albemarle Home Care is also working to develop a North Carolina Collaborative to Improve End-of-Life Care, in conjunction with medical schools, health care organizations, and others throughout the state. According to Director Kay Cherry, the keys to success in such endeavors are "persistence, passion, and patience."

•The Minnesota Partnership to Improve End-of-Life Care is being developed by three large health care systems: Allina Health Systems, Health Partners, and Fairview Systems. Together, the three systems cover 85 percent of Minnesotans. According to participants, Minnesota has a history of organizations collaborating to improve public health. The partnership is strengthened by the involvement of physicians and executives who champion end-of-life care.

The three have managed to overcome some potential barriers to collaboration, including concerns about recognition, payment and cost issues, oversight and audit, governance of the collaborative, and the need to have a common focus for effort. The group resolved finance and oversight issues by enlisting the Area Agency on Aging to be its fiscal agent. The coalition's board of directors will include two representatives from each partner and the fiscal agent.

Each partner is finding that it learns from others involved in the process. Ultimately, the group plans to bring end-of-life policy issues to public attention and to develop public education campaigns around improving end-of-life care.

• The New Hampshire Collaborative on End-of-Life Care is an organization of almost 70 individuals seeking to bridge the gaps between organizations involved in end-of-life care. It was created as the result of a 1997 survey that asked 2,500 health care professionals and other community members what they would do to improve end-of-life care. Over a six-month period, the group has undertaken 16 different improvement projects, focusing on issues such as improved advance care planning; increased awareness of cultural issues; improved communication among health care providers, patients, and families; improved service delivery to rural patients; and increased use of existing hospice and palliative care programs.

## Innovators Need to Know

What is easy and routine is what happens. Making improvements in just one local health care system can be a daunting task. However, together we can press for major policy change.

- Dying is, for the most part, publicly funded, and programs serving dying patients need to be accountable for the services they provide—or fail to provide.
- Political, economic and social forces affect the way end-of-life health care is provided. Individuals can work to make these forces more positive, based in the reality of end-of-life, not the myth or the stereotype.
- Innovators can push for change in their own communities—and at the state and federal level.
- There are many Web sites where advocates can exchange ideas and innovations.

## "The Agitator's Guide"

To keep efforts in perspective and to give you some thoughts on what you can do today, "The Agitator's Guide: Twelve Steps to Get Your Community Talking about Dying" by Americans for Better Care of the Dying is reprinted here.

1. Call your local paper's obituary writer. Ask him or her to say something about how a person lived during the last years or months—what did he or she do? What did the family do?

Summary of Recommendations from the National Task Force on End-of-Life in Managed Care (*continued*)

*Improve Access*
9. Reach out to patients and families as partners in end-of-life care.

*Develop and Evaluate Payment Methods*
10. Test new methods for aligning financial incentives with the provision of humane and effective care.
11. Ensure access by developing risk-adjustment strategies or other payment methods that properly compensate managed care providers and plans for the costs of caring for patients near the end of life.
12. Develop and study the effects of alternative reimbursement methods capable of enhancing coordination between managed care organizations and hospice programs.

Source: *Meeting the Challenge: Twelve Recommendations for Improving End-of-Life Care in Managed Care*

2. Write a letter to your U.S. representatives and senators. Urge them to have the Health Care Financing Administration sponsor demonstration programs in end-of-life care.

3. Call or write your local chamber of commerce. And talk to your employer, too, about ways to support family caregivers and protect their jobs during leave.

4. Talk to local churches or civic and volunteer groups. Together you can support those who are dying and their families through visits, transportation, meals, and even prayer groups.

5. Write letters to your local media. When articles or programs run about aging or death and dying, note your appreciation, point to gaps in coverage, and counter misleading anecdotes.

6. Talk to your doctors about advance care planning and pain control.

7. Ask for a report card. If your community has a comparison list of health plans, press the group to include something about caring for people who are very sick and likely to die. Do plans cover hospice? What do families say about symptom control? What about continuity of and access to care?

8. Ask local media to develop a series on how serious and eventually fatal illness affects people in your community.

9. Push your local health care system—even if it's only one doctor's office-to get involved in quality improvement efforts.

10. Write to your favorite television or radio show. Ask them to include stories about—or even just mention—people who are facing serious illness and death, and how they and their loved ones manage.

11. Keep pace with what's going on in the field. Americans for Better Care of the Dying advocates improved care of the dying and public policy that promotes such care. Our monthly print and electronic newsletter, *The Exchange*, reports on the field.

12. Read *Handbook for Mortals: Guidance for People Facing Serious Illness*. Donate copies to local churches, hospitals, or hospices—or give them to friends who need guidance and support.

### "Twenty Improvements in End-of-Life Care"

"Twenty Improvements in End of Life Care: Changes Internists Could Do Next Week!" is a list of ideas for clinicians to try.

1. Ask yourself as you see patients, "Would I be surprised if this patient died in the next few months?" For those "sick

enough to die," prioritize the patient's concerns—often symptom relief, family support, continuity, advance planning, or spirituality.

2. To eliminate anxiety and fear, chronically ill patients must understand what is likely to happen. When you see a patient who is "sick enough to die," tell the patient, and start counseling and planning around that possibility.

3. To understand your patients, ask:

- What do you hope for, as you live with this condition?
- What do you fear?
- It is usually hard to know when death is close. If you were to die soon, what would be left undone in your life?
- How are things going for you and your family? (Document and arrange care to meet each patient's priorities.)

4. Comprehensive and coordinated care often breaks down when providers don't have all the facts and plans. The next time you transfer a patient or a colleague covers for you, ask for feedback on how patient information could be more useful or more readily available next time.

5. Unsure how to ask a patient about advance directives? Try: "If sometime you can't speak for yourself, who should speak for you about health care matters?" Follow with:

- Does this person know about this responsibility?
- Does he or she know what you want?
- What would you want?
- Have you written this down?

6. To identify opportunities to share information with patients and caregivers, ask each patient who is "sick enough to die": "Tell me what you know about _____ [their disease]." Then: "Tell me what you know about what other people go through with this disease."

7. Most internists' practices have educational handouts on heart failure, COPD, cancer, and other fatal chronic illnesses to give to patients. Read them. If your handouts do not mention prognosis, symptoms, and death, exchange them for ones that do. Perhaps make *The Handbook for Mortals* and other resources available to your patients.

8. Some patients and their families are getting most of their information from the Internet. Log onto a patient-centered Internet site about an eventually fatal chronic illness to learn what is of interest to patients and families.

9. Is coordinating the care of your chronically ill patients taking up too much of your time? Call a local advocacy group (American Heart Association, American Cancer Society, etc.) for help, or consult with a care management service.

10. Discussing and recording advance directives with all your patients may take a while. How many patients over the age of 85 do you have? Start making plans with them. Expand to all who "are sick enough to die."

11. Use each episode in the ICU or ER as a "rehearsal." Ask the patient what should happen the next time. Be sure the patient has all necessary drugs at home and knows how to use them. Can you promise prompt relief from dyspnea near death? Tell the patient and family what's possible, and make plans together.

12. Ask your next patient who is "sick enough to die" whether anything happened recently regarding their medical situation for which they were unprepared. Work to anticipate the expectable complications and to have plans in place.

13. Since meperidine (Demerol) is almost the only opioid which has toxic metabolites and thus is contraindicated for chronic pain, banish meperidine from your prescribing and from the formularies where you work.

14. Very sick people will often be most comfortable at home or in nursing homes. Identify programs that are good at home care, send patients to those quality services, and work with them to fill the gaps your patients encounter.

15. Feedback on performance guides improvement. Find the routine surveys, administrative data, and electronic records that record symptoms, location of death, unplanned hospital or ER use, family satisfaction after the death, and other outcomes. Set up routines to get feedback on performance and improvement every month.

16. Except in hospice, most families never hear from their internist after a death. Change that! Make a follow-up phone call or set a visit to console, answer questions, support family caregivers, and affirm the value of the life just recently ended. At least send a card!

17. Working with very sick patients who die is hard on caregivers. Next week—and every week—praise a professional or family caregiver who is doing a good job.

18. We can't really change the routine care without changing Medicare. Contact your congressional representatives to ask for hearings, demonstration programs, research, and innovation to improve the Medicare program.

19. Some of our language really does not serve us well. Never say "There's nothing more to be done" or "Do you want

everything done?" Talk instead about the life yet to be lived and what *can* be done to make it better (or worse).

20. Patients and families need to be able to rely upon their care system. Consider what you can *promise* on behalf of your care system—pain relief, family support, honest prognosis, enduring commitment in all settings over time, planning for complications and death, and so on. Pick a promise that your patients need to hear and start working with others to make it possible to make that promise! Quality improvement strategies work.

## Resources

Americans for Better Care of the Dying
 P.O. Box 346
 Marvin Center
 Washington, DC 20052
 Phone: 202-530-9864
 caring1@erols.com
 http://www.abcd-caring.org

EPEC Project
 American Medical Association
 515 N. State Street
 Chicago, IL 60610
 Phone: 312-464-4979
 http://www.ama-assn.org/EPEC

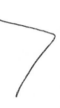

Last Acts Campaign
 Professional Outreach
 Ms. Karen Long
 Stewart Communications, Ltd.
 730 North Franklin, Suite 504
 Chicago, IL 60610
 Phone: 312-642-8652
 Fax: 312-642-1888
 karenl@stewcommltd.com

Last Acts has many work groups:

 Work Groups on Family, Workplace, Financing, Spirituality & Bereavement, Diversity
 Ms. Shawn Taylor Zelman
 Barksdale Ballard & Co.
 1951 Kidwell Drive, Suite 205

Vienna, VA 22182
Phone: 703-827-8771
Fax: 703-827-0783
szelman@bballard.com

Work Groups on Palliative Care, Professional Education, Institutional Innovation, Standards & Guidelines, Evaluation & Outcomes
Ms. Karen Long
Stewart Communications, Ltd.
730 North Franklin, Suite 504
Chicago, IL 60610
Phone: 312-642-8652
Fax: 312-642-1888
karenl@stewcommltd.com

Work Groups on Communications & Publicity
Mr. Ed Hatcher
Burness Communications
7910 Woodmont Avenue, Suite 1340
Bethesda, MD 20814
Phone: 301-652-1558
Fax: 301-654-1589
hatcher@burnessc.com

Work Groups on *Innovations in End-of-Life Care*, on-line journal and discussion forum
Ms. Anna Romer, Managing Editor
Center for Applied Ethics & Professional Practice
Education Development Center, Inc.
55 Chapel Street
Newton, MA 02458
Phone: 617-969-7100
Fax: 617-969-1569
intleoljournal@edc.org

Project on Death in America
Open Society Institute
400 West 59th Street
New York, NY 10019
General questions: pdia@sorosny.org
Web site questions: pdiamedia@sorosny.org
http://www.soros.org/death/

Midwest Bioethics Center
1021–25 Jefferson Street

Kansas City, MO 64105
Phone: 800-344-3829
Phone: 816-221-1100
Fax: 816-221-2002
bioethic@midbio.org
http://www.midbio.org

*Meeting the Challenge: Twelve Recommendations for Improving End-of-Life Care in Managed Care*, a report of the National Task Force on End-of-Life Care in Managed Care. Newton, MA: Educational Development Center, 1999.

# PART IV

# OPPORTUNITIES IN SPECIFIC DISEASES

# 13

# Alzheimer's and Other Dementias

## Opportunities to Honor Life

Roosevelt's admonition to "try something" holds true for organizations working to improve end-of-life care for patients with Alzheimer's and other dementing diseases (referred to as Alzheimer's throughout this chapter, since it is more prevalent). Yet when nothing seems to work, when patients are unresponsive, bed-bound, or wandering, when the caregivers own patience and skill have been tried, what else can be done? This chapter offers some descriptions and ideas for what might be done.

In his best-seller *The Notebook* (1996), Nicholas Sparks writes about one man's determination to remain connected to his wife of more than 50 years, even as her progressive dementia makes him a stranger to her. The couple has come to live in a nursing home, where they have separate rooms. Each night, the husband secretly goes to his wife and reads to her from a journal that chronicles their shared lives. As Noah Calhoun writes, "There are no monuments dedicated to me and my name will soon be forgotten, but I've loved another with all my heart and soul, and to me, this has always been enough."

The fictional character's dedication to his wife reflects the challenging reality many professional and family caregivers face as they deal with the long and slow progression of Alzheimer's. Despite the dehumanization Alzheimer's seems to cause, loved ones maintain a human and humane desire to stay connected. But the long and slow progression of Alzheimer's takes a toll on patients and families. Family caregivers may need additional emotional and social support as they care for loved ones in the end stages of these diseases.

Until the end of life, patients with Alzheimer's and other dementias need and deserve respect and compassion—and

> It is common sense to take a method and try it. If it fails, admit it frankly and try another. But above all, try something.
>
> —Franklin Delano Roosevelt

treatment to manage symptoms and maintain comfort. As one leading researcher explains, "I think that it's crucial to recognize that people with very advanced dementia are still sentient human beings who are aware of the environment and still require comfort measures and stimulation" (Volicer et al., 1999).

Health care organizations will increasingly face the needs of people dying of Alzheimer's, which is an ultimately fatal disease: It is the most common dementia and accounts for two-thirds or more of all dementia cases (Costa, 1996). Dementia is an acquired syndrome in which memory and cognitive function decline, eventually rendering patients completely dependent on others.

Even though all patients with dementia will eventually die without having ever returned to health, and even though most will die from the complications resulting from their dementia, health care providers and the general public often forget to view this disease as a fatal condition. Because patients with Alzheimer's may live with the disease for three to seven years, caregivers can find it difficult to recognize when a patient has reached a terminal stage of illness.

As the disease progresses, patients lose their ability to care for themselves and eventually become completely dependent on others, usually on family members—often, frail elderly spouses. The range, frequency, and severity of cognitive deficits and problem behaviors associated with dementia put these family caregivers under physically demanding and unremitting stressors. Providing care to an Alzheimer's patient can result in undesirable social role changes, depression and anxiety, and strained family relations; these caregivers often come to find that life is uncontrollable and overwhelming (Barnes et al., 1981; Morycz, 1985; Rabins et al., 1982; Williamson and Schulz, 1990; Zarit et al., 1980; Collins et al., 1994). Sherwin B. Nuland eloquently describes the life of many Alzheimer's caregivers when he writes, "It often seems as though the families of Alzheimer's patients are sidetracked from the broad sunlit avenues of ongoing life, remaining trapped for years, each in its own excruciating cul-de-sac" (Nuland, 1994).

Alzheimer's and other dementing diseases challenge the creativity and dedication of people who want to improve the quality of life for patients. A few innovative programs and policy initiatives already illuminate how to provide better care for end-stage dementias. The seven promises inherent in reliably competent care (discussed in chapter 2) apply directly to the care of dying dementia patients.

Using these promises, organizations would be able to develop and shape an ideal service program. Patients, families, and professional caregivers would find in their communities the social, medical, and emotional support essential to living with such a debilitating illness.

Organizations and individuals would work together to:

- Ensure competent care for related diseases
- Prevent premature disability
- Avoid skin breakdown and adverse drug events
- Maintain safety and comfort
- Make advance plans with family members for loved ones' eventual deterioration and likely complications
- Support family caregivers

The heart of such a program would be its ability and willingness to celebrate and honor the life coming to a close. Much remains to be done before this vision becomes a reality—but groups involved in breakthrough change can begin to sketch the outlines for this picture.

## In This Chapter

Few organizations have applied the Plan-Do-Study-Act model to improve care for dying dementia patients. Yet the success of this model in other areas of health care suggests that it can be applied to Alzheimer's care in a way that leads to reform and improvement. Teams that aim to improve care for Alzheimer's patients will need to use the approaches described elsewhere in this book and tailor them to the needs of dementia patients and their families. This chapter provides background information to guide quality improvement teams, specifically:

- Tailoring palliative care for dementia patients
- Knowing when a patient's prognosis might qualify for the Medicare hospice benefit
- Planning for deterioration and death
- Educating family caregivers and offering practical help
- Enhancing nursing facility practices
- Addressing difficult ethical issues, such as ending tube feeding or limiting family burdens

The chapter highlights the experiences of a few especially novel programs that have begun to examine the best ways to care for patients with dementia.

## Palliative Care and the Alzheimer's Patient

What does it mean to provide palliative care (described in detail in chapter 8) to Alzheimer's patients and their families? Essentially, the goal is to keep dying patients comfortable while supporting and comforting family and loved ones. Beyond the usual requirements of palliative care, Alzheimer's patients and their families need palliative care for two physical milestones that come near the end of life and that can overwhelm and distress families. These are a patient's markedly decreased appetite (and inability to eat) and a tendency to take to bed, where physiologic changes cause people to curl up in a fetal position.

As Alzheimer's patients near the end of life, their appetites decrease, or they begin to refuse food or to choke on it. Patients "forget" how to chew or how to swallow. Family caregivers can find this change quite difficult, challenging the very human desire to comfort and nurture others by offering food. Families may or may not want to offer artificial hydration and nutrition—or the patient may have expressed preferences in an advance directive. In either case, health care providers must address loved ones' concerns and fears.

More than patients with other diseases, Alzheimer's patients spend a substantial period at the end of life marked by being mostly unresponsive and bed-bound. At this stage, a patient can be positioned in a recliner; however, she will spend most of her time asleep, punctuated by rather aimless activity or moaning. Usually, this condition comes during or after substantial weight loss and is accompanied by a strong tendency for the legs to contract. Such a patient is "curled in a fetal position," with little muscle and little fat. The patient requires total nursing care, and avoiding skin breakdown is challenging. Such total care is difficult in part because the patient cannot respond in any meaningful way.

As Alzheimer's progresses through its series of dramatic and devastating changes, families learn to adjust to constant losses, living in an almost constant state of bereavement. Some model programs serve as guideposts for how to ease the necessary transitions and have pioneered methods that physically protect and comfort patients while maintaining their safety and supporting loved ones.

### Oregon Restraint Reduction Project

As their cognitive abilities deteriorate, many patients have a phase of very difficult behaviors that challenge both family and professional caregivers. Although the patient may still be able to walk and remains relatively strong, she can no longer make sense of the environment, or she responds inappropriately to caregivers. The patient endangers self or others through excessive activity, threatening or violent behavior, or wandering.

In the past, health care providers controlled such difficult behaviors with medications and/or restraints. At least in nursing facilities, restraint use has become uncommon, in part due to a strong federal effort to regulate this practice. Results from one three-year project by the Benedictine Institute for Long-Term Care (Rader, 1996) show what can be done to reduce the use of physical and chemical restraints, in part by looking at the root causes of patient behavior. This process can allow caregivers to avoid seemingly "rational" responses that are, in fact, counterproductive. Caregivers who take a different perspective on a patient's behavior can take planned and pur-poseful interventions.

The "reframing" methods were honed over months of trial and error. The accompanying instrument is a guide to this process. Teams interested in using the PDSA model to reduce or redirect troubling behavior may find this approach helpful. Using responses to this form, the caregiver team (which might include a family caregiver, home care aide, and nurse) considers how to modify the patient's environment, prevent the behavior, or limit its hazardous consequences. The team then comes up with a list of "changes to try." These changes are at the heart of a series of PDSA cycles during which the caregiver team tries to find effective and lasting solutions. The Oregon experi-ence found that caregivers could learn from their trials what was triggering troublesome behaviors and, through this pro-cess, could virtually eliminate chemical or physical restraints.

### Jacob Perlow Hospice

The Jacob Perlow Hospice program of Beth Israel Health Care System, based in New York City, completed a three-year pilot project (1993–95) to deliver the full range of hospice care and services to 124 patients with end-stage Alzheimer's and their families. In this time, the program provided a total of 17,358 days of home care. The project's primary goals were to:

- Increase access to hospice care through education and outreach
- Provide a full range of appropriate hospice home care and inpatient care services
- Create a model that would demonstrate the merit of hospice care for Alzheimer's patients and their families

Please fill out this form and return it to _____,

Answer questions you find pertinent. Thank you for taking the time.

To: The Care Conference Team

From: _____(Caregiver)

Date: _____

Name of Patient: _____

What questions do you have regarding this person?

What behavior, action, symptom, problem or talk have you observed in the resident which you would like addressed with/for him/her? (Please be specific).

If it is a behavior you noted, when did you first notice it? When does it mostly happen?

What do you think might be the reason for the behavior?

Why does this behavior concern you? (i.e., what effect does it have on the patient or those around him/her?)

Do you have intervention ideas (could be new ideas or interventions you/others have found to be helpful)?

Other observations about this resident that you would like to communicate to the care conference team or that you would like discussed at the care conference:

Figure 13.1 Reframing Behavior. Reprinted with permission of Joanne Rader.

Feeding and swallowing, pain control, and bowel and urinary management presented the most common significant problems for patients (and, consequently, their caregivers). To resolve these problems, nurses worked with family caregivers to develop coping strategies that enabled them to provide daily care.

Anxiety, exhaustion, and a sense of failure and blame proved to be the most frequent symptoms among family caregivers. Offering hospice services such as psychosocial and spiritual support to family caregivers helped to relieve some of their stress. Through hospice, families received other services, including practical assistance and education about the disease, pain assessment and management, and a way to find immediate help for problems and emergencies. Although such support cannot remove the burden of caring for a dementia patient at home, it can relieve the sense of isolation and despair families experience.

## Dementia Study Unit of the Bedford Veterans Hospital

Clinicians at the Geriatric Research and Education Clinical Center (GRECC) at the Edith Nourse Rogers Memorial Veterans Hospital in Bedford, Massachusetts, established a special unit for advanced dementia patients with whom to try new approaches, including palliative care. The Dementia Special Care Unit includes a 100-bed inpatient unit, an outpatient program, and an adult day care center.

The program's early research focused on treating infection as well as managing eating difficulties. The team found that the most intrusive medical interventions were not always in the patient's best interests, in part because they did not provide comfort (Volicer and Hurley, 1999). Researchers compared the effects of palliative care with the effects of more traditional care. "Conventional" approaches included antibiotics for fever, artificial feeding for inability to eat, and hospitalization for many complications. The "palliative care" approach avoided such interventions and focused on comfort and function. The study involved a small number of patients. Although those who received palliative care seemed to die a little more quickly, they seemed to have substantially better comfort care and much lower use of hospitals (Fabiszewski et al., 1990).

In the early 1990s, the team began to shift its focus from medical interventions to understanding psychiatric problems and behavioral issues of dementia patients. In addition, the group has begun to examine what it calls "resistiveness" to care. As researcher Ann Hurley explained (Volicer and Hurley, 1999), behavioral problems become more intense at different stages of dementia, and it is critical that professional and family caregivers respond appropriately.

Current research focuses on psychiatric problems and on understanding and managing disruptive behavior among these patients, as well as on reducing transfers to acute care settings (Innovations, 1999). The program is now developing ways to create appropriate meaningful activities based on psychiatric and behavioral assessment.

A current project is examining resistiveness to care, such as disruptive behavior, which seems to vary according to the stage of the disease. The team has developed a 13-point scale to measure and rate resistance, based on the presence, duration, and intensity of resistive behavior. The team is also studying interventions to prevent and decrease resistiveness. One important point is to help professional and family caregivers view the resistive behavior from another perspective, to recognize that if a patient is acting in a very troublesome manner, caregivers need to find the roots of the problem.

GRECC researchers stress the need for professional and family caregivers not to blame the victim, to step back from the view that Alzheimer's patients are aggressive or assaultive or obstreperous. The team uses a behavioral model that it calls "ABC: Antecedent, Behavior, Consequences." For example, the team described what happened during a nursing home consultation when a patient's bath-time acting out proved to be a reasonable response to undiagnosed metastatic cancer with bone fractures (Innovations, 1999).

Researchers emphasize the importance of continuity of care among Alzheimer's patients. Acute care settings can be very difficult not only for patients and loved ones but also for professional caregivers who are unaccustomed to the needs of Alzheimer's patients. Acute care settings, which sometimes involve restraints to prevent patients from wandering, can also be unsafe. And patients suffer the physical consequences of such hospitalizations, such as new pressure sores, contractures, and worsened nutritional status.


Knowing When a Dementia Patient
Is "Terminal"

Under current federal regulations (which some groups are trying to change), the Medicare hospice benefit (which is described at length in chapter 9) requires that a patient have a prognosis of less than six months. However, as explained in chapter 1, prognostication is quite uncertain for most dying people, and Alzheimer's is no exception. End-stage Alzheimer's patients can still live for an unpredictably long time because they do not develop the kinds of infection that commonly lead to death among these patients.

Because patients live for a long time with increasing disability, families (and, often, professional caregivers) find it hard to know when a person is in the last phase of illness. The Alzheimer's Association offers educational programs for families advising them of their right to choose hospice care. Medicare's hospice benefit is available to persons who live in nursing facilities provided that they are not relying on Medicare to support their nursing home costs and a hospice program has worked out the arrangements with the nursing facility. Enhancing the use of formal hospice programs is one direction for improvement activities for advanced dementia.

*Medical Guidelines for Determining Prognosis in Selected Non-Cancer Diseases* (Stuart, 1994) from the National Hospice Organizations recommends the following clinical criteria:

- Inability to dress independently
- Inability to bathe properly
- Inability to walk
- Consistent weight loss
- Lean body mass less than 70 percent of Ideal Body Weight
- Ability to say about six words (or less)
- Fecal and urinary incontinence
- Other serious medical problems

Exactly how to put these together or find other criteria is an ongoing challenge. A retrospective chart review of end-stage Alzheimer's patients at the Bedford GRECC (McCracken and Gerdsen, 1991) found that nurses generally recognized impending death. Their notes describing the dying process spanned from 5 to 38 days ahead of death.

The Bedford team has developed five levels of care (Innovations, 1999), an approach that tracks where patients are in the disease progress and helps to identify when patients are nearing the end of life. According to researcher Ann Hurley, RN, DNSc, "Each level of care is not only defined by what medical interventions are not applied, but by intensive care nursing interventions that are applied" (Innovations, 1999). Working with the unit physician, the nursing team negotiates a care level, which is then recommended to the family member. During a family conference, the family considers the recommendation—but is not forced to accept it. At this meeting, participants discuss advance care planning issues, such as the patient's more immediate prognosis, or the decisions the surrogate will need to make. Family members may have high expectations for the outcomes of medically aggressive treatment and may need more information about actual programs before making a decision.

The levels of treatment used at the GRECC are:

- *Level One:* Diagnostic workups, treatment of other medical conditions, transfer to acute care when necessary, CPR in the event of heart attack, and tube feeding
- *Level Two:* Less aggressive care, DNR status established; otherwise, same as Level One

- *Level Three:* DNR and no acute care transfer for medical management
- *Level Four:* Previous restrictions, as well as no workup or antibiotic treatment for life-threatening infections; anti-pyretics and analgesics for comfort
- *Level Five:* Supportive care, eliminating tube feeding

Despite the unpredictable course of the disease, the prognosis is usually clear enough for the patient who has lost weight, has low albumin, is not eating or is aspirating often, no longer speaks, and has taken to bed. These patients rarely live more than a few months, and their families can clearly benefit from supportive and palliative services. For instance, the program at the Bedford Veterans Hospital is set in a special care unit. Approximately 3,000 such units exist in nursing facilities and hospitals around the country. Groups aiming to try PDSA changes might begin by trying a few changes with a few patients in special care units, perhaps by working on advance care plans with five families and helping them understand crises that are likely to occur and how to plan for them. The group could then look at whether this approach improved family/proxy confidence or decision-making ability—and build another change cycle based on those results.

### On Lok Senior Health Services

The Program of All-Inclusive Care of the Elderly (PACE) administered by San Francisco's On Lok Senior Health Services provides comprehensive services to frail, nursing-home-eligible elderly living at home. (On Lok's program for developing comfort care plans is described in detail in chapter 3.) PACE's national standards now include attention to advance care planning, symptom control, and support near death. During the Breakthrough Series, the On Lok team worked to:

- Help professional caregivers recognize when a patient was at high risk of dying soon
- Develop comfort care plans
- Prepare families and staff for the patient's deterioration and death

Through staff education and ongoing training, as well as printed materials, On Lok staff were able to recognize when a patient was nearing death, to revise the plan of care, and to help staff and families to gain a sense that death was expected and that the dying was well supported.

Just as with other conditions, advance care planning gives patients, families, and professional caregivers a better chance to have the course unfold in the best possible way for each patient. If no one has thought through the merits of hospitalizing a patient with a fever, middle-of-the-night decisions made during a crisis will generally be to pursue the conventional course of calling the ambulance and starting the sequence of emergency room evaluation and hospitalization. If, instead, family and professional caregivers had thought through the merits, perhaps the disruption, fear, iatrogenic complications, and even the prolonged life would have been deemed not worth the effort.

The On Lok Senior Health Services, Jacob Perlow Hospice, and Bedford Veterans Hospital programs discussed above all have a strong dedication to advance planning for their dementia patients. They count it as a failure to have a patient's fever or other acute complication treated as an emergency. Instead, these are considered predictable events for which plans can be made.

Thinking ahead gives professional and family caregivers a plan for ways to support the patient and family in the patient's usual living situation. That decision might require having any number of specific plans in place:

- A hospice nurse or care manager who is able to visit promptly
- Readily available medications to reduce fever or secretions
- Discussions with funeral directors or memorial societies

The Washington Home in Washington, D.C., evaluated advance planning and discovered that documentation was "hit or miss." Many patients had good plans that were not readily available, while others had been overlooked in planning. The facility made it standard practice to put the current plan on the "bottom line" of the cover sheet (listing diagnoses and concerns), with a reference to the progress note that explained it, and to make review of the current advance plan part of the checklist of issues in the routine quarterly review. The repeat review showed that within one year, more than 90 percent of residents had a readily available advance care plan dealing with hospitalization, resuscitation, and surrogate designation.

The approaches to advance care planning for Alzheimer's patients are similar to those used for other patients (see chapter 5 for details). However, because Alzheimer's patients will become unable to make their own decisions, issues of competence may complicate discussions. Families need to do their best to represent the patient's own preferences whenever these are known. However, that can be a difficult task. Many families will know that "Mom would never have wanted to live this way," but they will not know what she would have wanted done, given that she is, in fact, living this way. Other families will be frankly overwhelmed by the caregiving or the costs that they face. Furthermore, as outlined below, society's conflicting and uncertain support for various courses of care leaves families uncertain as to how others will evaluate their choices. Nevertheless, clear plans and regular open discussions can prevent unnecessary emergency room visits, hospital admissions, or inappropriate care, so the best programs also make advance planning a central element.

### Supporting Family Caregivers

Although a variety of detailed schemes to characterize the stages of progressive dementias have been outlined in the literature, clinicians often categorize the course of a dementing disorder in terms of early, middle, and late states. A person in the early stage of dementia experiences personality and emotional changes, a mild memory deficit, and decreased ability to perform complex activities. During the middle stage, the dementia victim experiences increasing difficulty carrying out activities of daily living, moderately severe short- and long-term memory deficits, impairments in judgment, and behavioral disturbances. Late-stage dementia includes loss of awareness of surroundings, severe communication deficits, immobility, and total dependence on others. Throughout the disease process, family caregivers are responsible for the supervisory and direct care needs of the impaired person and interactions with the broader social and health care networks necessary to keep the impaired person in the community.

Family caregivers differ widely in the level and type of care-related strain they experience, and only a limited relationship exists between the severity of the patient's disease and the caregiver's subjective perceptions of burden or strain. Many factors seem to influence how family caregivers respond to the caregiving role.

As organizations have come to understand the negative effects of caregiving on family members, some have developed interventions that target caregivers. Direct comparisons of interventions are difficult due to differences in treatment philosophies, populations served, frequency and duration of interventions, content of interventions, peer versus professional intervention agents, home or community-based treatment, outcome measures, and level of analysis of the research studies from these interventions. Nevertheless, the research to date has yielded a rich knowledge base from which to develop future interventions (Bourgeois et al., 1996). Interventions typically include a wide range of services:

- Individual counseling to address emotional and psychological problems
- Group counseling that includes other caregivers in similar situations
- Information and referral, such as educational programs or skills training to enhance coping and problem-solving skills and patient management

While the approaches to caregiver interventions are quite diverse, all tend to be similar to those available to other groups requiring formal and informal support services to cope with psychological and/or physical disabilities.

Individual Counseling

Individual counseling is available primarily through outpatient clinics and care management services. In most cases, dementia patients and caregivers have access to a variety of follow-up services that help to ensure continued community residence. Nursing or social work professionals typically guide caregivers and other family members to support services, such as support groups, day care, and respite and long-term care, shortly after diagnosis. Some programs include family meetings to help all family members learn to meet the common goal of caring for the patient.

Individual counseling sessions are helpful when an individual caregiver faces a particularly challenging event or period of time in the disease. Some research suggests that daughters and daughters-in-law who were primary caregivers made greater gains in psychological functioning and well-being when receiving individual counseling as compared to group counseling. Group interventions seem to have produced greater improvements in caregivers' social supports; both models seem to improve caregivers' ability to cope with stress. Overall, the counseling literature supports treatments for narrowly defined problems when therapy is conducted with individual caregivers.

### Support Groups

Support group interventions are based on the assumption that given the appropriate knowledge of the patient's disease, the services available, and the opportunity to discuss common problems and fears with other caregivers, all would be better equipped to meet the challenges they face. In addition, family support group interventions are designed to offer families emotional support, enhance their coping skills, and provide them with general information. Professionals or trained peers can lead such groups, which can be ongoing or time-limited.

Although the administrative specifics of support groups vary, they all share an ultimate goal of educating families about dementia and promoting supportive relationships between families in similar situations. Support groups can meet on any number of schedules: weekly or bimonthly; for one hour or two; and for several weeks or months. Groups can be open to all caregivers or only to specific categories of caregivers, such as children, siblings, or spouses. Most research on support groups has examined the effect of group participation on at least one measure of caregiver distress (e.g., caregiver burden, depression, feelings of loneliness, locus of control, emotional competence, family impact) and/or on caregiver knowledge about dementia. Overall, the research suggests that support group interventions provide needed information about the disease and disease processes, psychological gains, and informal support networking for caregivers who are receptive to this kind of assistance.

### Respite Care

The idea behind respite care is that caregivers who have some periods of relief from this task might be better able to manage. Research tends to show that caregivers appreciate time away from caregiving and report that they feel less emotionally and socially isolated, have higher self-esteem, and experience more control over their own lives. Respite care includes daily attendance at adult day care; short-term, in-home companion services; and long-term institutionalization.

The perceived benefits yield insignificant differences on standardized measures of burden, depression, stress, and social support. The modest effects of respite interventions may be related to the amount of time spent in the respite settings. Researchers report that the median annual use of in-home respite care is 63 hours, that of day care is 10 days, and that of nursing home respite care is 11 days (Lawton et al., 1989).

Caregivers often wait too long or until a crisis occurs before using any services, including respite. Caregivers may be reluctant to seek out respite care, especially those who see it as a "transition from home to institution, thereby increasing the likelihood of institutionalization" (Scharlach and Frenzel, 1986).

Caregivers have vastly different opportunities to get relief from caregiving, yet the burden of care remains as long as the patient is not institutionalized permanently. The modestly positive effects of respite programs appear to increase as participation continues over time, even when patients are reported to have a decline in cognitive functioning.

### Skills Training

Skills training can have positive results for caregivers and for patients. When caregivers practice and use skills to resolve real-life problems, researchers report significant changes in outcome measures directly related to those skills.

For instance, researchers trained caregivers to develop and implement patient behavior change programs and monitored treatment effects across time (Pinkston et al., 1988). Training programs included didactic instruction, role-play, corrective feedback, and data collection designed to improve caregiver skills in areas such as patient assessment; identification, definition, and quantification of problem behaviors; and the development and implementation of individual intervention programs. In addition to significant changes in about three-quarters of targeted patient behaviors (of whom four-fifths maintained changes for six months after treatment), Pinkston reported changes in standard measures of patient mental status and independent functioning and caregiver burden (Pinkston and Linsk, 1984).

Another group of researchers taught caregivers more effective problem-solving strategies as well as ways to increase the pleasant activities in their lives. These caregivers experienced less stress and depression and improved morale compared to caregivers in a control group (Pinkston et al., 1988).

The literature also reflects evidence of the effects on long-term maintenance and generalization (e.g., for relaxation training, education and skills training, and patient-focused treatments).

### Comprehensive, Multicomponent Interventions

Caregivers have vastly different needs at various points in their lives as caregivers. In addition, no single intervention seems to address all of the needs caregivers are likely to have. To fill this gap, many programs now take a comprehensive, multifaceted approach to caregiver support by offering a range of community services and specific caregiving interventions. Programs have included elements such as: four-hour weekly respite care, weekly caregiver-focused health care visits, education, and monthly support group meetings. When compared to a control group receiving conventional community nursing care of the patient, caregivers reported an improved quality of life.

Multicomponent interventions blanket caregivers with a diversity of services in the hopes that a combination will meet a caregiver's unique needs at the appropriate time. Examples of effective programs include an outpatient clinic program offering psychiatric, medical, social work, nursing, and architectural advice to individual caregivers that resulted in increased caregiver satisfaction with their ability to cope with the patient's physical and mental health.

### Improving Nursing Facilities

Although nursing facilities seem to be roundly disliked and regulated, more than a quarter of people who live to age 65 will use a nursing facility for long-term care. Self-interest alone would seem to motivate teams to provide better care for Alzheimer's patients in nursing facilities.

A number of facilities have been quietly implementing innovations to enhance the environment both for those who live there and for those who serve them. This seems a natural place for vigorous quality improvement. The concerned caregiving team is already in place, measurement of effects is often easy, and opportunities for improvement abound. With encouragement from senior leadership, a little time for the caregiving team, and protection from adverse publicity regarding the data gathered, nursing homes could undoubtedly make major gains. Making those gains widespread will also require attention to ways to spread the news of innovations that make a real difference, since there are few forums for presenting what has been learned within the field.

The Washington Home, mentioned above, housed a hospice program. The caregiving teams in each program began to realize that they had some special expertise not shared by the other program. Not only did this lead to referring some dying cancer patients in the nursing home to hospice; it also led to skilled and experienced nursing home nurses serving as consultants to the hospice team when they started learning to support families as dementia patients died at home.

## A Caution about Controversial Ethical Issues

Quality improvement works best when there is widespread agreement on the aims to be pursued. Some potential aims are probably too controversial for teams to take on without caution and thought, perhaps especially when the society is quite ambivalent about the ethics involved. For example, many patients (before dementia) and their families (now) may think that it would be better not to live for long with dementia, but a team should probably avoid aiming specifically to accomplish that end. While one study from the Bedford VA showed that good hospice care had a small effect on shortening life, that was not the aim of the project. The project aimed to provide good, comprehensive support.

Whether and how to provide artificial nutrition has been a strikingly important example of societal anxieties. Artificial nutrition has not actually been shown to prolong life or to improve its quality—but it has not been shown to engender overwhelming harms, either. Some people see artificial feeding as something like "chicken soup," a potent symbol of caring. Others see it as "depending on a machine" and therefore find it fully offensive. Others are conflicted themselves. The more than 50 appellate court cases make it clear that the courts support good decision-making practices with regard to whether artificial feeding should be forgone. Thus, it is quite legitimate to develop programs to support good decision making by families and clinicians. However, the uncertainty and divisiveness over whether artificial nutrition is or is not part of a generally good end-of-life course for dementia patients makes it unlikely that a care program should aim to achieve low or high rates of use.

Another area of societal discomfort is the degree to which families should be expected to "care for their own." How much burden is it reasonable to expect spouses, children, and others to take on? Some feel that there is no reasonable limit, except for abject impossibility of doing more. Others feel that society should protect people from having to impoverish themselves or lose out on the chance to live their own life because of the dementing illness of a family member. Again, within the bounds of societal support (e.g., Medicaid), families and programs have substantial discretion, and good decision making is generally supported as worthwhile. However, the lack of societal consensus means that institutions should avoid actually aiming to protect families or to impose more burdens upon them.

In general, quality improvement by caregiving teams works best if their aim is broadly held to be a good thing, and venturing into areas where there are strong and contentious ethical issues should be done with substantial caution. Enabling patients (in advance) or families (now) to understand and act on their options usually is not contentious.

### Innovators Need to Know

- The usual elements of good end-of-life care also make sense in shaping programs that serve patients with advanced stages of dementia.
- Although prognostication is uncertain, many patients could make use of the Medicare hospice benefit or of hospice programs.
- Advance planning is often quite important, and improvement activities are often effective.
- Family caregiver support is often a high-yield improvement strategy.
- Nursing facilities offer a fertile arena for improvement work.
- Some values issues are sufficiently controversial that improvement teams should be cautious and thoughtful about selecting aims that endorse a particular point of view.

### Resources

Alzheimer's Association
  919 N. Michigan Avenue, Suite 1000
  Chicago, IL 60611
  Phone: 800-272-3900
  http://www.alz.org

*Alzheimer's Caregiving Strategies*, a CD-ROM developed by the U.S. Department of Veterans Affairs. To order, contact:
  HealthCare Interactive, Inc.
  P.O. Box 19646
  Minneapolis, MN 55419
  Phone: 612-824-2622
  Phone: 888-824-3020
  http://www.hcinteractive.com/

Alzheimer's Disease Education and Referral Center
   National Institute on Aging
   P.O. Box 8250
   Silver Spring, MD 20907-8250
   Phone: 800-438-4380
   Phone: 301–495-3311
   Fax: 301-495-3334
   E-mail adear@alzheimers.org
   http://www.alzheimers.org/

*Dirty Details: The Days and Nights of a Well Spouse*, by Marion Deutsche Cohen. Philadelphia: Temple University Press, 1996.

*Hard Choices for Loving People: CPR, Artificial Feeding, Comfort Measures Only, and the Elderly Patient*, by Hank Dunn. Herndon, VA: A&A Publishers, 1994. (To order bulk copies, call 703-707-0169.)

*Hospice Care for Patients with Advanced Progressive Dementia*, edited by Ladislav Volicer and Ann Hurley. New York: Springer Publishing, 1998.

*Individualized Dementia Care*, by Joanne Rader. New York: Springer Publishing, 1995.

*The 36-Hour Day*, 3d ed., by Nancy L. Mace, MA, and Peter V. Rabins, MD, MPH. Baltimore: Johns Hopkins University Press, 1999.

Interview with Ladislav Volicer and Ann Hurley, 1999: "Resources and Tools" on the *Innovations in End-of-Life Care* Web site: http://www2.edc.org/lastacts/resources.asp

# Opportunities to Improve Care for Cancer Patients

**14**

Many of the improvements in end-of-life care over the past 20 years began with attempts to improve the care of cancer patients. As the hospice movement began to promote a more holistic approach to care of the dying, health care providers applied hospice techniques to cancer patients farther from death and to patients with noncancer diagnoses. Today, people who suffer from a range of terminal illnesses benefit from practices first developed in cancer treatment and symptom management. For instance, although hospice originally focused on the needs of terminally ill cancer patients, its efforts to reduce cancer pain have driven the routine and aggressive use of opioids for serious pain. Much of what is known about medical management for symptoms such as dyspnea, terminal agitation, and bowel obstruction comes from efforts to relieve these symptoms in cancer patients. Treatment modalities such as long-acting opioids, transdermal drug delivery systems, and palliative radiation and chemotherapy have been developed primarily to meet the needs of cancer patients.

Cancer holds a unique place in medicine in general and in American society in particular. Medicine has waged war against cancer, and our language surrounding cancer treatment reflects this battle. Indeed, in the 1970s, the government declared war on cancer and directed millions of dollars to find ways to prevent and cure the disease. Like warriors, people whose cancer is cured or in remission are "survivors"; others "lose the battle" and die, generally following a rather predictable path to death.

Cancer has a special terror for many people. When cancer is diagnosed late in disease or is widespread, patients inevitably die. Cancer can seem to come from anywhere—lifestyle, envi-

> Even if you're on the right track, you'll get run over if you just sit there.
>
> —Will Rogers

ronmental hazards, workplace hazards, or genetic weaknesses. Unseen enemies can be frightening, especially when one cannot hide.

Cancer is the second leading cause of death in adults in the United States. In 2000, more than a half million men and women are expected to die of cancer. Lung, colon, breast, and prostate cancer are expected to account for more than half of these deaths (Greenlee et al., 2000). While research to prevent and control cancer continues, the number of cancer deaths has risen over the years and may continue to do so as the graying of America continues.

Although hospice programs serve many patients who are dying of cancer, a large majority of cancer patients continues to die in hospitals and nursing homes, without the benefit of hospice and palliative care. Of the 2.27 million people who died in 1993, only 256,900 received hospice services (Christakis and Sachs, 1996). The National Hospice Organization reports that in 1998, hospice served 540,000 patients (NHO, 1998), or about 23.17 percent of the 2.33 million deaths that year (NCHS, 1999). In fact, the National Center for Health Statistics reports that of the 2.28 million people who died in 1994, 55 percent were in hospitals and 19 percent were in nursing facilities. Almost all who die with hospice care die at home (IOM, 1997).

Hospice referrals come late in the course of the disease; in 1995, the median length of hospice stay was only 29 days. Some patients come to hospice in the final days or hours of their lives, making it almost impossible for hospice to learn enough about patients and families to provide quickly and smoothly the kinds of supportive care needed.

### In This Chapter

Earlier chapters featured improvement strategies for particular symptoms or problems, all of which bear some relationship to cancer. This chapter looks at a few ideas that are specific to cancer care, and readers are referred to earlier chapters for suggestions on pain and symptom management, advance care planning, continuity of care, and spirituality and bereavement. Here we highlight:

- Using quality improvement strategies to improve symptom management
- Setting "checkpoints" during the course of treatment to review patient goals and preferences
- Appreciating the benefits of doing "nothing"

- Measuring quality of life as an end point of treatment
- Increasing culturally appropriate end-of-life care
- Reducing the number of hospital deaths
- Increasing referrals to hospice

## Use Quality Improvement Strategies as a Way to Improve Patient Care

Despite advances in cancer treatment and symptom control, pain remains an undertreated symptom for many cancer patients, along with fatigue and dyspnea. Organizations can use the suggestions highlighted throughout this book as a starting point to improve care of dying cancer patients. Improvement teams can work to train health care providers about the usefulness of early referral to hospice and palliative care, the importance of pain assessment and treatment, approaches to advance care planning, and ways to support patients, families, and loved ones.

Significant progress has been made in treating cancer pain. New medications and delivery systems have been developed to improve efficacy and compliance. Advocacy has increased for the appropriate, aggressive use of opioids and for increased physician education about pain management (IOM, 1997; AHCPR, 1994). There are high expectations that pain can be controlled in the vast majority of patients. But significant challenges remain. For reasons described throughout chapter 3 (on pain), groups must attend to the ongoing problem of uncontrolled pain among some cancer patients.

Despite standards for cancer pain management (Zech et al., 1995; AHCPR, 1994), many studies report inadequate treatment (Portenoy, 1992; Du Pen, 1999; Institute of Medicine, 1997). Many physicians lack knowledge about the fundamentals of pain management (Sloan et al., 1998; Cleeland et al., 1986). Elderly and minority patients with cancer pain are at particular risk for receiving inadequate pain management (Cleeland et al., 1997). Patients, physicians, and caregivers continue to fear addiction (IOM, 1997). Physicians worry about regulatory discipline for prescribing opioids (Joranson and Gilson, 1988; IOM, 1997). Lack of understanding about pain management can lead to unfortunate, inaccurate associations between pain control and assisted suicide (for example, the proposed Lethal Drug Abuse Prevention Act of 1998).

Like pain, fatigue is so common at the end of life that it has been seen as a natural consequence of dying, with relief an infrequent option. Fatigue, which can so reduce quality of life, has not been seen as a symptom to be diagnosed, researched, or treated. Yet fatigue is one of the most common and debilitating symptoms in the final months and days of cancer patients' lives (Kuuppelomaki and Lauri, 1998; Cleary and Carbone, 1997; Vogelzang et al., 1997; Coyle et al., 1990).

Although fatigue may be caused by undiagnosed depression (another symptom frequently and incorrectly dismissed as an obvious, and untreatable, companion to terminal illness), other factors may contribute to it. Side effects of medication, sleep deprivation, and inadequate nutrition can cause fatigue, yet their effect may be reduced through interventions tailored to an individual's preferences and disease course. Patients and families, as well as providers, might want to check a Web site devoted to cancer fatigue: http://www.cancerfatigue.org, where visitors can post questions to oncology nurses; learn more about the causes, symptoms, and management of cancer fatigue; and search for educational events in their communities.

Often provider and family education is appropriate, but education alone rarely leads to quality improvement. Only when participants are already motivated to change is there an eagerness to learn that translates into changed behavior. Even so, education can be a useful step in enhancing provider knowledge and skills. Quality improvement teams can work to train physicians and nurses on the need for ongoing pain assessment and aggressive responses to intolerable pain intensity levels.

Many Breakthrough Series teams developed training programs to address problems such as pain and symptom management. In addition, many professional associations and public agencies are developing curricula on end-of-life care, including state-of-the-art pain management. For instance, the Department of Veterans Affairs has launched a systemwide program titled "Pain as the Fifth Vital Sign" and is funding a faculty leader program to develop end-of-life care curricula.

Other professionals, including nursing home administrators and accreditation surveyors, need to learn more about appropriate pain and symptom management. Anecdotes describe nursing homes in which opioids are never administered. Imagine the care provided to patients with severe pain in such institutions: Either pain goes untreated or patients are admitted to hospitals. This problem occurs when some nursing home staff fear that increased use of opioids and psychotropic medications, along with the decreased use of more aggressive (albeit futile) measures, will increase the number of deaths and create suspicion that death was hastened. The fear of being vulnerable to citations and claims of poor care actually causes these groups to provide poor care.

Health care professionals, like patients and families, need to distinguish between developing tolerance to, physical dependence on, and addiction to pain medications. There must be an expectation of "medical equanimity"—that is, an expectation that issues of pain and pain medications, especially opioids, will be addressed in a manner that does not increase patients' and families' worries or fears (Ferrell, 1991).

Many cancer patients are debilitated by fatigue. Despite the dearth of research on relieving fatigue, organizations can apply the Plan-Do-Study-Act model to improving care of patients who are overwhelmed by fatigue. For instance, teams might begin by regularly assessing patients for their fatigue level and its effect on their quality of life. Providers might discuss fatigue and ways to cope with it, then document recommended treatment and its effect.

In the course of improving care for dying cancer patients, organizations can begin to focus on accountability. Teams might consider making—and keeping—promises to patients and families. (Sample promises are described in chapter 2.) As groups test new ways to deal with old problems, leaders can establish ways to measure compliance.

Improvement teams will find many ways to measure quality improvement for pain management; for instance, they can measure the daily percentage of patients with pain intensity below 4 (on a 0-to-10 scale); the assessment of pain every shift (or more often) in hospital or other inpatient settings; the time between pain assessment and medication administration; and compliance with the WHO ladder for pain management.

Process measures for education might include attendance at mandatory educational programs; a passing score on a knowledge/attitude assessment examination; or documented continuing education credits in end-of-life care.

## Set Checkpoints to Reevaluate the Treatment Plan

Treatment protocols drive many cancer treatment regimens. To be a "good" patient or a "good" doctor, one may follow the directions for the next test or round of chemotherapy without stopping to evaluate the real cost or benefit to the patient. Some patients may need "permission" from their doctors or their families to take the time to weigh the benefits and burdens of their treatment. Building checkpoints into the schedule of visits gives patients permission to change the course of treatment, creating an expectation that periodic reevaluations are, in fact, part of what good patients and good doctors do.

Some patients, families, and physicians feel that they are "giving up" if they consider stopping a treatment course once it has begun, even if the treatment is doing more harm than the good that is expected (or hoped for). If checkpoints are set out in advance, they become part of the plan, not a "giving up" of the plan.

Checkpoints allow time and opportunity for patients and physicians to discuss alternatives to the painful (and inaccurate) "There's nothing more that I can do for you" conversations. Instead, treatments can be evaluated, overall goals revisited, and plans made to achieve those goals.

Checkpoints could be part of all chemotherapy and radiation therapy protocols. Improvement teams could document and review patient-provider discussions and any decisions that result. Leaders could offer feedback to clinicians regarding their compliance and adequacy of documentation.

### Don't Just Do Something—Stand There!

Sometimes the best course of action is no action—or, at least, stopping long enough to really think through what should be done. Many interns have been offered this pearl of wisdom from senior residents encouraging them to stop and think during moments of crisis. Stopping and doing nothing is especially important in caring for patients at the end of life. Assessing pain and symptoms, ensuring comfort, and providing support requires a good bit of "standing there" with patients and families. Yet "doing nothing" is deceptively difficult—think about how hard it is to stand in silence during lulls in conversation.

Physicians say to patients, "You can have chemotherapy, get radiation, or do nothing." In our "take charge, can do, never say die" culture, which reveres independence and grit, "nothing" can be seen as surrender, defeat, or lack of will. Other times, physicians ask patients and families if they want "everything" done (especially in conversations about attempted resuscitation). The unspoken opposite is often assumed to be "nothing" instead of "everything but attempted resuscitation."

Physicians, nurses, patients, and families can all benefit by understanding that each option represents something and that no option is truly "nothing." Pain and symptom management is valuable for preserving comfort and function. Reaching personal goals and completing unfinished business is intense work. Saying goodbye is terribly difficult. Patients, families, and health care professionals must learn that "standing there" may be the best thing to "do." Physicians and other health care workers must consider this when explaining treatment options, especially when these are not likely to offer any benefit while creating further burdens. Surely it would be better to say, "You can have chemotherapy, get radiation, or decide to focus on living life fully, for all the time you get."

## Measure Quality of Life as an End Point of Treatment

Oncology has definite end points: life span, remission rates, rates of tumor growth and regression. For patients at the end of life, quality of life remains an important concern. Before providers recommend additional cancer therapies, their human costs and potential benefit should be considered, especially when a patient is near the end of life. Quality of life as an outcome should be important as providers and families evaluate treatment options.

Teams can regularly evaluate quality of life during and after treatments for cancer rather than relying only on superficial patient satisfaction measures. As many Breakthrough Series teams learned, other measures, such as pain relief or perception of suffering, are also useful ways to gauge the quality of care.

## Increase Culturally Appropriate End-of-Life Care

As in so much of American life, the needs of dying patients who are racial and ethnic minorities, women, or poor have not been adequately addressed (Cleeland et al., 1997). Even hospice, which has successfully cared for thousands of cancer patients, has served primarily the white middle class (Brenner, 1997). Lifelong lack of access to preventive and curative services makes it difficult to persuade some patients that palliative care is more than "no treatment." Health care institutions' lack of minority staff may discourage patients and families from seeking or accepting available services. Health care professionals must be trained to meet the needs of patients and families in settings or cultures that are unfamiliar to them.

## Reduce the Number of Hospital Deaths

When asked, many people say they want to die at home, in the comfort of a familiar place with loved ones. More than half of very elderly and seriously ill patients express their desire to die at home (Lynn et al., 1997), but a disturbing study revealed that the number of hospital beds, not patient and family preference, was the most influential factor in determining the site of death (Pritchard et al., 1998). Although some people with cancer will die "suddenly," most are more likely to experience a decline (hours, days, weeks) before their deaths (IOM, 1997). This period of decline may lead to hospital transfer for evaluation or for care that is becoming too intensive to be rendered by the primary caregiver. Some people may experience a decline in health while already in the hospital.

Patients, families, and physicians may fail to plan for these declines, thereby ensuring that a trip from home to hospital will occur for lack of other means to maintain safety and comfort. Health care systems often lack clear, easily implemented procedures to enable transfer of patients from hospital to home with necessary services when death appears imminent or inevitable. Patients, families, and health care professionals may not recognize or believe that death is approaching, so treatments are continued without discussion of the impending death and where it should take place.

Cancer deaths in hospital should be reduced, and monitoring should be performed to verify that transfers are appropriate. Charts should be reviewed of all transfers occurring within 24 hours of death. Compliance with patient and family preferences, patient status, readiness of destination (hospital bed or oxygen in the home, for example), and plan for continuity of care should be documented and monitored to reduce the likelihood of inappropriate transfer.

### Innovators Need to Know

The challenges in improving end-of-life care for cancer patients are complex and interrelated. Treatment checkpoints will be useless if "doing nothing" or "giving up" is the only alternative to staying the course. Undesired in-hospital deaths will not decrease unless alternatives are readily available. Underserved populations will enroll in hospice only if hospices address the needs of these populations. Even so, innovators in end-of-life care can begin to change the field by improving its elements.

- Cancer continues to hold a special place in our culture— one in which people can be immobilized by their fears and misconceptions.
- Most work in improving end-of-life care has been done with cancer patients, so there is an array of information from which to draw.

- Innovators can use basic strategies described throughout this book to improve care for cancer patients and their families.


## Resources

American Alliance of Cancer Pain Initiatives
    1300 University Ave., Room 4720
    Madison, WI 53706
    608-265-4013
    Fax 608-265-4014
    www.aacpi.org

*Calvary Hospital: A Model for Palliative Care in Advanced Care,* by
    James E. Cimino, MD, and Michael Brescia, MD. Order from:
    Palliative Care Institute
    Calvary Hospital
    1740 Eastchester Road
    Bronx, NY 10461
    http://www.cancerfatigue.org
    Web site devoted to understanding, preventing, and coping with cancer fatigue, a debilitating symptom of disease and side effect of treatment.

National Hospice and Palliative Care Organization
    1700 Diagonal Rd., Suite 300
    Alexandria, VA 22314
    703-243-5900
    www.nho.org

# Depression and Delirium

**15**

Depression in dying patients is often dismissed as a natural reaction to knowing that one's life is ending. Although sadness and grief are normal reactions to such news, these emotions usually give way to others. Clinical depression, however, does not "give way"; instead, it plagues sufferers with guilt, self-doubt and blame, hopelessness, and loneliness. While those who are sad can have times in which they are content and able to enjoy life, those who are depressed are unable to engage in life or to find moments of pleasure. Depression can deplete a person's quality of life as much as any other disease.

Like most people, clinicians often think that they too would be depressed knowing they had a life-threatening disease. This belief leads some clinicians to disregard or not recognize depression in their dying patients. Cancer patients rarely receive antidepressants, although as many as 20 percent may be clinically depressed (Vachon, 1998). Left untreated, depression causes significant emotional harm, reduces the ability to participate fully in life, reduces the ability to comply with other medical treatments, and can contribute to other medical problems (Strouse, 1997).

Delirium is another common medical complication among dying patients; estimates suggest that anywhere from 25 to 85 percent of dying patients experience delirium at some point in the last year of life. Delirium may be a side effect of some pain medications, and it may be caused by other common end-of-life problems, such as dyspnea, dehydration, and cachexia. Delirium creates terrible distress for patients, families, and professional caregivers.

Both depression and delirium are treatable causes of suffering at the end of life. Although it can be difficult to distinguish

Tell me about despair,
   yours, and I will tell
   you mine.
Meanwhile, the world goes
   on.
   —Mary Oliver, "Wild Geese"
   *New and Selected Poems*

between the two, providers can learn to screen and treat patients accordingly.

Strategies to improve screening and treatment include adding common assessments to intake forms, requiring depression screening for dying patients, tracking screening rates and prescribing practices, and setting goals for practice improvement. With these steps, organizations take a critical move in improving the lives of thousands of patients and their families.

## In This Chapter

Few organizations have engaged in quality improvement measures that address depression among dying patients. Consequently, this chapter focuses on more general issues, with the hope that teams might engage in relevant quality improvement activities. This chapter provides:

- An overview of depression and delirium
- A simple yet effective depression screening method
- Strategies to educate patients and families
- Ideas for quality improvement projects

## About Depression

Depression is sometimes described as the "common cold" of mental illness, affecting more than 11 million Americans each year (NAMI 1996). However, unlike the usual cold, depression is a serious illness, one that takes a physical, mental, emotional, and economic toll on its victims and those who love them.

Depression can be fatal. It is the strongest risk factor for suicide, and experts suggest that of the approximately 30,000 people who commit suicide each year, more than 90 percent have a mental illness or addiction (Moscicki, 1997). It can kill in less direct ways, too, by causing patients not to comply with other medical treatments and by disrupting sleep and eating patterns, further compromising the health of already vulnerable people.

The good news is that such suffering can be alleviated: Medication and psychotherapy, usually in combination, relieve depression for almost 80 percent of those who seek treatment.

Common symptoms include:

- Changes in appetite
- Changes in sleep—either sleeplessness or waking too early

- Changes in sexual habits
- Feelings of guilt, hopelessness, and worthlessness
- Fatigue
- Physical complaints, usually gastrointestinal
- Inability to enjoy once-pleasurable activities
- Withdrawal from others
- Thoughts of suicide

Depressed people often lack the insight they might ordinarily have—insight that would otherwise help them cope with their problems. Depressed people usually withdraw from others; for dying patients, who may already feel isolated, this additional isolation can be devastating. Life can, indeed, feel bleak and hopeless.

Certain medical illnesses, such as cancer and heart disease, can cause symptoms similar to those of depression—decreased appetite, loss of energy and sex drive, loss of sleep, and fatigue. Doctors should be encouraged to look at these symptoms as signs of depression and to question patients about their mood. Family members can sometimes describe changes in the patient's well-being, mood, or usual coping ability.

The following factors can predispose people for depression:

- Social isolation
- Recent losses
- A tendency to pessimism
- Socioeconomic pressures
- A history of mood disorders
- Alcohol or substance abuse
- Previous suicide attempt(s)
- Poorly controlled pain

*Source*: AHCPR, 1994

Depression, overlooked in most adults, is virtually ignored in elderly patients. In part, this is because providers do not screen patients for depression; in part, it results from misinformation and misunderstanding about depression. Some older patients who are depressed may simply believe that this is just how life is, that they should simply bear their unhappiness. Others may feel too ashamed to discuss feelings of depression, believing depression to be a character flaw, or blaming themselves for their symptoms. Some may be concerned about the cost of treatment, which some insurance policies do not cover. Others may not realize that medications commonly prescribed to older people or to those with heart disease can cause depression. Still others view it as part of the normal aging process.

Doctors and others may mistake depression for early symptoms of dementia, or, like their elderly patients themselves, may view depression as a normal part of aging. However, because suicide rates increase with age—and the highest rates occur in white men over the age of 65 (Moscicki, 1997)—depression among the elderly is truly a risk factor for suicide.

Although depression increases the risk of suicide for all people, among terminally ill patients, hopelessness appears to be an important predictor of suicidal thoughts (Chochinov et al., 1998). Patients may look at their illnesses realistically—they may know their prognosis, their treatment, and so on—and yet still remain hopeful. Hopeless patients, on the other hand, have no desire to continue living. Among the hopeless, there is an absence even of anger—one typical reaction to illness—as well as an inability to engage in life. In a study of almost 200 terminally ill patients, the degree of hopelessness was correlated more highly with suicidal thoughts than was the level of depression.

Depression is best treated through a combination of psychotherapy and antidepressant medications. The newest generation of antidepressants—including Prozac, Zoloft, and Effexor—have fewer side effects than do earlier generations of antidepressants. Medications commonly prescribed for depression are the tricyclics, selective serotonin reuptake inhibitors (SSRIs), and norepinephrine and serotonin reuptake inhibitors (NSRIs). Doctors should be aware that cancer patients and old or frail patients may require lower doses of antidepressants to achieve results.

Should teams decide to screen more dying patients for depression, they must know how to provide appropriate treatment or make referrals. Teams of providers, including mental health professionals, can provide "depression consults," much as pain experts consult for pain, to educate colleagues and families.

Providers can recommend a treatment trial to patients. For example, a physician might prescribe an antidepressant for six weeks. Other drugs can be effective in patients for whom six weeks is too long to wait, or those for whom a quick improvement is essential to well-being. Psychostimulants often work within 24 to 48 hours.

The accompanying chart indicates which antidepressants are most effective for relieving specific symptoms. Because tricyclics are often used as adjuvant therapies, and not in therapeutic doses, they are not included in this list.

Table 15.1 Physical Symptom and Distress-Driven
Approach to Choosing an Antidepressant in
Adult Cancer Patients

| Distressing symptom | SSRI | Stimulant |
| --- | --- | --- |
| Fatigue | ++ | +++ |
| Insomnia | — | — |
| Pain | + | ++ |
| GI upset | — | + |
| Opioid side effects | ++ | ++ |
| Constipation | ++ | ++ |
| Loss of appetite | +/– | + |
| Akathisia | — | — |
| Anxiety | + | + |
| Dry mouth | ++ | ++ |

— no effect or avoid

+ least effect

+++ greatest effect

+/– mixed results

Adapted from Passick et al. (1997). *Depression in cancer patients:
Recognition and treatment.*

## About Delirium

Delirium may develop quickly; its severity may fluctuate over
the course of the day. Various medical conditions and some
medications may induce delirium.

Major symptoms of delirium include:

- Restlessness, anxiety, sleep disturbances, and irritability
- Rapidly changing course
- Short attention span
- Altered arousal
- Disturbance of the sleep-wake cycle
- Affective symptoms, such as anger and sadness
- Altered perceptions, such as hallucinations, visions, and
  illusions
- Disorganized thinking and incoherent speech
- Disorientation to time, place, or person
- Memory impairment

*Source*: Breitbart and Sparrow, 1998

Many seriously ill and dying patients experience "meaningful
delirium," in which they have visions or see long-dead family
members. Such hallucinations can be very comforting, not only

to patients but also to caregivers. Unfortunately, comforting hallucinations can sometimes quickly become terrifying ones, and health care professionals need to be alert to the importance of treating or managing delirium.

Like depression, delirium puts the dying at risk for other physical problems. With delirium, patients are at increased risk for dehydration, malnutrition, untreated pain, pressure ulcers, and a host of other problems. Rates of delirium increase with the severity of illness—and near the end of life—meaning that in the final days of life, when delirium takes the form of terminal restlessness or agitation, it may not be reversible.

Delirium and dementia share similar symptoms. Unlike dementia, delirium can sometimes be reversed, permitting patients to be awake, alert, calm, and coherent. But reversing delirium can be a long process, especially in people who are very sick or old.

Clinicians may find it hard to differentiate between depression, dementia, and delirium. In fact, doctors may overlook delirium almost half the time, either because they do not see the symptoms during brief encounters with patients or because the symptoms are attributed to age or dementia. Dementia may be long-standing but, in mild cases, not evident, complicating the diagnosis and treatment of either depression or delirium.

Because delirium, like depression, is a treatable cause of suffering at the end of life, quality improvement teams can work with clinicians to promote assessment and treatment. As with the strategies described in earlier chapters (on pain, dyspnea, and so on), teams can develop projects that increase assessment, educate clinicians and families, and track patient improvement.

One quality improvement activity is simply to assess and treat patients for delirium. As with depression, begin by selecting a unit, team, or ward on which to begin such assessments, which include the following elements:

- Use a physical examination for evidence of other conditions, such as sepsis, dehydration, or organ failure.
- Review all medications and note those that might induce delirium.
- When necessary, use laboratory tests that can reveal metabolic imbalances.

Obviously, for patients in the final stage of life, the goal is to avoid further invasive procedures. Still, by assessing all patients in a particular ward or unit, current practice patterns—and deficiencies—will become clear, and strategies for improvement can begin to be developed.

Patients with delirium are often treated with haloperidol, which is used most often for hallucinations. Thioridazine and chlorpromazine are also used. Lorazepam may be used with haloperidol to sedate an agitated patient rapidly.

### Screen Patients for Depression: "Are You Depressed?"

Rates of depression are so high among the general population that among the dying, screening for it should simply become a routine part of a checkup. Psychiatrist Harvey Chochinov recommends that doctors just ask patients: "Are you feeling depressed?" In studies he conducted with 197 patients receiving palliative care for advanced cancer, this single-item interview was as valid as other brief screening tools, such as the Beck Depression Inventory Short Form (Chochinov et al., 1997). Simply asking this question can begin an important conversation with patients.

An organization might decide to try improving depression screening rates for oncology patients or could begin with an even more specific group of patients—say, by screening all breast cancer patients for the next month. Chances are, anywhere from 10 to 20 percent of these patients will be depressed. The team could record how many patients are depressed, the treatment modalities tried, and their outcomes.

Teams can begin by:

- At initial and follow-up visits, asking patients about their mood
- Discussing symptoms of depression with patients and families
- Scheduling follow-up visits for patients who say they are depressed or who have symptoms
- Recommending treatment for patients who are depressed and, when appropriate, referring them for psychiatric care

How to manage such an endeavor? A team could aim to screen 5 or 10 patients each week for depression and could decide that within the following month, at least 90 percent of those who are depressed would be referred for treatment. Once broad screening measures are under way and the team has established a target level for follow-up, it can begin to measure outcomes. For instance, depressed patients could be scheduled for follow-up within one week of their initial visit. Follow-up for those who receive treatment can occur within another period of time—say, six to eight weeks.

Depression screening can be an early intervention, when patients are first diagnosed with a terminal illness. Screening can also become a routine part of the treatment plan. Rather than assume that a patient is depressed because he or she is dying, and consequently needs no treatment providers should assume that the patient is depressed *and* has a terminal illness— and that at least the depression can be treated.

### Suggestions for Quality Improvement

Although depression is a widespread problem, quality improvement endeavors to address it are less commonplace. Teams endeavoring to improve end-of-life care are in a good position to consider depression as a target area for improving care. One strategy might be to try out different screening instruments with dying patients. Another is to flag charts of dying patients and track whether they have been assessed for depression. Health care professionals can learn from mental health professionals about ways to raise the issue of depression with patients and families.

#### *Track Rates of Antidepressant Prescriptions*

An improvement team might establish a baseline for how it manages depression by reviewing medical records for the last 10 or 20 patients who died in the unit or hospice. Statistics suggest that several of these people will have been clinically depressed. In fact, did any patients have symptoms of depression? Were patients asked about their moods? Were any patients prescribed antidepressants?

A team could then set an aim that at least 80 percent of depressed patients would be treated. Begin to chart the rates at which antidepressants are prescribed, the number of patients referred to mental health professionals or support groups, and the number of patients who actually followed the referral.

Once an organization has a sense of its performance, setting aims becomes easy: for instance, that all end-of-life patients will be screened for depression and that all identified as being depressed are offered mental health counseling and/or antidepressant treatment, along with follow-up.

*Educate Providers on Suicide Risk Factors*

The U.S. Surgeon General describes suicide as a major public health problem, one that the federal government is working to reduce. These endeavors will eventually reach communities and clinicians. In the meantime, health care providers who work with dying patients need to be aware of the risk of suicide among depressed patients.

How can a quality improvement team address this issue? One way would be to heighten awareness among clinicians and patients about depression and how it raises the risk of suicide. Institution-wide in-service or training programs can help to raise awareness, as can an increased institutional commitment to diagnosing and treating depression and dementia.

Quality improvement teams can work with psychiatrists, psychologists, social workers, bereavement counselors, and the clergy to get important information to unit staff. A local suicide prevention group might be willing to provide training and resources for clinicians and patients.

Increased awareness of pain assessment and treatment (see chapter 3) has improved pain management for many patients. Similar endeavors aimed at increasing awareness of depression and suicide impression may benefit patients, too. Make staff aware of the suicide risk factors for terminally ill patients; adapt the following short list for use with patients and providers.

*Evaluate Suicidal End-of-Life Patients*

Once risk factors are known, staff members need to know how to evaluate suicidal patients. Dr. William Breitbart (1993) recommends the following steps for such evaluation:

1. Establish rapport with an empathic approach.
2. Obtain patient's understanding of illness and present symptoms.
3. Assess mental status.
4. Assess vulnerability variables and pain control.
5. Assess support system.
6. Obtain history of prior emotional problems or psychiatric disorders.
7. Obtain family history.
8. Record prior suicide threats, attempts.
9. Assess suicidal thinking, intent, plans.

## Suicide Risk Factors

*Knowing these risk factors might save a life:*

- Poorly controlled pain
- Previous suicide attempt(s)
- Family history of suicide
- Delirium
- Substance abuse
- Prior psychiatric diagnosis of depression
- Advanced disease
- Increasing age
- Disfiguring disease or surgery
- Poor social support

10. Evaluate need for one-to-one nurse in hospital or companion at home.
11. Formulate treatment plan, immediate and long-term.

*Source*: Adapted from W. Breitbart, Suicide risk and pain in cancer and AIDS patients, in C. R. Chapman & K. M. Foley (Eds.), *Current and Emerging Issues in Cancer Pain: Research and Practice* (pp. 49–65). New York: Raven Press.

### Comfort Delirious Patients and Their Families

In many cases, supportive care is the only treatment for delirium in the dying. Dr. William Breitbart (1993) recommends measures to address fluid and electrolyte balance, nutrition, vitamins, methods to reduce anxiety, disorientation, and education for family members. Patient anxiety may be lessened by creating a stable and secure environment—keeping patients at home, or surrounding those who are hospitalized with familiar objects.

Caregivers may become very alarmed when their loved ones become delirious. Patients with delirium may present a safety risk to themselves and others. Treating delirium requires several interventions, including supporting and reassuring patients and families. The patient may need to be moved to a safer environment. Strategies to reduce anxiety and disorientation include surrounding the patient with familiar objects, providing a clock and calendar, and encouraging family to remain present.

### Refer Patients and Families to Educational Resources

Patients and families may appreciate support groups and presentations that focus on mental health issues, including depression and delirium. Such programs can easily be tied to other programs on grief, loss, and bereavement. Programs can be offered periodically to patients and to loved ones and can provide information about depression and its treatment, the importance of recognizing depression at the end of life, and ways in which its treatment can improve the quality of a patient's life.

Many public and private organizations, including the National Institute of Mental Health, publish brochures, fact sheets, and videos about depression and its treatment. Several are listed at the end of this chapter.

Many helpful books about depression and its treatment have been written for lay audiences. Hospice and hospital patient libraries may want to add a few to their collections to recommend and lend to patients and their caregivers.

## Innovators Need to Know

- Although people who are told they have a terminal disease are likely to feel depressed and sad, clinical depression is not a healthy response to the diagnosis of terminal illness; depression is a treatable disease.
- Depression, which robs people of their ability to engage in and enjoy life, erodes the quality of life, impedes healing, and interferes with other medical treatments.
- Depression and delirium have distinct symptoms and treatments, although the two can be hard to distinguish.
- Asking patients "Are you depressed?" is a good indicator of how they feel and whether or not they need psychiatric help.
- People who are depressed are at increased risk for suicide and are more likely to request physician-assisted suicide.
- Other improvements include tracking prescriptions for antidepressants, educating patients and families about depression and delirium, and forging alliances with community-based mental health organizations.

## Resources

American Association for Geriatric Psychiatry
7910 Woodmont Avenue, Suite 1050
Bethesda, MD 20814-3004
Phone: 301-654-7850
Fax: 301-654-4137
http://www.aapgpa.org
Educational materials and resources on diagnosing and treating late-life depression, and depression in patients with dementia

American Psychological Association
750 First Street NW
Washington, DC 20002-4242
Phone: 202-336-5500
http://www.apa.org/
Resources for the public and professionals

AtHealth
Eastview Professional Building

1370 116th Avenue NE, Suite 201
Bellevue, WA 98004-3825
Phone: 425-451-4399
Phone: 888-ATHEALTH (888-284-3258)
Fax: 425-451-7399
E-mail: staff@athealth.com
http://www.athealth.com
Listings of psychiatrists and mental health professionals around
the country

D/ART—Depression: Awareness, Recognition, and Treatment
DEPRESSION
6001 Executive Boulevard, Room 8184, MSC 9663
Bethesda, MD 20892-9663
Phone: 800-421-4211
Sponsored by the National Institute of Mental Health; offers
publications for the public and professionals
Mental HealthNet
http://mentalhelp.net/
Extensive resources and links on the Web for professionals and
the public

National Alliance for the Mentally Ill
Colonial Place Three
2107 Wilson Boulevard, Suite 300
Arlington, VA 22201-3042
Phone: 703-524-7600
Phone: 800-950-NAMI
Fax: 703-524-9094
http://www.nami.org
Publications for the general public and professionals, with sup-
port groups nationwide and on the Web

# Offering End-of-Life Services to Patients with Advanced Heart or Lung Failure

## 16

Death is unpredictable for most patients—and even more so for patients who have advanced heart and lung failure. For most, death may come from one acute event or another, tomorrow or six months from now, or longer. Indeed, because they seem to come so often to the brink of death, only to be spared, it can be hard to accept that heart or lung failure will prove fatal. And patients and families can put off making important treatment decisions or discussing hopes, fears, and wishes for their lives.

Most people suffering from chronic, severe, and life-threatening diseases could benefit from comprehensive services that give patients and caregivers the resources and the confidence to manage symptoms, avoid emergency room admissions and frequent hospitalization, and remain in familiar and comfortable settings. Some programs around the country have begun to demonstrate how services would work for congestive heart failure (CHF) patients, and it seems that similar approaches would work for patients with other organ system failures, such as chronic obstructive pulmonary disease (COPD).

Under Medicare guidelines, however, most of these patients do not meet the enrollment criteria for hospice. Unlike cancer patients, for whom there is often a clear period of decline leading to death, CHF/COPD patients ordinarily have no clear period in which they are seen as dying. Instead, they slowly decline; episodes of being relatively functional and stable are punctuated by periodic life-threatening illnesses. Episodes of illness may well be appropriately treated with hospitalization and aggressive care.

Hospices wanting to expand services to include more patients with diseases like heart failure need to be willing to provide

A good heart is better than all the heads in the world.
—E. B. Lytton

what might seem like "aggressive" care, such as IV medication infusion and the occasional use of ER or ICU for symptom management. Doing this requires that hospices readjust their vision—and administration—to include patients who may live for many months or years with life-threatening illness.

## In This Chapter

Innovative programs nationwide have begun to develop programs tailored to the specific needs of patients with advanced heart or lung failure. These programs model what others can do to improve quality of care for these patients. This chapter describes:

- Tailoring end-of-life services to this patient population
- Providing integrated health care services
- Identifying and enrolling patients
- Training hospice staff how to care for heart and lung disease patients
- Educating patients and families on how to monitor symptoms and participate in treatment

## Offer Tailored End-of-Life Services to Patients with Advanced Heart or Lung Disease

By providing supportive end-of-life services to patients with advanced heart failure and lung disease, organizations can improve the quality of life for patients, in part by helping them manage symptoms, prevent exacerbations, and avoid stressful and frightening emergency room visits and hospitalizations. By teaching patients to manage their symptoms at home, programs give them greater control over their lives and some sense of mastery over their disease. By applying models of good end-of-life care to the treatment of late-stage heart disease, programs can help patients live well.

Hope Hospice in Florida achieved breakthrough results in improving access to hospice services for advanced cardiac disease patients. The team aimed to improve care for these patients by:

- Increasing cardiac patients cared for by hospice from 8 percent of total deaths to 30 percent
- Reducing hospital admissions and emergency room use

- Increasing caregiver confidence in caring for patients at home
- Increasing patient ability to cope with illness and deal with family concerns

The team followed the PDSA principle of starting with a small number of patients or clinicians with whom to test changes. For example, an emergency cardiac care medication kit for home use was initially tried with one cardiologist, four hospice nurses, and five cardiac patients. Over time, the team built on its success to include more patients; the team is now showing other Florida hospices how they, too, can meet the needs of these patients.

After a year of sustained activity, including outreach to area cardiologists and ICUs to increase hospice referrals, Hope found:

- It could maintain the level of increased referrals.
- Patients on comfort care protocols required fewer hospital days, home nursing visits, and after-hours responses.
- There were no ER visits or ER "near misses."
- Emergencies related to pain and shortness of breath could be managed at home.
- Patient and caregiver confidence in their own abilities increased.

Hope found that its program reduced inpatient hospital days for cardiac patients by 40 days per year, with projected annual savings of $45,680 for a population of seven patients.

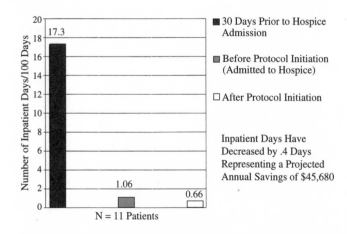

Figure 16.1 Reducing Cardiac Inpatient Days via Hospice Protocols. Reprinted with permission of Hope Hospice and Palliative Care, Fort Myers, FL.

Figure 16.2 Increasing Cardiac Referrals via Inpatient Facility via Educational Intervention. Reprinted with permission of Hope Hospice, Fort Myers, FL.

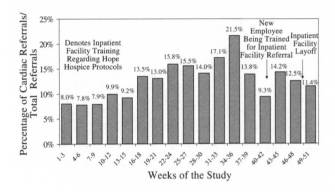

### ★★★A Model for Integrated Health Care Services: Kaiser Permanente Bellflower

The hospice model for care is based on integrated care delivery in which a multidisciplinary team works in concert to meet the diverse physical and psychosocial needs of dying patients. A similar model can be applied to end-of-life care for heart disease patients. A team at Kaiser Permanente Bellflower near San Diego developed a model among programs to improve care for patients with advanced heart disease.

The CHF Case Management Program at Kaiser Bellflower is an excellent model for others to follow in setting up care management programs for heart disease patients. In 1994, CHF was Kaiser Bellflower's third highest cause of hospital admission; in 1997, it was the seventeenth. The program has been expanded to cover the entire medical center.

Health care providers knew that fragmented care was not good for patients who experienced acute exacerbations of illness, saw many specialists, were frequently readmitted to acute hospitals and home health programs, and were seldom referred to hospice. (Of those who were, 26 percent died in their first week and 35 percent died in the next three weeks, limiting the time when hospice could provide supportive services for patients and families.)

A physician manager and case manager/nurse developed a program to improve care for heart disease patients. The program focused on four aims:

- Achieving an optimum quality of life for patients
- Providing patients with excellent care
- Preventing recurrent hospitalization and ER visits for CHF patients
- Helping to provide good end-of-life care

Between 1994 and 1997, 360 patients enrolled in the CHF program; of the 120 who have died, 80 percent were at home, and 30 percent were enrolled in hospice.

The CHF Case Management Program coordinates its services with:

- Hospice and palliative care
- Home health
- Mental health and social services
- Inpatient discharge planners
- All in- and outpatient services
- Primary care providers

Such integrated services require that each team member share information, an objective that requires teams to develop specific ways to routinely communicate about a patient's treatment and status.

## Ways to Identify and Enroll Patients

Most CHF patients are under the care of cardiologists or primary care physicians, who may or may not be aware of hospice programs and how they can serve cardiology patients. Outreach to cardiologists is one way programs can reach heart disease patients and work with them on end-of-life issues.

Teams have found many ways to identify patients and refer them to care management programs, primarily by working directly with hospital cardiology units, primary care doctors, and cardiologists. Using its computerized medical records, one team generated a list of all patients whose medical records included mention of heart disease. This list proved to be too broad, and the team tried a different tactic: A team member visited cardiologists, who reviewed their patient lists and identified patients who were not likely to be alive in a year.

### ★★★Community Hospitals Indianapolis

Community Hospitals Indianapolis provided end-of-life training sessions to staff in the hospital's CHF Clinic. Initial training sessions involved all clinic staff—nursing, dietary, pharmacy, and administrative—and educated them on general end-of-life care. Subsequent sessions included case reviews to discuss interventions for patients near the end of life and ways to approach advance care planning with them. Community Hospitals Indianapolis made end-of-life consultations to its CHF clinic, making its hospice staff available by beeper to:

- Pressing
- Squeezing
- Weight-Like
- Substernal
- Radiation
- Clenched Fist
- Dyspnea
- Nausea
- Vomitting
- Diaphoresis
- Like usual angina
- Post-exertion
- Cardiac diagnosis

Figure 16.3a Assessment of Chest Pain. Reprinted with permission of Hope Hospice, Fort Myers, FL.

- Cardiac
- Pneumonia
- Pneumothrax
- Pulmonary Embolism
- Thoratic Aortic Dissection
- Pericarditis
- Esophagitis
- Peptic Ulcer Disease
- Acute Cholecyatitis
- Herpes Zoster
- Chostrochronditis

Figure 16.3b Chest Pain. Reprinted with permission of Hope Hospice, Fort Myers, FL.

**Think:**
- Acute Dyspnea
- tachycardia
- Hx: DVT, PE, Malignancy, Immobilization

- *Pulmonary Embolism*

**No treatment desired:**
Call hospice MD
Initiate Palliative Care
- *MS neb, subc, iv, po*
- *Lorazepam*
- *Pentabarb*
- *$O_2$*

Figure 16.3c Chest Pain Assessment Protocol. Reprinted with permission of Hope Hospice, Fort Myers, FL.

- Consult with clinic staff, patients, and families
- Visit the clinic to assist its staff
- Assist in identifying which patients were "ready" for hospice referral
- Discuss end-of-life issues with cardiologists

### ★★★Hope Hospice

In its program, Florida's Hope Hospice also found cardiologists and primary care doctors reluctant to refer cardiac patients to hospice for fear that referrals were being made "too soon." However, Hope reviewed its data and found that the opposite was true: Between 1993 and 1995, 35 percent of its cardiac patients died within two weeks of referral, and 72 percent died within 90 days.

Hope used several strategies to increase cardiac referrals, including:

- Having daily discussions with discharge planners at local hospitals, telling them to refer patients who had an ejection fraction of 20 percent or less, were not candidates for surgery, and had recurrent hospital admissions and/or desired to avoid future hospitalization.
- Providing cardiologists and cardiac surgeons with referral information
- Having a hospice nurse liaison visit cardiology offices
- Collaborating with local hospitals to admit patients to hospice while still hospitalized

Hospice nurses are generally experienced and trained in oncology care. Hope Hospice provided its nurses training to assess and treat:

- Chest pain
- Cardiac pain
- Congestive heart failure
- Cardiac dyspnea

Samples of their teaching materials are presented in Figures 16.3a–f.

### Teach Patients to Monitor Symptoms and Participate in Treatment Planning

For some patients and families, learning how to manage the disease at home offers a sense of control and can improve

## Admission Orders to Hope Hospice–Cardiac

1. Admit to Hope Hospice.
2. Death certificate: I or covering physician will sign.
3. Do not resuscitate.
4. Diet as tolerated.
5. Dyspnea: O2 2–4 L prn.
6. Anxiety: Lorazepam (liquid or tabs) 0.5–1 mg po or sl q 4 prn.
7. Diarrhea: Imodium AD 2 mg after each loose stool to maximum 16 mg per 24 hours.
8. Constipation: Senokot-S 1–2 po qd prn constipation.
9. Fever: Acetaminophen 650 mg po or pr q 4 hours prn for temperature greater than 101°F.
10. Difficulty voiding: Foley/condom catheter prn; replace prn; irrigate with sterile saline prn; Lidocaine jelly 2 percent 10 cc prn for insertion.
11. Urinary symptoms: Urine reagent strips for urinalysis.
12. Nurse/pharmacist to instruct patient/family/caregiver in all aspects of medication administration and treatment modalities prn.
13. Hope Hospice physician to give orders in my absence.
14. Hospice physician may see patient at home.
15. See attached list for additional medications and orders.
16. Follow Hope Hospice protocol for chest pain.
17. For acute congestive heart failure follow cardiac chest pain protocol plus:
    _____ Furosemide 80 mg IV or
    _____ Furosemide _____ mg IV or
    _____ Other: _____.
18. Weigh every visit and prn CHF symptoms. If weight gain equal to or greater than 4 pounds give Furosemide _____ mg IV.
19. Cardiac comfort care kit.
20. Labs:
    _____ no labs
    _____ electrolytes, BUN/Creatinine before dobutamine
    _____ electrolytes, BUN/Creatinine q _____ months
    _____ INR q _____ months
    _____ Digoxin level q _____ months
    _____ Do not call normal labs to attending

Verbal orders received by: _____, RN.

Date _____

Physician: _____.

Date _____

| INR | a test of clotting | qd | daily | q4 | every 4 hours |
| BUN | a test of kidney function | po | by mouth | IV | intravenous |
| prn | as needed | sl | sublingual | | |

---

**Think:**

| | |
|---|---|
| • Acute Dyspnea | • *Pulmonary Embolism* |
| • tachycardia | • *Patient is a candidate for anticoagulation* |
| • Hx: DVT, PE, Malignancy, Immobilization | • *Call attending* |
| | • *O₂ 2-4 L/nc* |
| | • *Arrange for transport to hospital* |

Figure 16.3d Chest Pain Assessment Protocol. Reprinted with permission of Hope Hospice, Fort Myers, FL.

---

**Think:**

| | |
|---|---|
| •Pleuritic Chest Pain | • *Pneumonia* |
| •Pain Increased with Coughing Deep Breath | • *Pneumothorax* |
| | • *Pulmonary Embolism* |
| •Splinting of Chest | |

Figure 16.3e Chest Pain Assessment Protocol. Reprinted with permission of Hope Hospice, Fort Myers, FL.

---

**Think:**

| | |
|---|---|
| •Pleuritic Chest Pain | • *Pneumonia* |
| | • *Increased Temperature* |
| •Pain Increased with Coughing Deep Breath | • *Increased and Changed Sputum* |
| | • *Patient/Family Want Treatment* |
| •Splinting of Chest | |

Figure 16.3f Chest Pain Assessment Protocol. Reprinted with permission of Hope Hospice, Fort Myers, FL.

confidence in being able to manage problems. Breakthrough Series teams use daily phone calls to keep up with patients or remind them to take medications. Patients telephone with reports of symptom changes and are told what to do.

Ongoing training programs for patients and families allow them to feel confident in their ability to remain at home; support sessions with other patients and families reduce the isolation families often feel when caring for a very sick loved one.

Participants in Kaiser Bellflower's program weigh themselves daily and track other symptoms. If their weight changes (a sign that fluids are being retained), or they notice other troubling symptoms, patients call the case manager who works to stabilize symptoms.

Patients learn to recognize symptoms of heart failure, especially whether it is a "forward failure" or a "backward failure." Symptoms of forward failure, caused by an inadequate amount of blood being pumped to supply muscle activity, include weakness, lightheadedness, and fatigue. Backward failure, in which extra fluid cannot be pumped away, include lung congestion, shortness of breath, and swelling of the legs.

When patients first enroll in the program at Kaiser Bellflower, they are expected to call in daily for two weeks. Patients also receive an information package that contains detailed instructions about his or her treatment planning and daily routines, as well as relevant reading material.

Patients learn to report weakness and fatigue, especially in terms of how they are breathing. Difficulty breathing when lying down or at rest, waking at night unable to breathe, or feeling short of breath are all signs that something is wrong.

The routine is very simple. Each day they weigh themselves and report by telephone, answering these questions:

- What is your weight? Has it gone up or down?
- How is your breathing? Do you feel better sitting up or lying down, or does it make a difference?
- How are you feeling? Tired? Okay? Pretty good?
- Is there any swelling? If so, where?
- How much furosemide are you taking? Do you need to adjust it, or add a zaroxolyn?

The team has also tried out monthly group meetings of patients and a monthly newsletter. Group meetings give patients and family caregivers a chance to learn from and support one another. Presentations by health care professionals keep patients up-to-date on symptom management, emotional and psychosocial concerns, medications, and treatment concerns.

The team from the Palliative CareCenter of the North Shore used phone calls to help patients make the transition from daily nursing visits to daily phone calls. Along the way, patients kept a daily journal recording symptoms and medications. When the Palliative CareCenter first began its program, patients required several daily in-home nursing visits. During the first eight weeks of enrollment, one patient received 39 phone calls, many of these to remind her to take her medication. In that period, the patient, who had been requiring hospitalization every few days, had no exacerbation of symptoms.

### Provide Cardiac Comfort Care Kits

Patients treated at home often feel more secure knowing that medications are readily available to them or to their at-home care team. Hope Hospice developed a Cardiac Comfort Care Kit, which included the full range of medication a cardiac patient might need and which ensured that patients and caregivers could readily handle crises as they occurred. The kits contain approximately $80 worth of medications sealed in single-use, tamper-proof packages.

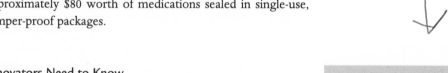

### Innovators Need to Know

The health care community may find many barriers as it works to develop comprehensive care management programs for people with advanced heart disease. Currently, Medicare does not reimburse programs for many of the supportive services these patients require; instead, organizations rely on charity and foundation funding to develop programs for patients. While Medicare reform continues to be debated in Washington, teams around the country can apply rapid-cycle change to problems in care for patients with heart disease and begin to make real reform happen sooner, not later.

- Comprehensive care management provides the medical and psychosocial services needed by patients with advanced heart or lung disease.
- Heart disease patients who learn basic self-care techniques can learn to manage some of their problems at home, avoiding the symptoms that often lead to emergency room visits and repeated hospitalizations.

| Cardiac Comfort Care Kit |
| --- |
| NTG 0.4 mg—1 bottle |
| Morphine 10 mg/5 cc UD #2 |
| Morphine inject 10 mg #2 |
| Furosemide 40 mg #4 |
| Furosemide 100 mg IV #2 |
| IV/subcutaneous access kit |
| Lorazepam 0.5 mg #5 |
| Naproxen 500 mg #2 |
| Sucralfate 1 gm/10 cc #2 |
| Maalox Plus 30 ml UD #2 |
| Normal saline 2.5 ml UD #4 |
| Compazine 10 mg po #2 |
| Compazine 25 mg PR #2 |
| ASA 325 mg #1 |
| Pentobarbital suppository 60 mg #4 |

- Blending the best of palliative medicine with the best of medical and disease management can help these patients enjoy a richer life during their final years.

### Resources

*On-Line Resources*

An ongoing conversation among clinicians and managers trying to improve care for advanced heart and lung disease is found at http://growthhouse.net/chf-copdnet. The site includes resource materials, search capabilities, and a way to use it as a listserv (sending communications directly to users' e-mail addresses). Major findings from the recent Breakthrough Collaborative on Advanced Heart and Lung Disease can be found at this site as available.

http: // www.cheshire-med.com /programs /pulrehab /rehinfo. html: This site offers extensive information materials from the Cheshire Medical Center (NH) pulmonary rehabilitation program.

*Standards for the Diagnosis and Care of Patients with Chronic Obstructive Pulmonary Disease.* American Thoracic Society. AJRCCM 152: S77-120. Order through http://www.thoracic. org/researchframe.html.

*Veterans Health Administration Clinical Practice Guideline for the Management of Persons with COPD or Asthma.* Available at http://www.va.gov (click on "Medical," then on "Clinical practice guidelines").

*Published Works*

*Agency for Health Care Policy and Research Clinical Practice Guidelines. Heart Failure: Evaluation and Care of Patients with Left-Ventricular Systolic Dysfunction.* AHCPR Publication No. 940612. June 1994. Rockville, MD: U.S. Department of Health and Human Services. Full text is at http://www.ahcpr.gov. Also available free from 1-800-358-9295.

*Living with Heart Disease*, by Marie R. Squillace and Kathy Delaney. Los Angeles: Lowell House, 1998.

*Management of End-Stage Heart Disease*, by E. A. Rose and L. W. Stevenson. Philadelphia: Little, Brown, 1998.

*Success with Heart Failure: Help and Hope for those with Congestive Heart Failure*, by Marc A. Silver and Jay N. Cohn. New York: Insight Books, 1998.

Rich, M. W., et al. (1995). A multidisciplinary intervention to prevent the readmission of elderly patients with congestive heart failure. *New England Journal of Medicine, 333*, 1190–95.

Stevenson, L. W., Massie, B. M., & Francis, G. S. (1998). Optimizing therapy for complex or refractory heart failure: A management algorithm. Proceedings of the Advanced Heart Failure Group meetings. *American Heart Journal, 135*, S293–309.

Wagner, E. H. (1998). Chronic disease management: What will it take to improve care for chronic illness? *Effective Clinical Practice, 1*, 2–4. Full text is at http://www.acponline.org/journals/ecp/augsep98/cdm.htm.

# Conclusion

*Getting Started*

## 17

Between the guiding principles of Yoda and the Little Engine That Could, organizations dedicated to improvement will find reality: Improvement can happen, no matter where a group begins. Most Breakthrough Series teams found that opportunity abounded—and that the need for improvement was irrefutable. Many innovators in end-of-life care work for large organizations and institutions, in which change is under way—albeit at a relaxed or even glacial rate. For innovators intent to improve quality quickly and in ways that patients and families can experience almost immediately, this chapter describes proven methods for launching improvements or for accelerating the rate of change. The basic steps are these:

Do, or do not. There is no "try."
—Yoda, *The Empire Strikes Back*

I think I can, I think I can . . .

*The Little Engine That Could*

1. Find out where the problems are—name them!
2. Find colleagues willing to engage in improvement projects.
3. Inform institutional leadership.
4. Set an aim.
5. Choose a simple measure.
6. Start with small-scale changes most likely to be effective.
7. Start to test changes with small numbers of people.
8. Ask for help and support whenever necessary.

## 1. Find Out Where the Problems Are—
   Name and Define Them

Teams in any Breakthrough Series quickly learn that they need not engage in long and arduous studies to gather evidence that an organization needs to improve some aspect of the care it provides. What is more important is to be able to pinpoint why change is needed and to name or define the need quickly and in simple terms.

Teams find that there are two ways to avoid additional research and to demonstrate why change is needed: Either use existing information or gather a limited amount of new information.

Examples of existing information include:

- Complaints about aspects of care
- Notes about persistent problems from the ethics committee
- Health care providers' own experiences trying to access certain services for dying patients
- Hospital or public health data about location of death
- Sentinel events in home care and hospice that demonstrate system problems

Some teams find that they really have no readily available data—and that national data and studies are not sufficient evidence for change in their own organizations. In such situations, teams collect a limited amount of information to describe how their organizations care for the dying. Chapter 2 describes many tools and strategies for collecting limited data on patients or in areas in which problems are likely. Teams can conduct basic chart reviews or arrange postdeath interviews with families and loved ones. For instance, a team might interview five family caregivers and ask them about their loved ones' deaths: Were patients in pain? Did families know where to turn or whom to call for help? What was the worst thing that happened? What was the best?

Teams can also interview health care providers to learn more about their experiences in caring for dying patients. Can they describe the system from a patient's perspective? Do they believe that the care given is the best possible? How would they describe an ideal system? What would need to change to make their own system ideal?

Another way to identify opportunities for improvement is to compare an organization or community to programs that are widely viewed as being examples of superlative care. This book is full of stories about organizations that excel in some aspect of care for the dying. How far would one's organization have to push to provide a similar level of care? Breakthrough Series teams frequently found that the gap between what they *believed* to be true about their organizations and what was actually true was quite stark and pointed to an immediate need for change.

This kind of information should be summarized in a one-page document that can be used to convince others that change is essential—and that it will improve the way the organization cares for the dying.

### 2. Find Colleagues Willing to Engage in Improvement

No matter how intelligent, experienced, creative, or energetic he or she is, no one person can create breakthrough change. Such work requires a multidisciplinary team (such as those described in chapters 2 and 11).

Colleagues willing to push for change can be easy to find. Innovators should talk to:

- The oncology nurse who is continually raising issues of informed consent
- The physician who is known for communicating well with patients and families
- The social worker who always seems to handle the tough cases
- The chaplain whom the nursing staff call first if there is an issue in end-of-life support
- The "sandwich generation" administrator who is a caregiver for a sick parent

These are examples of the people who will care about improving end-of-life care and who will devote time to make improvement happen. Teams can find support and resources from community organizations, the faith community, or voluntary groups focused on particular diseases.

It only takes two people to begin improving their own practices, organizations, or programs. As they begin to recruit a team, they must be sure to recruit:

- A day-to-day leader who can keep the improvement process moving
- A systems leader who can provide the resources and connections in the care system
- Technical expertise in the area targeted for improvement

Chapter 2 discusses details about building a team—and chapter 11 describes essentials for maintaining one.

### 3. Inform Institutional Leadership

Many innovators are not among senior management. In such cases, teams find it is essential to let senior administrators know about the improvement project, why it is important, and how it will enhance care for dying patients. When talking to senior leaders, most teams find it helpful to outline:

- Reasons for launching the project
- The project's goals
- How the project fits with the organization's mission and current priorities
- When results and findings will be reported

Some teams find that in early stages of their work, leadership may be unwilling to commit significant resources to the work. Once teams show progress and demonstrate the feasibility of making the change a routine practice, leaders are more willing to consider ways to support the improvements.

If senior leaders resist the idea of making breakthrough changes, team members should ask about objections and find ways to allay concerns. Some organizations, for instance, do not want to earn a reputation for being "a good place to die." Right now, health care organizations can find it difficult to put a positive spin on such a claim. Worse, they cannot (or do not) manage the financial risks inherent in caring for patients who are extremely sick and dying. In such cases, innovators might discuss the benefits of being known as an organization that manages pain quickly and meets the needs of family caregivers. In the face of persistent objections, keep efforts small and low-profile until there is reason or opportunity to ask leaders to reconsider the project.

### 4. Set an Aim

Setting an aim is critical to achieving breakthrough change. Teams need to be sure they choose specific, numeric, and feasible aims that signify recognizable improvement. Focusing on an aim is an essential step in creating change. A team might have a general sense that it wants to improve comfort care for all dying patients who come to its hospital or nursing home— but limits the aim initially to state that all patients with advanced heart disease will have a comfort care plan in place for at least 90 days before death.

Throughout this sourcebook, aims from other organizations are featured. These can be adapted to fit the needs of other organizations. Stating an aim offers a starting point for the team, one from which members can begin to build consensus about where to begin and which changes to try.

## 5. Select a Simple Measure

Selecting a simple measure is also critical for achieving break-through change. Teams need to choose one or two simple indicators that can track progress and improvement. Aim statements often point to measures (see Table 17.1).

Measures need to be meaningful—and must also provide compelling evidence to the team and to other providers. Whichever improvement indicators a team uses should be elements that patients, families, and providers agree are important to good care. Patients are not likely to care or appreciate that a team complies with a protocol—but will be glad to hear that it has successfully managed pain for 9 out of 10 patients in the last week.

At the outset, teams should collect a limited amount of data before the intervention or improvement begins. This need not be baseline data gathered from the charts of every patient over an extended period. Instead, teams can start with all patients on one unit on Tuesday and Friday, or with six patients each week for one month.

Some people will insist on having more baseline data before a change can begin. Teams do well to avoid the trap of collecting even more information simply to establish a baseline. In such cases, teams can agree to collect the data when changes begin—a point at which the baseline is still likely to hold steady for a few weeks before change occurs.

## 6. Start with Changes That Are Feasible and Likely to Be Effective

A key to future success is selecting initial changes that are feasible. Some teams are tempted by the idea of large-scale improvement projects—but feasibility and moderation are sometimes more useful when a project begins. Teams should

### Table 17.1 Sample Aims and Measures

| Aim | Measure |
|-----|---------|
| Increase by 50 percent the patients or their families who say their wishes were known and followed | Weekly percentage of a sample of 10 families of patients designated as end-of-life who strongly agree with the statement that their wishes were known and followed. |
| Decrease by 30 percent the patients with any day with an incidence of pain greater than 4 (out of 10) | Percentage of patients with any documentation of pain greater than 4, by bedside chart check at morning rounds |

begin by making changes that are likely to be effective and will quickly begin to improve patient care—and start with providers who want to participate in the improvement effort.

Teams can look to other organizations for ideas for change. This book and the resources listed throughout are excellent places to find ideas. Often, organizations have similar problems—and similar solutions.

In organizations in which a team identifies a laundry list of change ideas, set priorities. There are many strategies for managing and reducing pain—but only a few of these are likely to lead to breakthrough change. Begin by testing these, and save others for future projects.

### 7. Start to Test Changes with a Limited Number of People

The sooner a team tries changes, the more confident it will be that accelerating change is possible. The greatest pitfall in improvement is delaying the test for one more round of data collection, or for the next committee meeting to receive approval for rolling out the change to the entire organization. Begin testing on a small scale.

The best way to start is to try changes on one or two patients, during one afternoon or one shift. This kind of change is something that can be done "by next Tuesday." Willing team members can test the change on their own patients.

When teams begin to test changes, they also need to make plans: what is likely to happen, what the results might be, how these results can be measured and described. For example, if the change involves an advance care planning process, and the measure is family statements that their wishes were known and followed, ask the first family right after the first discussion whether or not they feel their wishes are known to the staff. Continue to study the results. Ask the physician and nurse who participated how the process went and how it could be improved in the future. Do not wait until the process has gone badly for six patients to modify the intervention!

Teams can then continue testing on ever larger samples and begin to study their results. Along the way, teams can document what they are learning and share it with others: Post a graph on the staff bulletin board to document the number of advance care planning discussions held in the clinic that week. Tell others about the results of interviews with family caregivers. Even if the changes tested show no result in the first few weeks of a project, resist the temptation to abandon the work or hide the results. Instead, use this as a chance to do a little detective work to determine whether the changes are really taking place (Is the protocol being used? Are the discussions really occurring?), then modify the plan as needed. If, over a month or six weeks, the indicators remain unchanged, then the team should consider trying other changes or using another measure or indicator to test for improvement.

Learning to test on a small scale is an unfamiliar concept in health care. Be patient and keep trying. Rapid-cycle change is a convincing and safe way to bring innovation into health care organizations.

### 8. Ask for Help Whenever Necessary

A striking aspect of health care is the resistance to collaboration. Yet getting support from others is an excellent way to jump-start an improvement effort. Whether or not a team is having difficulty getting started, members should consider looking outside the organization for colleagues and resources.

- Find another organization in the community (health care, senior care, advocacy, public education) interested or invested in improving end-of-life care, and investigate the idea of working together. Collaboration at this level increases the chances that improvement efforts will have widespread effect.
- Use an e-mail listserv or bulletin board on the Web to connect with others around the work and to find new ideas or answers to tough questions—or just to know that many others are involved in similar efforts.
- Attend national or regional meetings of organizations working on improving end-of-life care. Team members may be surprised by the number of colleagues nationwide who care about and struggle with similar problems.
- Invite an expert to visit the organization, to give grand rounds, or to meet with the team. New ideas are usually welcome—and the credibility offered by a national expert can raise awareness of the importance of the team's work.
- Visit another organization that is known for its outstanding end-of-life care. If a personal visit is impossible, talk to staff at the organization about their work: Find out about their successes, barriers and how they were overcome, other approaches to universal concerns. Visits and talks can be inspiring and can build confidence that better practice is possible. The team members can gather detailed information about the "how to's" from peers in other organizations—physician to physician, nurse to nurse, so-

cial worker to social worker. Such exchanges can provide a focus for improvement work and can stimulate creative thinking about adapting others' ideas and strategies to improve care elsewhere.

### Innovators Need to Know

Do not be daunted by a few obstacles. The system we have created is the one in which the people we love—and we ourselves—will come to die. That alone should be reason enough (selfish or self-serving though it might seem) to do a better job.

Establish a vision of a better system of care for people at the end of life, and continue to work toward it, even if that work seems incremental or inconsequential. Care for individual patients can be improved quickly—but the better system in which to provide the care will not appear overnight. Cultural change might take a generation to complete. But that change can begin today, one person at a time and one family at a time, until excellent and reliable care becomes the norm, not the result of some strange luck in which one happens to become gravely ill in the right city, with the right doctors, at the right time. Luck should not be the standard by which we measure health care—and organizations dedicated to improving that care soon discover that when luck runs out, patients suffer.

# Appendix: Instruments

## Instruments to Measure Quality

Limited research has been done to date that examines the quality of care for seriously ill patients and their families. Important first steps toward quality improvement involve collecting descriptive information on current care practices with existing instruments. Descriptive information should include measures that reflect important aspects of medical care, along with evidence that the measure(s) is related to a valued outcome or end point.

### Defining Measures for Quality of Care

The article "Measuring Quality of Care at the End of Life: A Statement of Principles" (Lynn, 1997) suggests 10 measures for improving the quality of care at the end of life. (See next page.)

In this appendix we have provided reports on four of the suggested domains from the commentary in the *Journal of the American Geriatrics Society* (*JAGS*, 1997). These reports include suggested instruments that you can use to measure these domains.

The domains included in this section are:

- Pain and physical symptoms
- Survival time and aggressiveness of care
- Spiritual/religious needs
- Grief/bereavement

Both the "Pain and physical symptoms" and "Survival time and aggressiveness of care" sections include copies of some of the suggested instruments.

Following these reports we have provided a list of suggested instruments to measure the additional domains listed in the *JAGS* commentary. Along with the title of the instrument you will find a citation for the journal in which it was published. Most instruments can be obtained and used by simply contacting the main author of the publication.

In the last section of this appendix you will find references for multidimensional instruments, along with copies of two instruments in this domain. These instruments provide examples on how to measure and examine relationships among a variety of outcome measures. This section also contains an excellent Web site reference for "The Toolkit"—a site dedicated to providing explanations, suggestions, references, and examples for measuring a variety of domains specific to end-of-life care.

The American Geriatrics Society developed this statement of principles, signed by 41 organizations, regarding domains in which to measure quality of care at the end of life:

1. *Physical and emotional symptoms.* Pain, shortness of breath, fatigue, depression, fear, anxiety, nausea, skin breakdown, and other physical and emotional problems often destroy the quality of life at its end. Symptom management is regularly deficient. Care systems should focus on these needs and ensure that people can count on a comfortable and meaningful end of their lives.
2. *Support of function and autonomy.* Even with the inevitable and progressive decline of fatal illness, much can be done to maintain personal dignity and self-respect. Achieving better functional outcomes and greater autonomy should be valued.
3. *Advance care planning.* Often, the experience of patient and family can be improved just by planning ahead for likely problems so that decisions can reflect the patient's preferences and circumstances rather than be a response to crises.
4. *Aggressive care near death*—site of death, CPR, and hospitalization. Although aggressive care is often justified, most patients would prefer to have avoided it when the short-term outcome is death. High rates of medical interventions near death should prompt further examination of provider judgment and care system design.
5. *Patient and family satisfaction.* The dying patient's peace of mind and the family's perception of the patient's care and comfort are extremely important. In the long run, we can hope that the time at the end of life will be especially precious, not merely tolerable. We must measure both patient and family satisfaction with these elements: the decision-making process, the care given, the outcomes achieved, and the extent to which opportunities were provided to complete life in a meaningful way.
6. *Global quality of life.* Often a patient's assessment of overall well-being illuminates successes and shortcomings in care that are not apparent in more specific measures. Quality of life can be good despite declining physical health, and care systems that achieve this should be valued.
7. *Family burden.* How health care is provided affects whether families have serious financial and emotional effects from the costs of care and the challenges of direct caregiving. Current and future pressures on funding

health care are likely to displace more responsibility for services and payment onto families.

8. *Survival time.* With pressures on health care resources likely to increase, there is new reason to worry that death will be too readily accepted. Purchasers and patients need to know that survival times vary across plans and provider systems. In conjunction with information about systems, satisfaction, and the other domains listed here, such measures will allow insights into the priorities and trade-offs within each care system.

9. *Provider continuity and skill.* Only through enduring relationships with professional caregivers can patient and family develop trust, communicate effectively, and develop reliable plans. The providers must also have the relevant skills, including rehabilitation, symptom control, and psychological support. Care systems must demonstrate competent performance on continuity and provider skill.

10. *Bereavement.* Often health care stops with the patient's death, but the suffering of the family goes on. Survivors may benefit with relatively modest intervention.

Instrument A.1 Standards of Patient Care: Palliative Care Standards of Practice, Community Memorial Hospital, Menomonee Falls, WI

Definition: Palliative care is defined as the active total care given to patients when a disease is not responsive to known curative or stabilizing treatment

Purpose: To meet the unique needs with attention to spiritual/cultural diversity and age-specific differences of each patient throughout the continuum of their illness, affirming life, but regarding dying as a normal process

| Standards of Care | Assessment | Frequency/ Duration | Intervention | Frequency/ Duration |
|---|---|---|---|---|
| Patients are informed of their right to quality of life as per their perception. | Assess the patient's desire for information | On admission to palliative care and ongoing. | Consult Palliative Care Nurse/Care Conference | As necessary |
| | | | Life Planning Questionnaire | |
| Patient will be involved in life planning that reflects their hopes and desires. | Assess patient knowledge/ understanding of the disease process. | On admission and ongoing | Provide Palliative Care Brochure | As necessary |
| | | | Provide other resources to facilitate life planning goals. —Symptom Management —Disposition —Financial —Disease Process —Spiritual/ Emotional | |
| The patient/family individual psychosocial needs will be met | Coping/ adjustment done: —Physical issues —Social concerns —Family concerns —Economic issues | On admission and ongoing as needed | Discuss assessment with the Palliative Care Consultant Team Consult appropriate resources | As necessary |

(continued)

| Standards of Care | Assessment | Frequency/ Duration | Intervention | Frequency/ Duration |
|---|---|---|---|---|
| Patient's religious/spiritual resources will be utilized in their care | Spiritual/Cultural Wellness Assessment | On admission to Palliative Care and ongoing. | Consult Chaplain or other religious/ spiritual leader. | As necessary |
| | | | Provide with written resource materials (i.e., Care Notes) | |
| | | | Bereavement Care —Mail sympathy card —Mail End-of-Life Survey —Chaplain to follow up and continue with bereavement care | |
| Patient and family will be able to express their understanding about the normal events of the dying process. | Assess the patient/family knowledge of the dying process. | Terminal stage of Palliative Care and as needed | Consult the Palliative Care Consultant for assistance with symptom management needed and a plan for providing the family with education related to the disease progression. | Terminal stage of Palliative Care and as needed |
| | | | Provide the Palliative Care Booklet | |
| | | | Provide additional appropriate resource materials related to symptom management. | |
| Patient's can expect to have their physical symptoms reduced and effectively managed | Assess for presence of symptoms that need management | | | |

| Standards of Care | Assessment | Frequency/ Duration | Intervention | Frequency/ Duration |
|---|---|---|---|---|
| | *Pain*: The Pain Management Record | See the Pain Management Record | Set pain goal with patient | As needed and applicable |
| | | | Discuss with physician and/or pharmacist pharmacological interventions. | |
| | | | Implement non-pharmacological interventions. Educate patient and family on how to manage side effects. | |
| | *Nausea/Vomiting*: Quality-of-life impact (0–4 scale) | As needed | Set goal | As needed and applicable. |
| | | | As above, consult physician and pharmacist. Implement non-pharmacological intervention. Educate patient/family on expectation for control and preventative measures | |
| | *Shortness of breath*: Assess patient's perception of presence, cause of SOB, and physical symptoms demonstrated | As needed and applicable | Discuss with physician and pharmacist pharmacological interventions | As needed and applicable |
| | | | Implement non-pharmacological intervention. Educate patient/family on impending signs of death. | |

(*continued*)

| Standards of Care | Assessment | Frequency/ Duration | Intervention | Frequency/ Duration |
|---|---|---|---|---|
| | *Anxiety*: Determine if cause is fear, pain, or psychological issues. | As needed and applicable | Provide pharmacological and nonpharmacological interventions (i.e., relaxation, massage, music, etc.) | As needed and applicable |
| | *Agitation*: Determine behavior type and cause. | As needed and applicable | Provide pharmacological and nonpharmacological interventions (i.e., oxygen, urinary catheter, delirium tree) | As needed and applicable |
| | | | Instruct patient/family on cause and expected behavior after intervention | |
| | *Delirium*: Assess utilizing the "High-Risk Patient/Patient with Mental Status Changes Questionnaire." | As needed and applicable | Follow the delirium tree | As needed or applicable. |
| | | | Maintain safety/environmental orientation needs (See Nursing Appendix or Delirium Manual) | |
| | | | Palliative Care Intervention | |
| | | | Instruct patient/family on cause, treatment, and expected outcome | |
| | *Constipation*: Assess per Bowel/ Constipation Protocol. | As needed or applicable | Utilize Bowel/Constipation Protocol | As needed or applicable |
| | *Diarrhea*: Assess for cause and associated symptoms. | As needed or applicable | Support with fluids, medical management, and skin care | As needed or applicable |

| Standards of Care | Assessment | Frequency/ Duration | Intervention | Frequency/ Duration |
|---|---|---|---|---|
| | *Skin Breakdown*: Assess per Skin Standard | As needed or applicable | Implement Standard of Care for skin | As needed or applicable |
| | *Nutrition/ Hydration*: Assess problems such as: <br> • anorexia <br> • dysphagia <br> • weight loss <br> • taste <br> • ascites <br> • cachexia <br> • dry mouth | As needed or applicable | Dietary consult <br><br> Medical management with medication <br> • Artificial support <br> • IV fluid <br><br> Tube feeding <br><br> Withdrawal of artificial support (see brochure) | As needed or applicable |
| | *Activity Intolerance*: Assess for immobility fatigue weakness | As needed or applicable | Physical therapy consult <br><br> Prioritize and pace activities <br><br> Planned set periods <br><br> Activities tolerated | As needed or applicable |
| | *Bladder Dysfunction*: Assess for: <br> • incontinence <br> • change function | As needed or applicable | Offer urinary catherization <br><br> Offer toileting schedule <br><br> Medical management with medications | As needed or applicable |

*(continued)*

Reviewed and Approved By:

| | | | |
|---|---|---|---|
| Unit Representative | Date | Practice Council Chairperson | Date |

| | | | |
|---|---|---|---|
| Other Discipline/Department | Date | Vice President Nursing | Date |

Other Discipline/Department _____ Date

Other Discipline/Department _____ Date

Other Discipline/Department _____ Date

*Source:* Community Memorial Hospital, Menomonee Falls, Wisconsin

References

American Board of Internal Medicine. (1996). *Caring for the dying: Identification and promotion of physical competency*. Educational Revenue Document and Personal Narratives.

Fine, Perry G., MD. (1997). *Palliative medicine primer: Pharmacologic management of symptoms in advanced and terminal diseases*. Vista Care.

Stearns, N., Lauria, M., Hermann, J., & Fogelberg, P. (1993). *Oncology social work: A clinician's guide*. American Cancer Society.

Midwest Bioethics Center Committee Consortium. (1997). *Pathways improving care for the seriously ill and dying: Guidelines for hospitals*.

## Instruments to Assess Pain
## and Physical Symptoms

Pain can be a difficult health measure to obtain because it relies on the subjective answer of the individual experiencing pain. While this is also true for other health measures like depression or grief, the difference is that pain is thought of as the actual agent for cause, whereas depression and grief are considered responses to an agent. Outside factors like personal characteristics or environmental conditions can also influence pain measurements, making the task of quantifying it even more challenging.

Most survey instruments contain measures for both pain and physical symptoms. Traditionally pain is measured in terms of sensation and intensity or through describing a person's emotional reaction to the pain. Measurements of physical symptoms may be easier to define, since we often use concrete measures involving the frequency or change in a specific symptom (e.g., shortness of breath or changes in appetite).

The instrument to assess pain included in this appendix is the On Lok Senior Health Services Pain Assessment instrument. Additional instruments that assess pain include:

- McGill Pain Questionnaire (Melzack, 1975), Short-Form Pain Questionnaire (Melzack, 1987). Measures subjective pain experience using sensory, affective, and evaluative word descriptors. The short form of the McGill Pain Questionnaire includes 11 questions referring to sensory experience of pain and the pain rating index of the long version as well as a visual analogue scale.
- The Memorial Pain Assessment Card (MPAC) (Fishman et al., 1987). An 8.5-by-11-inch card designed to provide a rapid evaluation of pain intensity, pain relief, and psychological distress. The scale includes eight pain intensity descriptors and three visual analogue scales that measure pain intensity, pain relief, and mood.

### Additional Instruments That Measure Pain and Physical Symptoms

- Edmonton Symptom Assessment System (Bruera et al., 1991). Consists of nine 100mm visual analogue scales for pain, activity, nausea, depression, anxiety, drowsiness, appetite, shortness of breath, and sensation of well-being. Instrument is designed to collect symptom data twice a day and then to transfer data to a symptom assessment graph.

Guidelines for Using Pain Assessment Tool

1. This pain assessment tool can be used for any participant. For every participant who is deemed a hospice case, it is imperative that he should have an initial pain assessment.

2. In assessing the intensity of pain, the nurse will determine if the participant can use the numerical scale. If not, the participant can use the simple descriptive scale. If the participant is still unable to use either scale, the nurse should use the Wong/Baker Faces and/or the nonverbal scale.

1. Have you had any pain in the past 24 hours?
2. Where is the pain? Does it radiate?
3. What is the intensity of the pain? Use the appropriate pain scale (see Figure A1 and Table A1)
4. How long have you had this pain?
5. What aggravates or relieves the pain?
6. What is the impact on your functional ability and quality of life?
7. What is your personal goal for pain relief? (use appropriate scale)
8. What was the worst pain in the past 24 hours? (Use any of the four scales below, Figure A.1.)

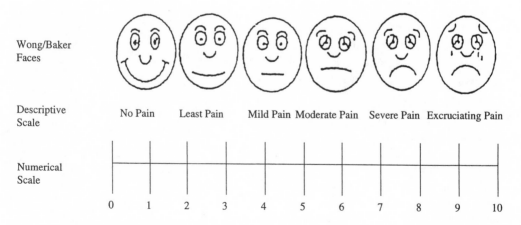

Figure A.1 Pain Assessment Scales

Figure A.1 (*cont.*): Nonverbal Scale of Pain Intensity

| Observation | Criteria | Points |
|---|---|---|
| Emotion | Smiling | 0 |
| | Anxious/irritable | 1 |
| | Almost in tears | 2 |
| Movement | None | 0 |
| | Restless, slow decreased movement | 1 |
| | Immobile, afraid to move | 2 |
| Verbal Cues | States no pain | 0 |
| | Whining, whimpering, moaning | 1 |
| | Screaming, crying out | 2 |
| Facial Cues | Relaxed, calm expression | 0 |
| | Drawn around mouth and eyes | 1 |
| | Facial frowning, wincing | 2 |
| Positioning/ | Relaxed body | 0 |
| Guarding | Guarding/tense | 1 |
| | Fetal position, jumped when touched | 2 |

9. Have you used any pain medication in the past 24 hours?
10. If yes, which medication?
11. Are you satisfied with the level of pain control with this medication? (Figure A.2)

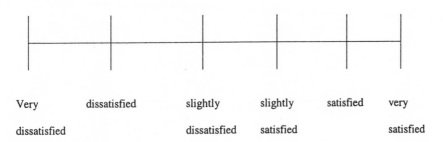

Very          dissatisfied          slightly          slightly          satisfied          very

dissatisfied                              dissatisfied          satisfied                              satisfied

Figure A.2 Verbal/Visual Scale

Conclusion of assessment:

1. If the participant has no pain, mild pain, or is satisfied with the current pain management, the nurse will conclude with:
   - "Thank you. I will check with you again in one week."
2. If the participant has moderate or severe pain or is dissatisfied with the current pain management, the nurse will conclude with:
   - "I will speak with the doctor today and we will make a change in your treatment plan."
3. Follow-up plans:
   - Follow-up for moderate pain will occur in the next two or three days.
   - Follow-up for severe pain will occur the next day.

Guidelines for documentation in chart:

1. Presence and location of pain
2. Intensity of pain. Indicate which scale is used.
3. If medication is used and, if so, which medication
4. Participant level of satisfaction
5. Follow-up plan

SLIDE

Instruments to Assess Survival Time and
Aggressiveness of Care

There are very few instruments available to assess survival
time or the aggressiveness of care. Measurements of aggressiveness of care are usually collected through chart-based documentation and include things like the timing of DNR orders, timing
of important decisions about life-sustaining treatment, time
spent using aggressive treatment prior to death, and medical
care in the last 48 hours of life. The use of patient interviews
is important in this domain because they capture the patient's
preferred approach to care and the extent to which that approach is being followed.

This appendix includes the Aggressiveness of Care Plan Discussion Documentation Sheet. Additional instruments that assess survival time and aggressiveness of care include the Support Team Assessment Schedule (Higginson et al., 1992), a
comprehensive tool that tracks a number of domains and is to
be completed by medical staff and patient.

### Instrument A.3. Aggressiveness of Care Plan Discussion Documentation Sheet

Dr. _____: _____ (# ___-___-___)
meets the criteria for discussion of prognosis and treatment plan. Please complete the following:

What is the goal of this       ☐ Cure            ☐ Prolong life
admission?                     ☐ Palliate        ☐ Provide hope
                               ☐ Other: _____

What is this patient's chance of surviving *one year*?_____%
                               ☐ Don't know

What does this patient think is his or her chance of surviving one year? _____%
                               ☐ Don't know              ☐ Patient has altered mental
                                                            status

Have you discussed prognosis with this patient?
☐ Yes
☐ No ⟹ Why not? (choose all applicable)
☐ Patient does not want to know
☐ Fear of psychologically harming the patient
☐ Preserving hope
☐ Family does not want patient to know
☐ Patient has altered mental status
☐ Physician time constraint
☐ Other _____

Place an X on the line below that best describes this patient's wishes with respect to a care plan

that focuses on survival prolongation versus on comfort

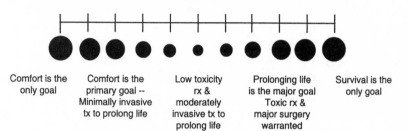

| Comfort is the only goal | Comfort is the primary goal -- Minimally invasive tx to prolong life | Low toxicity rx & moderately invasive tx to prolong life | Prolonging life is the major goal Toxic rx & major surgery warranted | Survival is the only goal |

To achieve further longevity at this time, which treatments would this patient be willing to receive?

☐ Major surgery      ☐ Short term ICU care

☐ Toxic chemotherapy      ☐ Protracted ICU care

☐ Transfusions      ☐ Mechanical ventilation

☐ Hemodialysis      ☐ Resuscitation

☐ Don't know

Signature: _____ Today's date: ___/___/___

Social Worker

☐ Patient unable to communicate →Stop

Appropriate surrogate decision maker is:

_____

Phone # _____

Advance directive: ☐ Patient does not want ☐ Provided materials to complete ☐ On chart ☐ Not on chart

Patient would like further discussion with physician concerning:

_____

_____

_____ Signature:

_____

Reprinted with permission of Neil Wagner, UCLA Medical Center, Los Angeles, CA

Instruments to Assess Spirituality

Measurements of spirituality involve identifying factors that
give meaning to one's life and how these factors correlate to a
person's health. Religious measures often differ from spiritual
measures in that they include a measurement of one's participation in either institutional or noninstitutional religious services.
Religious measures may also include an examination of the
relationships between an individual and others in their common
place of worship (e.g., social support) and how this relationship
impacts their general well-being.

*PROPOSAL*

Health care providers should also be concerned about how
well they are meeting the spiritual and religious needs of their
patients. Measures of this include such things as examining how
well a patient's spiritual and/or religious needs are documented,
implemented, and followed.

*Instruments to Assess Spirituality*

- Functional Assessment of Chronic Illness Therapy (FACIT).
  Self-administered survey tool that measures spiritual well-
  being as it relates to medical populations. Originally de-
  signed to assess the spiritual domain of quality of life.
  Current versions include measuring the spiritual domain
  of physical well-being, functional well-being, social/family
  well-being, and relation with the doctor.
  Information about FACIT is available from:
  Center on Outcomes, Research and Education
  Evanston Northwestern Healthcare
  Evanston, Illinois
  Phone: 847-570-1735

- Meaning in Life Scale (ML) (Warner and Williams, 1987).
  A 15-item interviewer administered scale to measure how
  worthy life is for an individual. The ML examines meaning
  in life beyond the dimensions of satisfaction and well-
  being through considering purpose in life, belief systems,
  and statements of faith as they relate to these dimensions.
- Herth Hope Index (VandeCreek et al., 1994). A 12-item
  interview with three dimensions including temporality
  and future, positive readiness and expectance, and inter-
  connectedness. Each domain contains four items measured on a 1–4 Likert scale.

## Instruments to Assess Grief

The grief process is multifaceted and cannot be measured through a short set of questions. Good survey instruments for grief should include measurements for how well or how poorly the individual is able to go through the process of grief.

Instruments that assess grief include the Grief Resolution Index (GRI) (Remondet and Hanson, 1995). This index is designed to identify those individuals who are experiencing prolonged psychological distress associated with the death of a spouse. This index provides a good indication of how well an individual was able to go through the process of grief. It is able to predict both short-term and long-term adjustment to the death of a spouse.

## Additional Instruments to Measure Quality

The following are suggested instruments for the other domains suggested in the *JAGS* commentary:

### *Patient and Family Satisfaction*

- FAMCARE (Kristjanson, 1993). 20-item scale that asks family members to list indicators of quality of palliative care from their perspective and the patient's perspective.

### *Global Quality of Life*

- McGill Quality of Life Questionnaire (Cohen et al., 1995). 20-item scale to measure quality of life at the end of life.

### *Family Burden*

- Caregiver Strain Index (CSI) (Robinson, 1983). Measures objective measures of burden and has been shown to predict the psychological and physical well-being of the caregiver.

### *Provider Continuity and Skill*

- Picker-Commonwealth Survey of Patient Centered Care (Cleary et al., 1991). Parts of this 61-item scale can be used to capture continuity within an organization. The survey is designed to identify the patient's experience of hospitalization based on patient-specific reports.

## Multidimensional Instruments

The following instruments that measure multiple aspects of care are included in this appendix:

- HealthPartner's Comfort Assessment Tool: Examines the relationship between pain, suffering, and coping
- Palliative Services Referral Form: Referral form to document dimensions of pain, respiratory distress, psychosocial, pastoral care, and hospice information

The following are additional instruments that measure multiple aspects of care:

- Modifications of instruments from the SUPPORT Study: Study that examined a variety of domains and outcomes specific to end-of-life care. Journal supplement provides copies of chart review instruments and summaries of questionnaires used throughout the study. Here, we provide a composite chart review instrument for inpatients and an after-death instrument for interviewing a surviving family member.

### Internet Resources

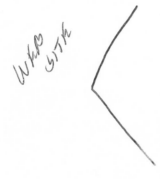

- The Toolkit: http://www.medicaring.org. Web site that provides bibliography of instruments to measure the quality of care and quality of life for dying patients and their families (originally collected and organized by a group led by Joan Teno, MD, now at Brown University). Includes on-line access to survey instruments designed for the "middle manager" who wants to measure how well the organization is caring for dying patients, consider organizational strengths and opportunities for improvement, and examine how these measures impact quality improvement.

### User's Guide and Fact Sheet for HealthPartner's Comfort Assessment (Instrument A.4)

- The obligation of health care providers to relieve human suffering stretches back to antiquity, but little attention is explicitly given to the problem of suffering in health care education, research, or practice.
- Suffering can occur not only during the course of a disease but also as a result of its treatment

- To be successful in relieving suffering requires an understanding of what suffering is and how it relates to care at the end of life.

*Key Components of the Comfort Assessment*

- Pain assessment
- Suffering
- Physical suffering
- Spiritual suffering
- Personal/family suffering caused by
  - Loss of enjoyment of life
  - Concern for your loved ones
  - Unfinished business
  - Fear of the future
- Assessment of patient's subjective ratings using a 0–10 scale
- A Comfort Index is calculated by subtracting the suffering score in any category from the coping score
- Negative values are areas that warrant particular attention, as they indicate where suffering is greater than the patient's ability to cope with his or her suffering.
- The Comfort Assessment can be administered by any member of the interdisciplinary team

*Key Findings to Date*

- More patients experience suffering than pain (92 percent vs. 72 percent)
- 61 percent of patients reported their highest level of suffering as "severe" in at least one category
- 59 percent of patients rate their ability to cope with suffering as high
- The most severe suffering was observed in the Personal/Family category
- 37 percent of patients had a negative Comfort Index score on their initial assessment in at least one area
- Improvements were noted in 70 percent of the negative Comfort Index scores on follow-up Comfort Assessment

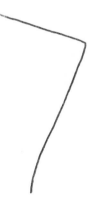

*What Do Staff Report about Comfort Assessment Tool?*

- 75 percent indicated a high level of added value
- Having the assessment on a piece of paper made it easier to ask questions

- Helps to zero in on specific areas I can help with
- Questions provided the opportunity to explore areas that might not have been addressed because it's easy to remain focused on relief of physical symptoms
- Suffering and pain are perceived as different entities by patients.
- You don't know if a patient is suffering unless you specifically ask.
- Interventions can help connect people to people and to their spiritual dimension.
- Many patients believe they have a significant capacity to cope with suffering.

## About Use of Comfort Assessment Tool

Please feel free to adapt this tool to your environment. Our only request is that you acknowledge HealthPartners, Minneapolis, MN, as the original source.

Instrument A.4a. HealthPartners Comfort Assessment Instrument. Reprinted with permission of HealthPartners, Minneapolis, MN.

| **HealthPartners** Continuing Care Department  883-6877 8100 34th Avenue South PO Box 1309 Minneapolis, MN 55440-1309 <br><br> **COMFORT ASSESSMENT**  Page 1 of 2 | Patient Name: <br><br> Medical Record #:  (label) |
|---|---|

Person Answering Questions: _____     Staff Initials: _____

*Pain*

1. On the diagram, shade in the areas where you feel pain. Put an X on the area that hurts most.

Right    Left    Left    Right

2. Please rate your pain by circling the one number that best describes your pain...

...at its worst in the past 24 hours

0  1  2  3  4  5  6  7  8  9  10
No Pain                         Pain as bad as you can imagine

...right now

0  1  2  3  4  5  6  7  8  9  10
No Pain                         Pain as bad as you can imagine

3. | Indicate the pattern of pain: ❑ Constant  ❑ Intermittent  ❑ Brief  ❑ No Pattern |

4. Indicate the character/quality of pain which applies:

| **Bone** | **Visceral** | **Nerve** |
|---|---|---|
| ❑ Worse with movement | ❑ Squeezing | ❑ Burning |
| ❑ Muscle aching | ❑ Deep | ❑ Tingling |
| ❑ Heavy | ❑ Pressing | ❑ |
| Sharp/Shooting | | |
| ❑ Dull | ❑ Crushing | ❑ |
| Throbbing | | |
| ❑ Steady | ❑ Cramping | ❑ |
| Numbness | | |
| ❑ Tender to pressure | ❑ Bloating | ❑ Light |
| touch painful | | |
| | | ❑ Itching |

5. What level of pain is acceptable?

0  1  2  3  4  5  6  7  8  9  10
No Pain                         Pain as bad as you can imagine

6. Symptoms other than pain that cause you problems:

❑ Shortness of Breath  ❑ Fatigue      ❑ Anxiety    ❑ Insomnia
❑ Nausea               ❑ Constipation  ❑ Other

7. Circle the one number that describes how, during the last 24 hours, **your symptoms have interfered with your comfort.**

0  1  2  3  4  5  6  7  8  9  10
Does Not Interfere                Completely Interferes

Distribution: White: Medical Records    Yellow: Home Chart    Pink: Staff Copy
©HealthPartners, Inc. 1998

Instrument A.4b.

| COMFORT ASSESSMENT | Page 2 of 2 | Patient Name:   (label) |
| | | Medical Record #: |

*Suffering*

### *Physical*

8. How much are you suffering due to your symptoms?

    0 1 2 3 4 5 6 7 8 9 10
    No Suffering       Extreme Suffering

### *Spiritual*

9. How much are you suffering from spiritual distress?

    0 1 2 3 4 5 6 7 8 9 10
    No Suffering       Extreme Suffering

    ❑ Can't get to place of worship     ❑ Concern about unknown/death
    ❑ Clergy doesn't visit     ❑ Unresolved spiritual issues
    ❑ Distress/conflict with belief system     ❑ Other

- - - - - - - - - - - - - - - - - - - - - - - - - - - - - - - - - - - - - - - - - - - - -

### *Personal or Family Distress*

10. How much are you suffering due to loss of enjoyment of life?

    0 1 2 3 4 5 6 7 8 9 10
    No Suffering       Extreme Suffering

    ❑ Regular Routines     ❑ Socializing
    ❑ Hobbies     ❑ Other

- - - - - - - - - - - - - - - - - - - - - - - - - - - - - - - - - - - - - - - - - - - - -

11. How much are you suffering due to your concern for
    your loved ones?    ❑ Financial
                     ❑ Emotional

    0 1 2 3 4 5 6 7 8 9 10
    No Suffering       Extreme Suffering

12. How much are you suffering due to unfinished business?

    0 1 2 3 4 5 6 7 8 9 10
    No Suffering       Extreme Suffering

13. How much are you suffering due to your fear of the future?

    0 1 2 3 4 5 6 7 8 9 10
    No Suffering       Extreme Suffering

14. Do you want any help in these areas? (check those that apply)
    ❑ Physical     ❑ Spiritual     ❑ Personal Distress     ❑ Family Distress

15. What is your biggest concern?

    - - - - - - - - - - - - - - - - - - - - - - - - - - - - - - - - - - - - - - - - - -

    - - - - - - - - - - - - - - - - - - - - - - - - - - - - - - - - - - - - - - - - - -

16. How would you rate your ability to cope with suffering?

    0 1 2 3 4 5 6 7 8 9 10
    Not Able to Cope       Good Ability to Cope

17. What, if anything helps you to reduce or cope with your suffering?

    - - - - - - - - - - - - - - - - - - - - - - - - - - - - - - - - - - - -

- - - - - - - - - - - - - - - - - - - - - - - - - - - - - - - - - - - - - - - - - - - - -

| Continuing Care Department | Comfort Assessment | Signature/Title: |
| | | Date:            Time: |

Instrument A.5 Referral Model Parkland Health and Hospital System for referral of oncology patients to palliative care. Reprinted with permission, Parkland Health & Hospital System, Dallas, TX.

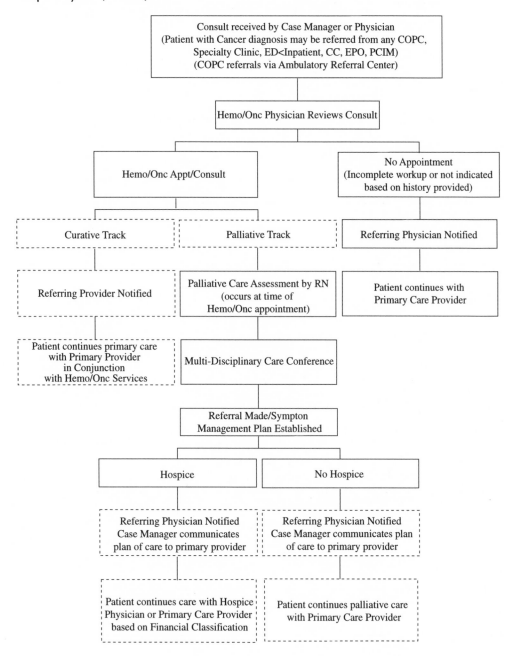

Instrument A.6 Parkland Palliative Services Referral Form. Reprinted with permission, Parkland Health & Hospital System, Dallas, TX.

<table>
<tr><td colspan="5" align="center">Parkland Health & Hospital System<br>Dallas, Texas<br><br>Palliative Services<br>Referral Form</td></tr>
<tr><td colspan="2">Department Requesting Referral:</td><td>Referring Physician/Pager#:</td><td>Date of Referral:</td><td>Patient's Age</td></tr>
<tr><td colspan="2">Diagnosis:</td><td>Date Diagnosed:</td><td colspan="2">Patient's Phone Number: (    )</td></tr>
<tr><td colspan="5">Brief History:</td></tr>
<tr><td colspan="5"></td></tr>
<tr><td colspan="5"></td></tr>
<tr><td colspan="5">DNR:      Yes       No</td></tr>
<tr><td colspan="5">Current Medications:</td></tr>
<tr><td colspan="5"></td></tr>
<tr><td></td><td>Assessment</td><td>Intervention</td><td>Outcome</td><td>Follow-up</td></tr>
<tr><td>Pain</td><td>Location:<br><br>Current:<br>0 1 2 3 4 5 6 7 8 9 10<br><br>Goal:<br>0 1 2 3 4 5 6 7 8 9 10</td><td></td><td></td><td></td></tr>
<tr><td>Respiratory</td><td>Dyspnea:    Yes   No<br>O$_2$ Required:  Yes   No</td><td></td><td></td><td></td></tr>
<tr><td>Psychosocial</td><td>Service</td><td>Referral</td><td></td><td></td></tr>
<tr><td></td><td>ACS</td><td>Yes  No  N/A</td><td></td><td></td></tr>
<tr><td></td><td>Social Services</td><td>Yes  No  N/A</td><td></td><td></td></tr>
<tr><td></td><td>Psych</td><td>Yes  No  N/A</td><td></td><td></td></tr>
<tr><td>Pastoral Care:</td><td>Directive to Physician:   Yes No<br>Durable Power of Attorney:  Yes No<br>At Home DNR:        Yes No</td><td>Chaplain Referral:<br><br>Yes    No    Refused</td><td></td><td></td></tr>
<tr><td>Hospice</td><td>Primary Caregiver in Home:  Yes No<br>Name:</td><td>Hospice Referral:<br><br>Yes    No    Refused</td><td>Agency:</td><td></td></tr>
<tr><td>Other</td><td></td><td></td><td></td><td></td></tr>
<tr><td>Primary Care Provider</td><td colspan="2">Provider Name/Location:            Pager # :</td><td></td><td></td></tr>
<tr><td colspan="5">Comments:</td></tr>
<tr><td colspan="5"></td></tr>
<tr><td colspan="5">RN Signature/ID #:</td></tr>
</table>

Instrument A.7 End-of-Life Chart Review Instrument for
Inpatient Deaths, Center to Improve Care of the Dying,
Arlington, VA

Date _____

End-of-Life Chart Review—Administrative Information

SID#_____

Chart Abstractor # _____

Last Name, First Name, MI

_____/_____/_____   _____/_____/_____   _____
Date of Birth      Date of Death      Age

___M / F___   _____
Sex           Social Security Number

Race/Ethnicity:              Religion:

1. White/Caucasian           0. None (not religious)
2. Black/African American    1. Jewish
3. Asian or Pacific Islander 2. Orthodox Jewish
4. Other                     3. Catholic (Roman or Orthodox)
5. Hispanic                  4. Jehovah's Witness
6. Native American           5. Christian Scientist
7. Not documented            6. Seventh-Day Adventist
                             7. Protestant (and all other
                                Christian)
                             8. Other
                             9. Not documented

Insurance:

Private/commercial insurance
Medicare
Medicaid
Health Maintenance Organization (HMO)
No insurance/self-payment
Other insurance

Next of Kin: _____

Name _____

Relationship _____

Address _____

_____

Telephone # _____

Is a surrogate or health care proxy named? _____

Surrogate name _____

Relationship _____

Address (if different from next of kin) _____

_____

Telephone #_____

Date _____
End-of-Life Chart Review—Inpatient

SID # _____

Chart Abstractor # _____

_____/_____/_____     _____/_____/_____
Date of admission        Date of death

Diagnosis and Status _____

_____

DRG#

_____

Primary diagnosis, ICD-9 code

_____

Secondary diagnoses, ICD-9 codes

_____

_____

_____

Procedures, ICD-9 codes
0 = no, 1 = yes, 9 = not applicable. All information should be
obtained from progress notes and orders.

Were any of the following formal directives noted:
_____ Living Will _____ DPOAHC
_____ Values History _____ Medical Directive
_____ Any other advance directive/combined directives

Date of first formal advance directive chart documentation:
____/____/____
_____ Was a Do Not Hospitalize (DNH) order noted?

_____Is there any interpretation as to how the advance directive applies in the current situation in the physician's progress notes?

_____ Do Not Resuscitate (DNR) ___/___/___ (first date)
_____ Do Not Intubate (DNI) ___/___/___ (first date)
_____ Comfort measures only ___/___/___ (first date)
_____ Full code documented ____/___/___ (first date)


## Sentinel Decisions
*All information should be obtained from physician's progress notes and orders.*

| | Resuscitation | Vasopressors | Feeding Tubes and IV-enteral | Mechanical Ventilation | ICU |
|---|---|---|---|---|---|
| Decision to forgo made before entry to hospital (0 = no, 1 = yes) | | | | | |
| Discussion with patient (0 = no, 1 = yes) date | / / | / / | / / | / / | / / |
| Discussion with family or surrogate (0 = no, 1 = yes) date | / / | / / | / / | / / | / / |
| Decision to forgo made, accepting death, and documented in orders (0 = no, 1 = yes, 2 = not mentioned, 9 = N/A) | | | | | |
| date in progress notes | / / | / / | / / | / / | / / |
| date in orders | / / | / / | / / | / / | / / |
| 0 = no, 1 = yes, 9 = N/A | | | | | |

Resuscitation
_____ Patient resuscitated during or just before entry into the hospital
_____ Documentation of conflict between:
    _____ patient and surrogate
    _____ patient and physician
    _____ surrogate and physician
_____ Resuscitation forgone: date _____/_____/_____
_____ Resuscitation tried—heartbeat established, consciousness regained before death:
    date(s) _____/_____/_____
_____ Resuscitation tried—heartbeat established, no consciousness regained before death:
    date(s) _____/_____/_____

ICU
_____ Was patient in an ICU at the time of death or within the last 2 calendar days? (0 = no, 1 = yes)

Dates in an ICU (note admit and discharge dates) _____
Total number of days in an ICU _____
_____ Was discharge from ICU expecting death? (0 = no, 1 = yes, 9 = N/A)

## Symptoms/Problems
**Refer to progress and nursing notes for the day of death and the day before.**

| Symptom/Problem | Assessed? (0 = no, 1 = yes) | Plan of treatment documented? (0 = no, 1 = yes 9 = N/A) | Monitor or follow-up of treatment plan? (0 = no, 1 = yes, 9 = N/A) | Effective? (0 = no, 3 = partially, 4 = fully, 9 = N/A) |
|---|---|---|---|---|
| Pain/discomfort | | | | |
| Anxiety | | | | |
| Somnolence | | | | |
| Confusion | | | | |
| Agitation/restlessness | | | | |
| Shortness of breath | | | | |
| Cough | | | | |
| Congestion/secretion | | | | |
| Lack of appetite | | | | |
| Difficulty swallowing | | | | |
| Nausea/emesis | | | | |
| Diarrhea | | | | |
| Constipation | | | | |
| Incontinence | | | | |
| (type _____) | | | | |
| Fever | | | | |
| Itching | | | | |
| Decubitis ulcers | | | | |
| Fatigue | | | | |
| Other | | | | |

_____

0 = no, 1 = yes; for the day of death and the day before. Refer to progress notes.

\_\_\_\_ antibiotics
\_\_\_\_ family emotional needs are noted
\_\_\_\_ chaplaincy consult
\_\_\_\_ chemotherapy regimen
focus on palliation (not life prolonging) _____
\_\_\_\_ enteral tube (NG/peg/G)
\_\_\_\_ foley catheter
\_\_\_\_ intravenous fluid
\_\_\_\_ intravenous medication
\_\_\_\_ intubation
\_\_\_\_ narcotics (as noted in administrative records)
max narc dose, last full calendar day before death: _____
\_\_\_\_ physical restraints
\_\_\_\_ surgery in the OR type:
\_\_\_\_ ventilator

## Diagnostics

0 = no, 1 = yes; for the day of death and the day before. Refer to progress notes and orders.

\_\_\_\_ A line
\_\_\_\_ blood draws, #: _____
\_\_\_\_ Swan-Ganz
\_\_\_\_ x-rays

Patient ID#: _____

Date of Interview: ____/____/_____

Interviewer #: _____

After-Death Interview
1/12/2000 Version
From the *MediCaring* Project
The Center to Improve Care of the Dying

## Instructions for the Interviewer

- *When conducting this interview, read all lowercase text aloud.*
- *Instructions for interviewers are provided throughout the questionnaire in italic print. Words appearing in italics are meant to guide the interviewer and should not be read aloud.*
- *Instructions, written in lowercase letters, should be read aloud to the respondent to guide him/her in answering.*
- *Questions should be read in their entirety, exactly as written.*
- *Many of the questions are followed by ellipses (. . .) indicating that the interviewer should read the answer choices aloud to the respondent. Read all of the answer choices before pausing for a response. For yes/no questions, as well as a few select others, the answer categories should not be read. These questions will not be followed by an ellipsis, and the answer categories will appear in uppercase letters.*
- *The interviewer will often be expected to fill in personal information into survey questions. For instance, the patient's name is often inserted into questions. The interviewer will know to substitute specific information when a word written in capital letters is enclosed in parentheses:*
  - Was (PATIENT) able to make decisions in the last week of life?

Read As:

  - Was *Mr. Smith* able to make decisions in the last week of life?
- *At times, the name of the hospital in which the patient died should be inserted, or the date on which the patient died. The interviewer should be prepared with this information before beginning the interview.*
- *When lowercase words appear in parentheses, the interviewer should choose the appropriate word:*
  - Was (PATIENT) unconscious or in a coma all of the time during the last week of (his/her) life?

Read As:

- Was Mrs. Jones unconscious or in a coma all of the time during the last week of *her* life?
- *Words that are underlined should be emphasized when read. It is important to the meaning of the question that these words are read with emphasis.*
- *At times, optional words or phrases are provided in parentheses after a question. These words or phrases should be read only if the respondent requests further clarification. In all other cases, questions should be read as written, and no definition or clarification should be provided to the respondent.*
- *Circle the number corresponding to the answer chosen by the respondent. For fill-in or open-text answers, write in the appropriate information as stated by the respondent.*
- *Based on the answers to certain questions, it is sometimes logical to skip subsequent questions (a surrogate who reports no pain should not be asked about pain severity). Instruction on skips is generally provided within parentheses after a specific answer choice. If this answer is selected, move on to the question number indicated after that answer choice.*
- *At times, it is necessary to refer back to previous answers to determine if a questions or group of questions should be skipped or read. It is important that the interviewer familiarize him/ herself with the instrument before conducting interviews.*

## Oral Informed Consent for Telephone Survey

*Introduction*

> Hello, is this (SURROGATE)? This is (YOUR NAME) calling from (NAME OF PROGRAM). I am very sorry to hear of the loss of (PATIENT). I know that this is a difficult time for you, but I would like to do one final interview with you to find out what (PATIENT'S) care was like at the end of (his/her) life. We think that this is very important information in determining how well (NAME OF PROGRAM) is caring for patients and families. Is this a good time to speak with you? (IF Yes, CONTINUE. IF NOT, SCHEDULE ANOTHER TIME). Before I begin, I want to read you a few sentences to make sure that you have all the information about the study.

*Interviewer: Read the following to each respondent. Do not proceed with the interview until the points have been heard by the respondent and all questions and concerns have been answered.*

- The study that I am asking you to participate in will provide important information about how well (NAME OF PROGRAM) is doing in providing care for seriously ill patients and their family members.
- Your participation in these data collection efforts is very important to the success of this study.
- I will be asking questions about your health and the health care services that you have received from (NAME OF PROGRAM).
- You are free to decide not to participate at all in the interview or you may stop at any time. You are free to refuse to answer any question or group of questions. You will continue to receive the best care possible whether or not you decide to participate in this questionnaire.
- Your answers will be kept strictly confidential and will be used only for the purpose of this study.
- Your individual responses will not be shared with any of your health care providers from (NAME OF PROGRAM).

May I begin?

Yes ............................................1 (Continue)

No ...........................................2 (Thank them for their time)

---

*Rescheduled Interview Date:* _____

*Introduction:* Let me begin by asking a few questions about (PATIENT'S) death and the time since we last spoke with you on (DATE).

1. According to our records, (PATIENT) died on (DATE). Is this correct?

   Yes ...........................................................................................................................1

   No ............................................................................................................................2

   ____/____/____ DATE

2. Was (PATIENT) in the hospital since we spoke last on (DATE)?

   Yes ...........................................................................................................................1

   No ............................................................................................................................2

3. About how many days was (he/she) in the hospital? _____ days

4. Was (PATIENT) in the intensive care unit or critical care unit?

   Yes ...........................................................................................................................1

   No ............................................................................................................................2

5. About how many days was (he/she) in the intensive care unit or critical care unit?
   _____ days

6. Since we last spoke, did anyone call 911 to get emergency care for (PATIENT)?
   Yes.................................................................................................................1
   No ..................................................................................................................2

7. Since we last spoke, did (PATIENT) go to the emergency room?
   Yes.................................................................................................................1
   No ..................................................................................................................2

8. Was (PATIENT) in a nursing home or other long-term care facility since we spoke last on (DATE)?
   Yes.................................................................................................................1
   No ..................................................................................................................2

9. Did (PATIENT) stay in a hospice facility since we last spoke?
   Yes.................................................................................................................1
   No ...........................................................................................................2 (11)

10. For about how many days did (PATIENT) stay in the hospice facility?
    _____ DAYS

11. Was outpatient hospice involved in the care of (PATIENT) since we last spoke, so that a hospice worker helped to care for (him/her) at home?
    Yes.................................................................................................................1
    No ...........................................................................................................2 (13)

12. For about how many days did (PATIENT) get outpatient hospice care?
    _____ DAYS

13. Where did (his/her) death take place?
    Hospital (ICU Unit) ......................................................................................1
    Hospital (other) ...........................................................................................2
    Patient's own home.......................................................................................3
    Nursing home or other long-term care facility ...........................................4
    Inpatient hospice..........................................................................................5
    Family member's home .................................................................................6
    Other home ..................................................................................................7
    Other.............................................................................................................8
    In transit to medical facility.........................................................................9
    Don't know...................................................................................................+

14. Do you think that (ANSWER TO 13) was where (PATIENT) would have most wanted to die?
    Yes..........................................................................................................1 (16)
    No ..................................................................................................................2

15. What would have allowed (PATIENT) to die at (his/her) preferred place of death?

_____

_____

_____

_____

16. Since we spoke with you last, was there ever a problem with the transfer of information about (PATIENT'S) medical treatment from one care setting to another?
    Yes..................................................................................................................1
    No ...................................................................................................................2

*Introduction*: Now I would like to ask you some questions about (PATIENT'S) last three days of life.

17. During the last three days, did (PATIENT) have a resuscitation effort? (That is, was CPR done when (his/her) heart stopped)?
    Yes..................................................................................................................1
    No ...................................................................................................................2
    Don't Know .....................................................................................................+

18. During the last three days, was (PATIENT) attached to a respirator or ventilator (that is, a machine that helps breathing)?
    Yes..................................................................................................................1
    No ...................................................................................................................2

19. During the last three days, was (PATIENT) fed through a tube?
    Yes..................................................................................................................1
    No ...................................................................................................................2

20. During the last three days, did (PATIENT) receive dialysis (or, artificial kidney treatments)?
    Yes..................................................................................................................1
    No ...................................................................................................................2

21. During the last three days, did (PATIENT) receive oxygen at home?
    Yes..................................................................................................................1
    No ...................................................................................................................2

22. Do you know about continuous positive airway pressure, or CPAP, machines?
    Yes..................................................................................................................1
    No ............................................................................................................ 2 (24)

23. During the last three days, did (PATIENT) use a CPAP machine for oxygen at home?
    Yes..................................................................................................................1
    No ...................................................................................................................2

24. Was (PATIENT) unconscious or in a coma all the time during the last three days of (his/her) life?

Yes ............................................................................................. 1 (82, p.22)

No ............................................................................................................ 2

Don't Know ................................................................................... + (82)

25. Could (PATIENT) communicate in some way during the last three days of life?

Yes ............................................................................................................ 1

No ............................................................................................................ 2

26. Was (PATIENT) able to make decisions in the three days of life?

Yes ............................................................................................................ 1

No ............................................................................................................ 2

27. How difficult was it for (PATIENT) to tolerate the physical symptoms and problems (he/she) experienced? Was it . . .

very difficult ............................................................................................ 1

somewhat difficult .................................................................................... 2

not very difficult ...................................................................................... 3

not at all difficult .................................................................................... 4

28. How difficult were the emotional symptoms and problems (he/she) experienced? Were they . . .

very difficult ............................................................................................ 1

somewhat difficult .................................................................................... 2

not very difficult ...................................................................................... 3

not at all difficult .................................................................................... 4

*Introduction*: The following questions are about (PATIENT'S) last three days of life.

29. During the last three days, what were the three most troublesome symptoms for (PATIENT)?

1. _____

2. _____

3. _____

*Interviewer: Use symptoms 1–3 to answer the following series of questions:*

30. How often did (he/she) have (SYMPTOM 1)? Was it . . .

occasionally ............................................................................................ 1

about half of the time ............................................................................ 2

most of the time ...................................................................................... 3

all of the time .......................................................................................... 4

31. How severe was the (SYMPTOM 1) on average? Was it . . .

not at all severe ...................................................................................... 1

moderately severe .................................................................................... 2

extremely severe ...................................................................................... 3

32. How much did the (SYMPTOM 1) distress or bother (him/her)? Would you say . . .

not at all ................................................................................................................1

a little bit ...............................................................................................................2

somewhat ...............................................................................................................3

quite a bit ..............................................................................................................4

very much ..............................................................................................................5

33. Did (PATIENT) tell you directly about his/her (SYMPTOM 1)?

Yes .........................................................................................................................1

No ..........................................................................................................................2

34. Did someone on (PATIENT'S) health care team talk with you or (PATIENT) about how (SYMPTOM 1) would be treated?

Yes .........................................................................................................................1

No ..........................................................................................................................2

Don't Know ...........................................................................................................+

35. Did someone on (PATIENT'S) health care team tell you or (PATIENT) about the medicine or treatment for (SYMPTOM 1) in a way that you understood?

Yes .........................................................................................................................1

No ..........................................................................................................................2

36. Did someone on (PATIENT'S) health care team tell you or (PATIENT) how (SYMP-TOM 1) would be treated if it got worse?

Yes .........................................................................................................................1

No ..........................................................................................................................2

37. Was there any time during the course of illness that (PATIENT'S) health care team did not do everything they could to help control (his/her) (SYMPTOM 1)?

Yes .........................................................................................................................1

No ..........................................................................................................................2

38. Did (PATIENT) ever need immediate assistance from the health care team because the (SYMPTOM 1) got so bad?

Yes .........................................................................................................................1

No ..........................................................................................................................2

39. Did (PATIENT) ever have to wait too long for a treatment to relieve (SYMPTOM 1) to be given to (him/her)?

Yes .........................................................................................................................1

No .................................................................................................................. 2 (40)

39B. IF yes: how long was the wait? _____

40. How often did (he/she) have (SYMPTOM 2)? Was it . . .

occasionally ...........................................................................................................1

about half of the time ............................................................................................2

most of the time ....................................................................................................3

all of the time ........................................................................................................4

41. How severe was the (SYMPTOM 2) on average? Was it . . .

    not at all severe..................................................................................................1

    moderately severe..............................................................................................2

    extremely severe.................................................................................................3


42. How much did the (SYMPTOM 2) distress or bother (him/her)? Would you say . . .

    not at all..............................................................................................................1

    a little bit............................................................................................................2

    somewhat............................................................................................................3

    quite a bit...........................................................................................................4

    very much...........................................................................................................5


43. Did (PATIENT) tell you directly about his/her (SYMPTOM 2)?

    Yes......................................................................................................................1

    No .......................................................................................................................2


44. Did someone on (PATIENT'S) health care team talk with you or (PATIENT) about how (SYMPTOM 2) would be treated?

    Yes......................................................................................................................1

    No .......................................................................................................................2

    Don't Know ....................................................................................................... +


45. Did someone on (PATIENT'S) health care team tell you or (PATIENT) about the medicine or treatment for (SYMPTOM 2) in a way that you understood?

    Yes......................................................................................................................1

    No .......................................................................................................................2


46. Did someone on (PATIENT'S) health care team tell you or (PATIENT) how (SYMPTOM 2) would be treated if it got worse?

    Yes......................................................................................................................1

    No .......................................................................................................................2


47. Was there any time during the course of illness that (PATIENT'S) health care team did not do everything they could to help control (his/her) (SYMPTOM 2)?

    Yes......................................................................................................................1

    No .......................................................................................................................2


48. Did (PATIENT) ever need immediate assistance from the health care team because the (SYMPTOM 2) got so bad?

    Yes......................................................................................................................1

    No .......................................................................................................................2

49. Did (PATIENT) ever have to wait too long for treatment to relieve (SYMPTOM 2) to be given to (him/her)?

Yes ............................................................................................................. 1

No ...................................................................................................... 2 (50)

49B. IF yes: how long was the wait? _____

50. How often did (he/she) have (SYMPTOM 3)? Was it . . .

occasionally ................................................................................................ 1

about half of the time ................................................................................. 2

most of the time ........................................................................................ 3

all of the time ............................................................................................. 4

51. How severe was the (SYMPTOM 3) on average? Was it . . .

not at all severe ......................................................................................... 1

moderately severe ..................................................................................... 2

extremely severe ....................................................................................... 3

52. How much did the (SYMPTOM 3) distress or bother (him/her)? Would you say . . .

not at all ..................................................................................................... 1

a little bit ................................................................................................... 2

somewhat .................................................................................................. 3

quite a bit .................................................................................................. 4

very much .................................................................................................. 5

53. Did (PATIENT) tell you directly about his/her (SYMPTOM 3)?

Yes ............................................................................................................. 1

No ............................................................................................................... 2

54. Did someone on (PATIENT'S) health care team talk with you or (PATIENT) about how (SYMPTOM 3) would be treated?

Yes ............................................................................................................. 1

No ............................................................................................................... 2

Don't Know ............................................................................................... +

55. Did someone on (PATIENT'S) health care team tell you or (PATIENT) about the medicine or treatment for (SYMPTOM 3) in a way that you understood?

Yes ............................................................................................................. 1

No ............................................................................................................... 2

56. Did someone on (PATIENT'S) health care team tell you or (PATIENT) how (SYMPTOM 3) would be treated if it got worse?

Yes ............................................................................................................. 1

No ............................................................................................................... 2

57. Was there any time during the course of illness that (PATIENT'S) health care team did not do everything they could to help control (his/her) (SYMPTOM 3)?

Yes ............................................................................................................. 1

No ............................................................................................................... 2

58. Did (PATIENT) ever need immediate assistance from the health care team because the (SYMPTOM 3) ever got so bad?

Yes.................................................................................................................................1

No ...................................................................................................................................2

59. Did (PATIENT) ever have to wait too long for treatment to relieve (SYMPTOM 3) to be given to (him/her)?

Yes.................................................................................................................................1

No ...................................................................................................................................2

59B. IF yes: how long was the wait? _____

*Introduction:*

60. How would you rate (PATIENT'S) overall quality of life during the last three days of (his/her) life?

Excellent........................................................................................................................1

Very good ......................................................................................................................2

Good ...............................................................................................................................3

Fair ..................................................................................................................................4

Poor..................................................................................................................................5

61. Between the time that (PATIENT) became sick and died, do you think that the sense of meaning in (his/her) life increased, decreased, or stayed the same?

Increased ........................................................................................................................1

Decreased........................................................................................................................2

Same..................................................................................................................................3

62. Would you say that (PATIENT) felt that (his/her) life became more valuable, less valuable, or stayed the same since (his/her) illness?

More valuable ................................................................................................................1

Less valuable..................................................................................................................2

Same..................................................................................................................................3

*Introduction:* The next set of questions is about religious or spiritual beliefs.

63. Did you feel that anyone on the health care team really understood what you and your family were going through?

Yes.................................................................................................................................1

No ...................................................................................................................................2

64. Did someone talk with you and/or (PATIENT) about your religious or spiritual beliefs in a sensitive manner?

Yes.................................................................................................................................1

No ...................................................................................................................................2

Don't Know ...................................................................................................................+

65. Did someone on the health care team suggest that you and/or (PATIENT) see a religious or spiritual leader?

Yes ...........................................................................................................1

No .....................................................................................................2 (66)

Don't Know ................................................................................... + (66)

65B. IF Yes: Was it at the earliest time it would have been helpful?

Yes ...........................................................................................................1

No ............................................................................................................2

Don't Know ..............................................................................................+

66. During the last three days, was there anything the health care team did that made it harder to practice your religious or spiritual beliefs?

Yes ...........................................................................................................1

No ............................................................................................................2

Don't Know ..............................................................................................+

66B. If Yes: Please tell me about it:

_____

_____

_____

_____

67. In (his/her) last three days, was (PATIENT) at peace and ready to die?

Yes ...........................................................................................................1

No ............................................................................................................2

Don't Know ..............................................................................................+

68. Did the (PLACE OF DEATH) setting interfere with (PATIENT) finding peace in (his/her) last three days?

Yes ...........................................................................................................1

No ............................................................................................................2

Don't Know ..............................................................................................+

69. Did a doctor really listen to you and (PATIENT) about your hopes, fears, and beliefs as much as you wanted?

Yes ...........................................................................................................1

No ............................................................................................................2

Don't Know ..............................................................................................+

70. Did the nurses really listen to you and (PATIENT) about your hopes, fears, and beliefs as much as you wanted?

Yes ...........................................................................................................1

No ............................................................................................................2

Don't Know ..............................................................................................+

*Introduction*: The next section is about <u>your feelings</u> about (PATIENT'S) last hospitalization and (his/her) death.

71. Did a member of the health care team talk to you about what would happen at the time of death?
    Yes.................................................................................................................1
    No ..................................................................................................................2

72. Did a member of the health care team talk with you about what it would be like for you after (PATIENT'S) death?
    Yes.................................................................................................................1
    No ..................................................................................................................2

73. Did a member of the health care team call you to see how you were doing after (PATIENT'S) death?
    Yes.................................................................................................................1
    No ..................................................................................................................2

74. Did a member of the health care team suggest someone you could turn to for help if you were feeling overwhelmed?
    Yes.................................................................................................................1
    No ..................................................................................................................2

*Introduction*: Now I am going to ask you some questions about your feelings about (PATIENT'S) medical care during the last three days of life. Please answer yes or no to the following questions.

75. Do you feel that more should have been done by the health care team to keep (PATIENT) free from pain during the last three days?
    Yes.................................................................................................................1
    No ..................................................................................................................2
    75B. IF Yes: What do you think should have been done?
    _____
    _____
    _____

76. For symptoms other than pain, do you feel that more should have been done to keep (PATIENT) comfortable during the last three days?
    Yes.................................................................................................................1
    No ..................................................................................................................2
    76B. IF Yes: What do you think should have been done?
    _____
    _____
    _____
    _____

77. Did you or (PATIENT) want to be more involved in making decisions about (PATIENT'S) care during the last three days?
Yes.................................................................................................................1
No ..................................................................................................................2
No decisions made..........................................................................................3

78. Do you feel that you or (PATIENT) would have made different decisions about (his/her) care if the health care team had given you more information?
Yes.................................................................................................................1
No ..................................................................................................................2

79. Would you have liked the health care team to be more sensitive to your feelings?
Yes.................................................................................................................1
No ..................................................................................................................2

80. Did you feel that the health care team should have paid more attention to your wishes for (PATIENT'S) care during the last three days?
Yes.................................................................................................................1
No ..................................................................................................................2

81. Did you feel that the nurses were as helpful as possible in explaining (PATIENT'S) condition during the last three days?
Yes.................................................................................................................1
No ..................................................................................................................2

82. Do you feel that the doctors were as helpful as possible in explaining (PATIENT'S) condition during the last three days?
Yes.................................................................................................................1
No ..................................................................................................................2

83. Do you feel that (PATIENT'S) doctor provided you with enough information so that there were no surprises or unplanned medical events in (his/her) last three days?
Yes.................................................................................................................1
No ..................................................................................................................2

84. Was there any time during the last three days when it was not clear which doctor was in charge of (PATIENT'S) care?
Yes.................................................................................................................1
No ..................................................................................................................2

85. Did you have confidence in the doctors who took care of (PATIENT) during the last three days?
Yes.................................................................................................................1
No ..................................................................................................................2

86. Was (PATIENT) referred to specialists (he/she) needed at the right time during the last three days?

Yes.................................................................................................................................1

No ..................................................................................................................................2

None needed...................................................................................................................3

87. Were there any problems with bills, paper work, or anything else to do with (his/her) medical care during or after (PATIENT'S) last three days?

Yes.................................................................................................................................1

No ..................................................................................................................................2

87B. IF Yes: What were they?

_____

_____

_____

_____

88. During the last month of life, was there ever a time that medication or treatments that (PATIENT) needed were unavailable?

Yes.................................................................................................................................1

No ..................................................................................................................................2

88B. IF Yes: Tell me what happened:

_____

_____

_____

_____

*Introduction*: The next questions are about your overall opinion about (PATIENT'S) care in (his/her) last three days of life.

89. If you were to describe the overall treatment of (PATIENT) and (his/her) loved ones during (his/her) last three days, would you say it was excellent, very good, good, fair, or poor?

Excellent.......................................................................................................................1

Very Good .....................................................................................................................2

Good .............................................................................................................................3

Fair ...............................................................................................................................4

Poor...............................................................................................................................5

90. Did you trust that (SYSTEM) would provide the best medical care possible for (PATIENT)?

Yes.................................................................................................................................1

No ..................................................................................................................................2

91. Would you recommend (SYSTEM) for the care of a seriously ill friend or family member?

Yes ................................................................................................................... 1

No ..................................................................................................................... 2

91B. If No: Why not?

_____

_____

_____

_____

92. Was there something particularly helpful or thoughtful that the health care team did for (PATIENT) or (his/her) family?

_____

_____

_____

*Introduction:*

93. Did anyone on (PATIENT'S) health care team talk with you or (PATIENT), in a way that was easily understandable, about the likelihood that (PATIENT) would die near the time (he/she) did?

Yes ................................................................................................................... 1

No ..................................................................................................................... 2

94. How long before (PATIENT) died did you know that (he/she) was likely to die from his/her illness? Would you say . . .

one year or more .......................................................................................... 1

six months to one year ................................................................................ 2

three months to six months ....................................................................... 3

one month to three months ....................................................................... 4

days to one month......................................................................................... 5

less than seven days ..................................................................................... 6

I never knew, and the death was a surprise ............................................ 7

*Introduction*: Now I would like to ask you some questions about (PATIENT'S) final three days of life.

95. During the last three days, did anyone on (PATIENT'S) health care team tell you or (PATIENT) about choices for treatment in a way you could understand?

Yes ................................................................................................................... 1

No ..................................................................................................................... 2

Don't Know ................................................................................................... +

96. Did (PATIENT) have specific wishes or plans about the types of medical treatment (he/she) wanted or did not want when close to dying?

Yes ................................................................................................................... 1

No ........................................................................................................... 2 (99)

Don't Know ........................................................................................... + (99)

97. Did you or (PATIENT) talk with someone on (his/her) health care team about these wishes?

Yes ............................................................................................................................. 1

No ...................................................................................................................... 2 (99)

Don't Know ................................................................................................... + (99)

98. Did you or (PATIENT) and (PATIENT'S) health care team make a plan to ensure that (PATIENT'S) wishes for medical treatment were followed?

Yes ............................................................................................................................. 1

No ............................................................................................................................. 2

99. During (PATIENT'S) last three days, did (he/she) prefer a course of treatment that focused on extending life as much as possible, even if that meant more pain and discomfort, or on a plan of care that focused on relieving pain and discomfort as much as possible, even if that meant not living as long?

Extend life as much as possible .......................................................................... 1

Relieve pain or discomfort as much as possible ................................................. 2

Don't Know ................................................................................................... + (101)

100. To what extent were these wishes followed in the medical treatment (he/she) received in the last three days? Were they followed . . .

a great deal ............................................................................................................. 1

very much ............................................................................................................... 2

moderately .............................................................................................................. 3

very little ................................................................................................................. 4

not at all .................................................................................................................. 5

Don't Know ............................................................................................................ +

101. Did anyone on the health care team talk with you or (PATIENT) about whether or not to use resuscitation (or CPR) if (his/her) heart stopped?

Yes ............................................................................................................................. 1

No ............................................................................................................................. 2

102. Did anyone on the health care team talk with you or (PATIENT) about whether or not to use mechanical ventilation if (he/she) was no longer able to breath on (his/her) own?

Yes ............................................................................................................................. 1

No ............................................................................................................................. 2

103. Did anyone on the health care team talk with you or (PATIENT) about whether or not to use tube feedings or total parenteral nutrition if (he/she) was no longer able to eat for (him/her)self?

Yes ............................................................................................................................. 1

No ............................................................................................................................. 2

104. Did anyone on the health care team talk with you or (PATIENT) about whether or not to use intensive care?

Yes ............................................................................................................................. 1

No ............................................................................................................................. 2

105. Did anyone on the health care team talk with you or (PATIENT) about whether or not (he/she) would benefit from a transplant?

Yes.........................................................................................................................1

No .........................................................................................................................2

*Introduction:* The following questions ask about the last six months of (PATIENT'S) life.

*Interviewer: Read Option A if records indicate that the patient did not have a DPOAHC, and Option B if patient did have DPOAHC.*

106. A. Our records show that (PATIENT) did <u>not</u> have a Durable Power of Attorney for Health Care naming someone to make decisions about medical treatment if (he/she) could not speak for (him/her)self. Is this correct?

Yes.........................................................................................................................1

No .........................................................................................................................2

Don't Know ..........................................................................................................+

IF No: Did (PATIENT) complete a new Durable Power of Attorney for Health Care in the past six months?

Yes.........................................................................................................................1

If Yes: Who was named in that document as the Durable Power of Attorney?

_____

No .........................................................................................................................2

Don't Know ..........................................................................................................+

B. Our records show that (PATIENT) had a Durable Power of Attorney for Health Care naming someone to make decisions about medical treatment if (he/she) could not speak for (him/her)self. Is this correct?

Yes.........................................................................................................................1

No .........................................................................................................................2

Don't Know ..........................................................................................................+

If Yes: Were there any changes made to the document in the past six months?

Yes.........................................................................................................................1

No .........................................................................................................................2

*Interviewer: Read Option A if records indicate that the patient did not have a living will, and Option B if patient did have living will.*

107. A. Our records show that (PATIENT) did not have a Living Will giving direction for the kinds of medical treatment (he/she) would have wanted if (he/she) could not speak for (him/her)self. Is this correct?

Yes.........................................................................................................................1

No .........................................................................................................................2

Don't Know ..........................................................................................................+

If No: Did (PATIENT) complete a new Living Will in the past six months?

Yes.........................................................................................................................1

No .........................................................................................................................2

Don't Know ..........................................................................................................+

B.   Our records show that (PATIENT) had a Living Will giving direction for the kinds of medical treatment (he/she) would have wanted if (he/she) could not speak for (him/her)self. Is this correct?

Yes....................................................................................................................................1

No .....................................................................................................................................2

Don't Know ......................................................................................................................+

IF Yes: Were any changes made to the document in the past six months?

Yes....................................................................................................................................1

No .....................................................................................................................................2

Don't Know ......................................................................................................................+

*Interviewer: If respondent confirmed that patient does not have a durable power of attorney or living will, go on to question 110. If patient does have one or the other, ask:*

108.  Did you or (PATIENT) discuss (his/her) Living Will or Durable Power of Attorney for Health Care with anyone on (PATIENT'S) (MEDICARING PROGRAM NAME'S) care team?

Yes....................................................................................................................................1

No .....................................................................................................................................2

Don't Know ......................................................................................................................+

109.  What role did (PATIENT'S) Living Will or Durable Power of Attorney play in making medical decisions? Did it help a great deal, help a little, have no effect, cause some problems, or cause major problems?

It helped a great deal .......................................................................................................1

It helped a little................................................................................................................2

It had no effect.................................................................................................................3

It caused some problems ..................................................................................................4

It caused major problems.................................................................................................5

Don't Know ......................................................................................................................+

*Family Impact*

110.  In the past six months, did anyone in the family have to quit work or make any other major changes in his or her life to provide personal care for patient?

Yes....................................................................................................................................1

No .....................................................................................................................................2

Don't Know ......................................................................................................................+

111.  In the past six months, how difficult was it to obtain needed nursing and medical care? Was it . . .

extremely difficult.............................................................................................................1

very difficult......................................................................................................................2

somewhat difficult ............................................................................................................3

not too difficult.................................................................................................................4

not difficult at all ..............................................................................................................5

112. Have you had to use all or most of the family's savings as a result of (PATIENT'S ) illness?

   Yes...................................................................................................................1
   No .....................................................................................................................2
   Don't Know ..................................................................................................... +
   N/A.................................................................................................................4

113. Did (PATIENT'S) illness mean the loss of the major source of income for the family?

   Yes...................................................................................................................1
   No .....................................................................................................................2
   Don't Know ..................................................................................................... +

114. Have the costs of care for (PATIENT'S) illness required the family to move to a less expensive place to live?

   Yes...................................................................................................................1
   No .....................................................................................................................2
   Don't Know ..................................................................................................... +

115. Have the costs of care for (PATIENT'S) illness required putting off important medical care for anyone in the family?

   Yes...................................................................................................................1
   No .....................................................................................................................2
   Don't Know ..................................................................................................... +

116. Have the costs of care for (PATIENT'S) illness required putting off plans for education or otherwise greatly changed the plans for anyone else in the family?

   Yes...................................................................................................................1
   No .....................................................................................................................2
   Don't Know ..................................................................................................... +

117. Has anyone in the family become ill, or unable to function normally, in part because of the stress and strain of (PATIENT'S) illness?

   Yes...................................................................................................................1
   No .....................................................................................................................2
   Don't Know ..................................................................................................... +

# Resources

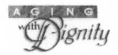

# FIVE WISHES™

*Five Wishes* is changing the way Americans talk about and plan for the care they want to receive at the end of life. *Five Wishes* has been featured twice on the NBC Today Show and is being distributed by hundreds of hospitals and hospices, churches and synagogues, doctor and law offices, and countless employers and retiree groups.

Why is *Five Wishes* so popular? There are many good reasons. It is easy to understand and simple to use. It speaks to people in their own language, not in "doctor speak" or "lawyer talk." It is the first living will to include not only the medical wishes but also the personal, emotional and spiritual wishes of seriously ill persons. And it helps families talk with their physician about a subject that before was too hard to face.

# ℱIVE WISHES

has captured the hearts and minds of Americans who want to maintain their human dignity and need help expressing their wishes. It is a gift to your family members and friends so that they won't have to guess what you want.

With the help of the American Bar Association Commission on Legal Problems of the Elderly, and the advice of experts in end-of-life care, *Five Wishes* was written to meet the legal requirements under the health decision statutes of 33 states and the District of Columbia.

## FIVE WISHES STATES

ℐf you live in the District of Columbia or one of the 33 states listed below, you can use *Five Wishes* and have the peace of mind to know that it meets your state's requirements under the law:

| | | | |
|---|---|---|---|
| Arizona | Idaho | Mississippi | Pennsylvania |
| Arkansas | Illinois | Missouri | Rhode Island |
| Colorado | Iowa | Montana | South Dakota |
| Connecticut | Louisiana | Nebraska | Tennessee |
| Delaware | Maine | New Jersey | Virginia |
| District of Columbia | Maryland | New Mexico | Washington |
| Florida | Massachusetts | New York | Wyoming |
| Georgia | Michigan | North Carolina | |
| Hawaii | Minnesota | North Dakota | |

ℐf your state is not one of the 33 states listed above, *Five Wishes* does **not** meet the technical requirements in the statutes of your state, and some doctors in your state may be reluctant to honor *Five Wishes*. However, you can still use *Five Wishes* to put your wishes in writing. This will be a helpful guide to your care providers. Most doctors and health care professionals understand that they have a duty to listen to your wishes no matter how you express them.

Talk to your doctor during your next office visit. Give your doctor a copy of *Five Wishes* and ask to have a talk about it. Make sure your doctor understands your wishes and will honor them. Ask him or her to urge other doctors treating you to honor them.

You have a legal and moral right to decide what kind of medical treatment you want or don't want when you are seriously ill and your death is expected. You also have a right to choose a person to make health care decisions for you when you are no longer able to speak or think clearly. *Five Wishes* helps you exercise these rights. But remember, your doctor needs to know, and be willing to follow, your wishes.

## HOW DO I CHANGE TO *FIVE WISHES*?

If you already have completed a living will or durable power of attorney for health care (such as a previous edition of *Five Wishes*), you may want to change over to the new *Five Wishes* instead. All you need to do to is fill out and sign your new edition of *Five Wishes* as directed in the instructions. This takes away any advance directive you had before. To make sure the right form is used, please do the following:

• Destroy all copies of your old living will and/or durable power of attorney for health care, or write "revoked" in large letters across the copy you have (notify your lawyer if he or she helped prepare those old forms for you),                          AND

• Tell your Health Care Agent, family members and doctor that you have filled out the new *Five Wishes*, and tell them what your wishes are.

## 1 The Person I Want To Make Health Care Decisions For Me When I Can't Make Them For Myself

If I am no longer able to make my own health care decisions, this form names the person I choose to make these choices for me. This person will be my Health Care Agent (or other term that may be used in my state, such as proxy, representative, or surrogate).

This person will make my health care choices if both of these things happen:
1) My attending or treating doctor finds that I am no longer able to make health care choices,
AND
2) Another health care professional agrees that this is true.

### PICKING THE RIGHT PERSON TO BE YOUR HEALTH CARE AGENT

Choose someone who knows you very well and cares about you, and who can make difficult decisions. Sometimes a spouse or family member is not the best choice because they are too emotionally involved with you. Sometimes they are the best choice. You know best. Make sure you choose someone who is able to stand up for you so that your wishes are followed. Also, choose someone who is likely to be nearby so that they are ready to help you when you need them.

Whether you choose your spouse, family member or friend to be your Health Care Agent, make sure you talk about your wishes with this person and that he or she agrees to respect and follow them.

Your Health Care Agent should be at least **18 years or older** (in Colorado, 21 years or older) and should not be:
- your health care provider, including owner or operator of a health or residential or community care facility serving you.
- an employee of your health care provider.
- serving as an agent or proxy for 10 or more people unless he or she is your spouse or close relative.

### The person I choose as my Health Care Agent is:

NAME

PHONE NUMBER

ADDRESS

CITY/STATE/ZIP

If this person
- Is not able or willing to make these choices for me,
- Is divorced or legally separated from me, OR
- This person has died,

### Then these people are my next choices:

SECOND CHOICE NAME

PHONE NUMBER

ADDRESS

CITY/STATE/ZIP

THIRD CHOICE NAME

PHONE NUMBER

ADDRESS

CITY/STATE/ZIP

1 of 8

I understand that my Health Care Agent can make health care decisions for me. I want my Agent to be able to do the following **(Please cross out anything you don't want your Agent to do that is listed below):**

- Make choices for me about my medical care or services, like tests, medicine, or surgery. This care or service could be to find out what my health problem is, or how to treat it. It can also include care to keep me alive. If the treatment or care has already started, my Health Care Agent can keep it going or have it stopped.

- Interpret any instructions I have given in this form or given in other discussions, according to my Health Care Agent's understanding of my wishes and values.

- Arrange for admission to a hospital, hospice, or nursing home for me. My Health Care Agent can hire any kind of health care worker I may need to help me or take care of me. My Agent may also fire a health care worker, if needed.

- Make the decision to request, take away or not give medical treatments, including artificially-provided food and water, and any other treatments to keep me alive.

- See and approve release of my medical records and personal files. If I need to sign my name to get any of these files, my Health Care Agent can sign for me.

- Move me to another state, to carry out my wishes. My Health Care Agent can also move me to another state for other reasons.

- Take any legal action needed to carry out my wishes.

- Apply for Medicare, Medicaid, or other programs or insurance benefits for me. My Health Care Agent can see my personal files, like bank records, to find out what is needed to fill out these forms.

- Listed below are any changes, additions, or other limitations on my Health Care Agent's powers:

_____
_____
_____
_____
_____
_____
_____
_____
_____
_____
_____
_____
_____
_____
_____
_____
_____
_____
_____
_____
_____

## If I change my mind about having a Health Care Agent, I will:

- Destroy all copies of this Part of the *Five Wishes* form, OR

- Write the word "Revoked" in large letters across the name of each agent whose authority I want to cancel and signing my name on that page, OR

- Tell someone, such as my doctor or family, that I want to cancel or change my Health Care Agent.

**2 of 8**

## 2 My Wish For The Kind Of Medical Treatment I Want Or Don't Want

I believe that my life is precious and I deserve to be treated with dignity. When the time comes that I am very sick and am not able to speak for myself, I want the following wishes, and any other instructions I have given to my Health Care Agent, to be respected and followed.

The instructions that I am including in this section are to let my family, my doctors and other health care providers, my friends and all others know the kind of medical treatment that I want or don't want.

### A. General Instructions

- I do not want to be in pain. I want my doctor to give me enough medicine to relieve my pain, even if that means that I will be drowsy or sleep more than I would otherwise.

- I do not want anything done or omitted by my doctors or nurses *with the intention of taking my life.*

- I want to be offered food and fluids by mouth, and kept clean and warm.

### B. Meaning of "Life-Support Treatment"

Life-support treatment means any medical procedure, device or medication to keep me alive. Life-support treatment includes: medical devices put in me to help me breathe; food and water supplied artificially by medical device (tube feeding); cardiopulmonary resuscitation (CPR); major surgery; blood transfusions; dialysis; and antibiotics.

If I wish to limit the meaning of life-support treatment, I write this limitation in the space below:

_____
_____
_____
_____
_____
_____
_____
_____
_____
_____
_____
_____
_____
_____
_____
_____
_____
_____

### C. If I am close to death:

If my doctor and another health care professional both decide that I am likely to die within a short period of time, and life-support treatment would only postpone the moment of my death (**choose one of the following**):

☐ I want to have life-support treatment.

☐ I do not want life-support treatment. If it has been started, I want it stopped.

☐ I want to have life-support treatment if my doctor believes it could help, but I want my doctor to stop giving me life-support treatment if it is not helping my health condition or symptoms.

## D. If I am in a coma and I am not expected to wake up or recover:

If my doctor and another health care professional both decide that I am in a coma from which I am not expected to wake up or recover, and I have brain damage, and life-support treatment would only postpone the moment of my death (choose *one* of the following):

☐ I want to have life-support treatment.

☐ I do not want life-support treatment. If it has been started, I want it stopped.

☐ I want to have life-support treatment if my doctor believes it could be helpful, but I want my doctor to stop giving me life-support treatment if it is not helping my health condition or symptoms.

## E. If I have permanent and severe brain damage and I am not expected to recover:

If my doctor and another health care professional both decide that I have permanent and severe brain damage, (for example, I can open my eyes, I can not speak or understand) and I am not expected to recover, and life-support treatment would only postpone the moment of my death (choose *one* of the following):

☐ I want to have life-support treatment.

☐ I do not want life-support treatment. If it has been started, I want it stopped.

☐ I want to have life-support treatment if my doctor believes it could help, but I want my doctor to stop giving me life-support treatment if it is not helping my health condition or symptoms.

## F. If I am in another condition under which I do not wish to be kept alive:

If there is another condition under which I do not wish to have life-support treatment, I describe it below. In this condition, I believe that the costs and burdens of life-support treatment are too much and not worth the benefits to me. Therefore, in this condition, I do not want life-support treatment. (For example, you may write "end-stage condition." That means that your health has gotten worse and you are not able to take care of yourself in any way, mentally or physically. Life-support treatment will not help you get better.)

(Please leave the space blank if you have none.)

_____

_____

_____

_____

_____

---

### IN CASE OF AN EMERGENCY...

If you have a medical emergency and ambulance personnel arrive, they may look to see if you have a **Do Not Resuscitate** form or bracelet. Many states require a person to have a **Do Not Resuscitate** form filled out and signed by a doctor. This form lets ambulance personnel know that you don't want them to use life-support treatment when you are in the process of dying. Please check with your doctor or with your local hospital, hospice, or health officials to see if you need to have a **Do Not Resuscitate** form filled out.

---

When you talk with your family, doctor, Health Care Agent, and priest, minister or rabbi about what you have chosen, you may feel that the above instructions do not express all of your wishes, or your own religious beliefs. Please use the space below to make very clear what you want, and under what conditions.

_____

_____

_____

_____

## Part B

I want to be treated with dignity near the end of my life as Part A of Five Wishes is followed. To be treated with dignity means that I would like people to do the things written in Part B when it can be done.

I understand that my family, my doctors and other health care providers, my friends, and others may not be able to do the things, or are not required by law to do the things written in Part B.

I do not expect my wishes in Part B to place new or added legal duties on my doctors or other health care providers.  I also do not expect these wishes in Part B to excuse my doctor or other health care providers from giving me the proper care asked for by law.

### 3 My Wish For How Comfortable I Want To Be

*(Please cross out anything that you **don't** agree with)*

- I do not want to be in pain. I want my doctor to give me enough medicine to relieve my pain, even if that means that I will be drowsy or sleep more than I would otherwise.
- If I show signs of depression, nausea, shortness of breath, or hallucinations, I want my caregivers to do whatever they can to help me.
- I wish to have a cool moist cloth put on my head if I have a fever.
- I want my lips and mouth kept moist to stop dryness.
- I wish to have warm baths often.  I wish to be kept fresh and clean at all times.
- I wish to be massaged with warm oils as often as I can be.
- I wish to have my favorite music played when possible until my time of death.
- I wish to have personal care like shaving, nail clipping, hair brushing, and teeth brushing, as long as they do not cause me pain or discomfort.
- I wish to have religious readings and well loved poems read aloud when I am near death.

### 4 My Wish For How I Want People To Treat Me

*(Please cross out anything that you **don't** agree with)*

- I wish to have people with me when possible. I want someone to be with me when it seems that death may come at any time.
- I wish to have my hand held and to be talked to when possible, even if I don't seem to respond to the voice or touch of others.
- I wish to have others by my side praying for me when possible.
- I wish to have the members of my church or synagogue told that I am sick and asked to pray for me and visit me.
- I wish to be cared for with kindness and cheerfulness, and not sadness.
- I wish to have pictures of my loved ones in my room, near my bed.
- If I am not able to control my bowel or bladder functions, I wish for my clothes and bed linens to be kept clean, and for them to be changed as soon as they can be if they have been soiled.
- I want to die in my home, if that can be done.

# 5 My Wish For What I Want My Loved Ones To Know

*(Please cross out anything that you **don't** agree with)*

- I wish to have my family members and loved ones know that I love them.
- I wish to be forgiven for the times I have hurt my family, friends, and others.
- I wish to have my family members and friends know that I forgive them for what they may have done to me in my life.
- I wish for my family members and loved ones to know that because of the faith I have,

I do not fear death itself. I think it is not the end, but a new beginning for me.
- I wish for all of my family members to make peace with each other before my death, if they can.
- I wish for my family and friends to think about what I was like before I had a terminal illness. I want them to remember me in this way after my death.
- I wish for my family and friends to look at my dying as a time of personal growth for everyone, including me. This will help me live a meaningful life in my final days.
- I wish for my family and friends to get counseling if they have trouble with my death. I want memories of my life to give them joy and not sorrow.

If anyone asks how I want to be remembered, please say the following about me:

_____

_____

_____

_____

The following person knows my funeral wishes: _____

If there is to be a memorial service for me, I wish for this service to include the following *(list music, songs, readings or other specific requests that you have)*:

_____

_____

_____

_____

**Add other wishes here** *(such as your wishes about donating any or all parts of your body when you die)*:

_____

_____

_____

_____

_____

_____

# SIGNING THE FIVE WISHES FORM

*Please make sure you sign your Five Wishes form in the presence of the two witnesses.*
*Make sure they sign their names in your presence. You <u>do not</u> need to have this form notarized unless you*
*live in Hawaii, Missouri, North Carolina or Tennessee (see below).*

I, _____ , ask that my family, my doctors and other health care providers, my
   <sub>Print Your Name</sub>
friends, and all others, follow my wishes as communicated by my Health Care Agent (if I have one and he or she is available), or as otherwise expressed in this form. If any part of this form cannot be legally followed, I ask that all other parts of this form be followed. I also revoke any prior health care advance directives of mine.

Signature: _____

Address: _____

_____

Phone #: _____     Date: _____

7 of 8

## WITNESS STATEMENT (2 witnesses needed):

I declare that the person who signed or acknowledged this form (hereafter "person") is personally known to me, that he/she signed or acknowledged this [Health Care Agent and/or Living Will form(s)] in my presence, and that he/she appears to be of sound mind and under no duress, fraud, or undue influence.

I also declare that **I am over 19 years of age and am NOT**:

- the individual appointed as (agent/proxy/surrogate/patient advocate) by this document,
- the person's health care provider, including owner or operator of a health, long-term care, or other residential or community care facility serving the person,
- an employee of the person's health care provider,
- financially responsible for the person's health care,

- an employee of a life or health insurance provider for the person,
- related to the person by blood, marriage, or adoption, and,
- to the best of my knowledge, a creditor of the person or entitled to any part of his/her estate under a will or codicil, by operation of law.

**Signature of Witness (1)** _____

Print Name of Witness    _____

Address                  _____

                         _____

Phone Number(s)          _____

**Signature of Witness (2)** _____

Print Name of Witness    _____

Address                  _____

                         _____

Phone Number(s)          _____

**If you are a resident of Hawaii, Missouri, North Carolina, or Tennessee**, you should have the following completed. If you live in any other state, you <u>do not</u> need to have the following completed.

### NOTARIZATION

STATE OF _____ )

                                        )ss.

COUNTY OF_____ )

On this _____ day of _____, 19/20_____ , the said _____
_____, and _____, known to me (or satisfactorily proven) to be the person named in the foregoing instrument and witnesses, respectively, personally appeared before me, a Notary Public, within and for the State and County aforesaid, and acknowledged that they freely and voluntarily executed the same for the purposes stated therein.

My Commission Expires:        _____
                              NOTARY PUBLIC

*Note:* This material is provided by permission of Aging With Dignity, which makes it available for reading only. Any further use beyond reading, including, but not limited to, photocopying and other similar reproduction requires the advance permission of Aging With Dignity, 215 South Monroe Street, Suite 620, Tallahassee, FL 32301, 850-681-2010. To obtain additional copies of the Five Wishes booklet, send your request to: Aging with Dignity, P.O. Box 1661, Tallahassee, FL 32302-1661. Aging with Dignity requests a donation of $4 per copy to defray printing and mailing costs, or $1 per copy for orders of 10 copies or more; checks or money orders can be made payable to Aging with Dignity.

Patient Name _____ Medical Record# _____

Checklist: To be completed by Communications Coordinator

**St. Thomas Health Services**
**Elements of Care Checklist**

I. Caregivers

    A. Responsible physician (be prepared to change if necessary)

    _____

    B. Communications coordinator (Person who will be responsible for continuity and consistency of information)

    _____

    C. House officer and/or physician-employed nurse clinician who will actively participate in coordinating communication

    _____

    D. Nursing staff members participating actively in communication (may change but the goal is consistency) (no more than three)

    _____

    _____

    _____

    E. Other involved staff (pastoral care [always], ethics, case manager, respiratory therapists, etc.,) (no more than three)

    _____

    _____

    _____

    F. Other consultants who may speak to the patient and/or family

    _____

II. Patient

    A. Advance directives

        1. Do they exist?    Yes        No

        2. Are they in the chart?    Yes        No

        3. If advance directives exist but are not in chart, what is being done to make them available?

    _____

    B. Has code status been discussed?    Yes        No

    C. Code Status—DNR        DNI        Neither

    D. Is patient competent?    Yes        No        Questionable

    E. If patient not competent, who is surrogate?

    _____

    (Designate if durable power of attorney for health care, otherwise may be more than one person)

    F. If patient incompetent, does family have internal dissension that will be a problem?    Yes
    No

    G. Is there family or team conflict? Describe it

    _____

    _____

    H. Plan to deal with conflict (consults to social work, ethics)

    _____

I.  Does the surrogate(s) know the patient's wishes and goals and are they able to articulate them?
    Yes        No
J.  Basic goals as minimal end point of therapy:
    _____

K.  Other complicating factors:
    _____

L.  Particular spiritual needs:
    _____

M.  Unusual communications problems and solutions (language difficulties, etc.):
    _____


Daily Checklist
(Filled out by individual present at physician discussion
with patient/surrogate)
_____

Date _____
Location (hospital unit) _____
_____

Has physician or representative (could be house officer or nurse clinician, as long as they clearly carry message of responsible physician) spoken to patient or surrogate family (if patient incompetent)   Yes        No

_____
Name of physician or representative

Other caregiver who was present at discussion (nurse, pastoral care, communications coordinator, etc.) For consistent message, one of team should always be present at this discussion.

_____

Current assessment of prognosis:
_____

Plan for next 24 hours (include symptom management):
_____

Chart documentation reflecting above?   Yes        No
New discussion regarding DNR status, withdrawal, or related end-of-life issues:
_____

Precepts of Palliative Care, Last Acts
Palliative Care Task Force

Palliative care refers to the comprehensive management of the physical, psychological, social, spiritual, and existential needs of patients. It is especially suited to the care of people with incurable, progressive illnesses.

Palliative care affirms life and regards dying as a natural process that is a profoundly personal experience for the individual and family. The goal of palliative care is to achieve the best possible quality of life through relief of suffering, control of symptoms, and restoration of functional capacity while remaining sensitive to personal, cultural, and religious values, beliefs, and practices.

Palliative care can be complementary to other therapies that are available and appropriate to the identified goals of care. The intensity and range of palliative interventions may increase as illness progresses and the complexity of care and needs of the patients and their families increase. The priority of care frequently shifts during this time to focus on the dying process with an emphasis on end-of-life decision making and care that supports physical comfort and a death that is consistent with the values and expressed desires of the patient.

Palliative care guides patients and families as they make the transition through the changing goals of care and helps the dying patient who wishes to address issues of life completion and life closure.

Palliative care has become an area of special expertise within medicine, nursing, social work, pharmacy, chaplaincy, and other disciplines. However, advances in palliative care have not yet been integrated effectively into standard clinical practice. The fundamental precepts of palliation should be a basic component of the attitudes, knowledge base, and practice skills of all clinicians.

The Last Acts Palliative Care Task Force believes that acknowledgment and incorporation of the following core precepts into all end-of-life care can serve as a starting point for needed reform.

## Respecting Patient Goals, Preferences, and Choices

*Palliative care:*

- Is an approach to care that is foremost patient-centered and addresses patient needs within the context of family and community
- Recognizes that the family constellation is defined by the patient and encourages family involvement in planning and providing care to the extent the patient desires
- Identifies and honors the preferences of the patient and family through careful attention to their values, goals, and priorities, as well as their cultural and spiritual perspectives
- Assists patients in establishing goals of care by facilitating their understanding of their diagnosis and prognosis, clarifying priorities, promoting informed choices, and providing an opportunity for negotiating a care plan with providers
- Strives to meet patients' preferences about care settings, living situations, and services, recognizing the uniqueness of these preferences and the barriers to accomplishing them.
- Encourages advance care planning, including advance directives, through ongoing dialogue among providers, patient, and family
- Recognizes the potential for conflicts among patient, family, providers, and payors, and develops processes to work toward resolution

## Comprehensive Caring

*Palliative care:*

- Appreciates that dying, while a normal process, is a critical period in the life of the patient and family, and responds aggressively to the associated human suffering while acknowledging the potential for personal growth
- Places a high priority on physical comfort and functional capacity, including, but not limited to: expert management of pain and other symptoms, diagnosis and treatment of psychological distress, and assistance in remaining as independent as possible or desired
- Provides physical, psychological, social, and spiritual support to help the patient and family adapt to the anticipated

decline associated with advanced, progressive, incurable disease

- Alleviates isolation through a commitment to non-abandonment, ongoing communication, and sustaining relationships
- Assists with issues of life review, life completion, and life closure
- Extends support beyond the life span of the patient to assist the family in their bereavement

### Utilizing the Strengths of Interdisciplinary Resources

*Palliative care:*

- Requires an interdisciplinary approach drawing on the expertise of, among others, physicians, nurses, psychologists, pharmacists, pastoral caregivers, social workers, ancillary staff, volunteers, and family members to address the multidimensional aspects of care
- Includes a clearly identified, accessible, and accountable individual or team responsible for coordinating care to assure that changing needs and goals are met and to facilitate communication and continuity of care
- Incorporates the full array of interinstitutional and community resources (hospitals, home care, hospice, long-term care, adult day services) and promotes a seamless transition between institutions/settings and services
- Requires knowledgeable, skilled, and experienced clinicians, who are provided the opportunity for ongoing education, professional support, and development

### Acknowledging and Addressing Caregiver Concerns

*Palliative care:*

- Appreciates the substantial physical, emotional, and economic demands placed on families caring for someone at home, as they attempt to fulfill caregiving responsibilities and meet their own personal needs
- Provides concrete supportive services to caregivers such as respite, round-the-clock availability of expert advice and support by telephone, grief counseling, personal care assistance, and referral to community resources

- Anticipates that some family caregivers may be at high risk for fatigue, physical illness, and emotional distress, and considers the special needs of these caregivers in planning and delivering services
- Recognizes and addresses the economic costs of caregiving, including loss of income and nonreimbursable expenses

## Building Systems and Mechanisms of Support

*Palliative care:*

- Requires an environment that supports innovation, research, education, and dissemination of best practices and models of care
- Needs an infrastructure that promotes the philosophy and practice of palliative care
- Relies on the formulation of responsible policies and regulations by institutions and by state and federal governments
- Promotes equitable and timely access to the full array of interdisciplinary services necessary to meet the multidimensional needs of patients and caregivers
- Demands ongoing evaluation, including the development of research-based standards, guidelines, and outcome measures
- Assures that mechanisms are in place at all levels (e.g., systems, direct care services) to guarantee accountability in provision of care
- Requires appropriate financing, including the development of new methods of reimbursement within the context of a changing health care financing system

| Employee Name | | Team | Preceptor | Date of Hire |
| --- | --- | --- | --- | --- |

| Date Done | Preceptor Signature | Upon completion of the Hospice Interdisciplinary Competencies, The Hospice Professional will have: |
| --- | --- | --- |
| 1) | 1) | 1) Articulated hospice philosophy, goals and objectives with emphasis on the meaning of palliative care and the meaning of quality of life. |
| 2) | 2) | 2) Demonstrated an understanding of the organization's communication systems and the different types, functions and physical layout of hospice sites. |
| 3) | 3) | 3) Assumed responsibility for personal professionalism, growth and development, and learning while completing the competency-based Initial Hospice Training. |
| 4) | 4) | 4) Articulated basic ethical principles and hospice's approach to decision making from an organizational and clinical perspective. |
| 5) | 5) | 5) Explained the Interdisciplinary Team (IDT) Case Management Process. |
| 6) | 6) | 6) Outlined the process of patient/family referral and admission. |
| 7) | 7) | 7) Reviewed end-stage disease process and related pain and symptom management. |
| 8) | 8) | 8) Demonstrated appropriate universal precautions techniques. |
| 9) | 9) | 9) Demonstrated an understanding of hospice nursing care. |
| 10) | 10) | 10) Demonstrated an understanding of hospice spiritual care. |
| 11) | 11) | 11) Demonstrated an understanding of hospice psychosocial care. |
| 12) | 12) | 12) Discussed grief and bereavement issues and participated in Bridges Program. |
| 13) | 13) | 13) Discussed the importance and utilization of hospice volunteers. |
| 14) | 14) | 14) Demonstrated appropriate death attendance and closure skills. |
| 15) | 15) | 15) Discussed the importance of accepting diversity in hospice. |
| 16) | 16) | 16) Articulated and demonstrated an understanding of providing and documenting patient care across settings, including reimbursement and regulatory issues. |
| 17) | 17) | 17) Discussed the utilization and referral procedure for ancillary services and departments. |
| 18) | 18) | 18) Discussed the role of hospice in community outreach efforts and services. |

*When complete please forward this page to the Institute. Keep a copy for yourself and submit a copy to your PFCC. Thank you.

| Hospice Clinical Competency #5 | Explain the Interdisciplinary Team (IDT) case management process. |
|---|---|

| Learner Objectives | Learning Activities/Evaluation | Date Objectives: Completed | Evaluated |
|---|---|---|---|
| I. Describe the function, process, and purpose of IDT and role of each member. | 1) Attend "IDT Case Management" session in Initial Hospice Training. | 1) _____ | 1) _____ |
| | 2) Read "Interdisciplinary Team Case Management" independent learning module. | 2) _____ | 2) _____ |
| | 3) Observe visits, as assigned, with all IDT members, including evening/weekend team members. | 3) _____ | 3) _____ |
| | 4) Observe interaction and collaboration of team members at IDT meeting and during work hours. | 4) _____ | 4) _____ |
| | 5) Explain purpose of the following components of IDT meeting: A) spiritual reflection B) announcements C) review of deaths D) admissions E) IDT care planning F) individual and team support | 5) _____ | 5) _____ |
| | 6) Read "Mr. M" case study & review with preceptor or team member. | 6) _____ | 6) _____ |
| | 7) Discuss IDT meeting, format of meeting, and benefits of IDT case management with preceptor or PFCC. | 7) _____ | 7) _____ |
| II. Review care planning process with preceptor. | 1) Identify steps in IDT care planning process with preceptor, including: A) initiate care plan B) review and update IDT care plans C) complete closure of care plan D) complete death summary/discharge summary to physician E) complete bereavement risk assessment | 1) _____ | 1) _____ |
| | 2) Participate in above steps of IDT care planning. | 2) _____ | 2) _____ |
| | 3) Explain your role in IDT care plan process, including: A) collaborate with admissions department to receive report on assigned patient. B) contact patient/family within 24 hours & initiate visits within 48 hours. C) collaborate with IDT members regarding changes in care plan between IDT meetings. D) initiate appropriate communication of patient/family changes to evening and weekend care team. E) incorporate discipline-specific issues in IDT care plan. | 3) _____ | 3) _____ |

# Glossary

*acetaminophen* an antipyretic (reducing fever) and analgesic (reducing pain)

*adjuvant therapy* treatment alongside the central treatment, usually aimed at reducing the risk of recurrence of cancer or at delaying onset of problems with widespread disease

*advance directive* a set of instructions, usually written, intended to allow a patient's current preferences to shape medical decisions during a future period of incompetence

*Alzheimer's disease* progressive mental deterioration manifested by loss of memory, ability to calculate, and visual-spatial orientation, along with confusion and disorientation

*analgesic* a compound capable of relieving pain by altering perception of pain without producing anesthesia or loss of consciousness

*antidepressants* agents used in treating/counteracting depression

*Balanced Budget Act* a 1997 act of Congress that has major, and as yet uncertain, effects on the financing of care through Medicare

*benzodiazepines* any of a group of tranquilizers that includes Valium

*bereavement* an acute state of intense psychological sadness and suffering experienced after the tragic loss of a loved one

*cancer* general term frequently used to indicate any of various types of malignant neoplasms, most of which invade surrounding tissues, may metastasize to several sites, and are likely to recur after attempted removal and to cause death of the patient. Some cancers can be effectively treated, especially if detected early. Most are eventually fatal.

*capitation* a mode of paying for health services by a fixed rate per person per unit of time, usually a month

*cardiopulmonary resuscitation (CPR)* restoration of cardiac output and pulmonary ventilation following cardiac arrest and apnea, using artificial respiration and manual closed-chest compression or open-chest cardiac massage

*case manager* a person, usually a social worker or nurse, who helps to coordinate the services needed for a patient with complex chronic illness, usually while living at home

347

*change concept* a general idea for how to accomplish improvement

*chaplain* an individual ordained or consecrated for religious ministry, specially trained to offer support, prayer, and spiritual guidance to patients and families

*chemotherapy* treatment of a disease by means of chemical substances or drugs; usually used in reference to cancer treatment

*chlorpromazine* an antipsychotic and tranquilizing agent with anti-emetic (preventing vomiting) and other effects

*chronic disease* an illness marked by long duration or frequent recurrence

*chronic obstructive pulmonary disease (COPD)* general term used for those diseases with permanent or temporary narrowing of small bronchi, in which forced expiratory flow is slowed, often called emphysema or bronchitis

*chronic pain* pain that may exist for months or years, rarely causing changes in heart rate or blood pressure but often causing loss of appetite, sleep disturbance, and depression

*codeine* an analgesic and cough suppressant; an opioid drug

*congestive heart failure (CHF)* inadequacy of the heart as a pump so that it fails to maintain adequately the forceful circulation of blood, with the result that congestion and edema develop in the tissues

*continuity* absence of interruption, a succession of parts intimately united

*continuous quality improvement* an approach to quality improvement in which past trials of change are used as the basis of future trials and something is always being tested for its effects on improvement

*curative* having healing or curing properties

*defibrillator devices* any device whose purpose is to restore the natural rhythm of a fibrillating heart (a heart undergoing rapid irregular contractions)

*dementia* the loss, usually progressive, of cognitive and intellectual functions, without impairment of perception or consciousness; caused by a variety of disorders, most commonly structural brain disease. Characterized by disorientation and impaired memory, judgment, and intellect. Often, Alzheimer's disease.

*delirium* an altered state of consciousness, consisting of confusion, distractibility, disorientation, disordered thinking and memory, defective perception, prominent hyperactivity, agitation, and autonomic nervous system overactivity; caused by a number of toxic structural and metabolic disorders

*demonstration project* organized implementation of a novel approach to providing care, with evaluation, and aimed at assessing the merits of widespread use of the approach

*diagnosis* the determination of the nature of a disease

*diagnosis related group (DRG)* the basis of payment for hospitalization in Medicare, in which a group of related conditions of similar average costs are paid this same fixed rate for almost all costs associated with a hospitalization (except physician's fees)

*dietitian* an expert in the practical application of diet in the prevention and treatment of disease

*"do not resuscitate" order (DNR)* an order dictating that an individual does not desire resuscitative measures in the case of failed breathing or cardiac arrest

*doula* originally, a layperson who helps a new mother through pregnancy and early infant care, and now a model being tested to use experienced volunteers to help persons facing serious illness

*dyspnea* shortness of breath, a subjective difficulty or distress in breathing, usually associated with disease of the heart or lungs

*electrocardiogram (EKG, ECG)* graphic record of the heart's integrated action currents obtained with the electrocardiograph

*emergency medical system* services specifically designed, staffed, and equipped for the emergency care of patients

*end of life* the period of time marked by disability or disease that is progressively worse until death

*equianalgesic conversions* the approximate dose of an opioid drug that is equal to one now being given. Essential for converting from one drug or route to another.

*ethics committee or consultant* a service of many hospitals and a few other care provider programs, which provides expertise on ethics issues and conflicts of values

*etiology* the cause of a disease

*evaluation and management services* a category of billing for physician services that focuses on understanding the patient's problems and arranging a care plan to help

*fatigue* that state, following a period of mental or bodily activity, characterized by a lessened capacity for work and reduced efficiency of accomplishment, usually accompanied by a feeling of weariness, sleepiness, or irritability

*fee-for-service* payments to health care providers based on each service provided

*fiscal intermediary* the company that receives bills for Medicare, evaluates their appropriateness, and issues payment on behalf of Medicare

*full risk capitation* the capitation payment to an insurer or provider is to pay for all covered services including hospitalization, and the organization that accepts capitation is at risk for all costs

*furosemide* a highly potent diuretic (drug to increase urination)

*health maintenance organization (HMO)* provider and insurer that accepts full risk capitation and aims, among other things, to be more efficient by emphasizing prevention

*hemodynamic* relating to the physical aspects of the blood circulation

*home health aide* person who assists ill, elderly, or disabled persons in the home, carrying out personal care and housekeeping tasks

*home health agency* an agency that offers home care services through physicians, nurses, therapists, social workers, and homemakers whom they recruit and supervise

*hospice* a care program that provides a centralized program of palliative and supportive services to dying persons and their families, in the form of physical, psychological, social, and spiritual care; such services are provided by an interdisciplinary team of professionals and volunteers who are available at home and in specialized inpatient settings

*hospital* an institution for the treatment, care, and cure of the sick and wounded, for the study of disease, and for the training of physicians, nurses, and allied health personnel

*hydration* the taking in of water

*hypersomnolence* excessive drowsiness

*hypoxemia* subnormal oxygenation of arterial blood, short of anoxia (absence or almost complete absence of oxygen from inspired gases, arterial blood, or tissues)

*IHI* the Institute for Healthcare Improvement; teaches quality improvement and coordinates the Breakthrough Series

*immediate t-bar placement* a one-step ventilator cessation with continued airway support

*innovation* a newly introduced practice or method intended to improve the current practice

*inpatient respite care* admission of a patient to a hospital, nursing facility, or inpatient hospice to allow the family to have a period without direct caregiving. Also, a payment rate for this service in the Medicare hospice benefit.

*inpatient symptom management care* admission of a patient to a hospital, nursing facility, or inpatient hospice to control symptoms. Also, a payment rate for this service in the Medicare hospice benefit.

*intensive care unit (ICU)* a hospital facility for provision of intensive nursing and medical care of critically ill patients, characterized by high quality and quantity of continuous nursing and medical supervision and by use of sophisticated monitoring and resuscitative equipment

*interim payment system (IPS)* a temporary and complex payment system under the Balanced Budget Act. Early effects have been particularly problematic for complex patients needing nursing facility care or home care.

*intractable pain* pain that is not easily managed, governed, or alleviated

*institutional review board (IRB)* a panel at each institution doing research on human subjects that reviews the risks posed to subjects and the consent process proposed

*long-term care facility* a facility that provides a range of health, personal care, social, and housing services to people who are unable to care for themselves independently as a result of chronic illness or mental/physical disabilities

*lorazepam* a benzodiazepine

*management information system* a data system for managing a care program, usually at least providing information needed for billings and collections

*Medicaid* a program of medical aid designed for those unable to afford regular medical service and financed by the state and federal governments in the United States

*medical power of attorney* authority to act for another regarding medical decisions

*Medicare* a U.S. government program of medical care especially for the aged and disabled

*meperidine* meperidine hydrochloride; a widely used narcotic analgesic that should have very limited use because it is short-acting but has long-lived psychotigenic metabolites

*minimum data set (MDS)* a set of data collected on a regular basis concerning all residents of long-term care facilities

*modality* a form of application or employment of a therapeutic agent or regimen

*morphine* the most commonly used opioid drug

*narcotic antagonist* an agent inhibiting the effect of narcotics on the central nervous system

*Nuremberg Code* agreement to protect patients involved in research. A cornerstone is the requirement for voluntary and informed consent.

*nurse practitioner* a registered nurse with at least a master's degree in nursing and advanced education in the primary care of particular groups of clients, capable of independent practice in a variety of settings

*nursing home* a facility for the care of individuals who do not require hospitalization and who cannot be cared for at home

*oncologist* a specialist in the study of the physical, chemical, and biological properties and features of cancers, including causation, pathogenesis, and treatment

*opioid* a drug possessing some properties characteristic of opiate narcotics but not derived from opium; the class of drug including narcotics such as morphine

*opiophobia* unreasonable fear of the potential effects of opioids, affecting clinicians as well as the public

*Programs for All-Inclusive Care of the Elderly (PACE)* a federal program offering elderly clients a range of health care services, transportation, food, and social activities, as well as physical, recreational, and occupational therapy

*pain assessment tool* a device, like a "face scale" or questionnaire, used to assess a patient's pain

*pain ruler* a pain assessment tool in which a patient marks severity of pain as a distance along a ruler

*palliative care services* services designed to provide relief of symptoms that interfere with quality of life when treatments won't change the time course of the illness

*Patient Self-Determination Act (PSDA)* a federal statute requiring patients to be informed of their authority to make certain medical decisions, under state law

*per capita rate, AAPCC* the rate paid for each patient, each month, in Medicare. AAPCC stands for "area average per capita cost," which is based on the average past utilization in that area and is adjusted only for age and gender. This payment system is set to change with the Balanced Budget Act, both to have somewhat more uniform payments across the nation and to adjust somewhat for illness status (risk adjustment)

*physician orders for life-sustaining treatment (POLST)* a physician order form that records patient preferences and treatment intentions; meant to enhance the appropriateness and quality of care and assist health care providers in honoring patients' treatment wishes

*primary care* care of a patient by a member of the health care system who has had initial contact with the patient

*prognostication* a forecast of the probable course and/or outcome of a disease

*prospective payment system (PPS)* comprehensive payment for an episode of care, on the basis of initial problems (see also Diagnostic Related Group, the PPS for hospitals)

*proxy* an individual who has been granted the authority or power to act on another's behalf *protocol* a precise and detailed plan for the study of a biomedical problem or for a regimen of therapy

*psychosocial* involving both psychological and social aspects

*psychostimulants* a medication with energizing or mood-elevating effects

*quantitative measures* measures that can be expressed in terms of definite numbers or amounts

*recreational/occupational therapy* a form of therapy that encourages and instructs manual activities for therapeutic or remedial purposes in mental and physical disorders

*resource utilization groups–version III (RUG-III)* classification of patients in nursing facilities by disability and other care needs, for the purpose of determining coverage and rates in the Medicare system

*routine home care* a daily rate in the Medicare hospice benefit; at least 80 percent of the Medicare beneficiary payment days must be at this rate

*sedative-hypnotics* medications that cause sleep or sleepiness

*skilled nursing facilities (SNF)* a residential facility that provides professional nursing around the clock, usually along with rehabilitation

*status quo* the existing state of affairs

*stroke* term denoting the sudden development of focal neurological deficits usually related to impaired cerebral blood flow

*supportive services* care services designed to help patient and family cope with the effects of illness and disability, rather than to alter the course of disease

*system leader* a chief executive officer, president, or other authoritative leader of a care system

*tachycardia* rapid beating of the heart, conventionally applied to rates over 100 per minute

*tachypnea* rapid breathing

*terminal extubation* the rapid cessation of mechanical ventilation and removal of the artificial airway, often followed by administration of humidified air or oxygen

*terminal weaning* a stepwise reduction of ventilatory support, leaving the artificial airway in place during the withdrawal of ventilation

*therapeutic* relating to the treatment, remediation, or cure of a disorder or disease

*thioridazine* an antipsychotic and tranquilizer, also useful for limiting nausea

*treatment modalities* methods of treatment

*tricyclics* tricyclic antidepressants; a group of related medications used to relieve depression and to enhance the effects of opioid analgesics, among other actions

*ventilator* a machine that takes over breathing for the patient, controlling the intake and expiration of air

# References

Agency for Health Care Policy and Research (AHCPR). (1994). *Clinical practice guideline: Management of cancer pain*. Rockville, MD: Public Health Service.

Ahmedzai, S. (1999). Palliation of respiratory symptoms. In D. Doyle, G. W. C. Hanks, & N. MacDonald (Eds.), *Oxford textbook of palliative medicine* 2nd Ed (pp. 583–616). Oxford: Oxford University Press.

Barnes, R. F., et al. (1981). Problems of families caring for Alzheimer patients: Use of a support group. *Journal of the American Geriatrics Society, 29*(2), 80–85.

Bernabei, R., et al. (1998). Management of pain in elderly patients with cancer. *Journal of the American Medical Association, 279*, 1877–82.

Billings, A. (1998). What is palliative care? *Journal of Palliative Medicine, 1*, 73–81.

Bourgeois, M. S., et al. (1996). Interventions for caregivers of patients with Alzheimer's disease: A review and analysis of content, process, and outcomes. *International Journal of Aging and Human Development, 43*, 35–92.

Breitbart, W. (1993). Suicide risk and pain in cancer and AIDS patients. In C. R. Chapman & C. M. Foley (Eds.), *Current and emerging issues in cancer pain: Research and practice* (pp. 49–65). New York: Raven Press.

Breitbart, W., & Sparrow, B. (1998). Management of delirium in the terminally ill, in Ian Maddocks (Ed.), *Progress in palliative care: Science and the art of caring, 6*(4).

Brenner, P. R. (1997). Managing patients and families at the ending of life: Hospice assumptions, structures, and practice in response to staff stress. *Cancer Investigation, 15*, 257–64.

Brescia, F. J., et al. (1992). Opioid use and survival in hospitalized patients with advanced cancer. *Journal of Oncology, 10*, 149–55.

Brody, H., et al. (1997). Withdrawing intensive life-sustaining treatment: Recommendations for compassionate clinical management. *New England Journal of Medicine, 336*, 652–57.

Bruera, E., et al. (1991). The Edmonton symptom assessment system (ESAS): A simple method for the assessment of palliative care patients. *Journal of Palliative Care, 7,* 6–9.

Buckman, R., & Kason, Y. (1992). *How to break bad news: A guide for health care professionals.* Baltimore: Johns Hopkins University Press.

Campbell, M. L. (1993). Case studies in terminal weaning from mechanical ventilation. *American Journal of Critical Care, 2,* 354–58.

Campbell, M. L., & Carlson, R. W. (1992). Terminal weaning from mechanical ventilation: Ethical and practical considerations for management. *American Journal of Critical Care, 1,* 52–56.

Campbell, M. L., & Thill, M. C. (1996). Impact of patient consciousness on the intensity of the do-not-resuscitate therapeutic plan. *American Journal of Critical Care, 5,* 339–45.

Campbell, M. L., et al. (1998). Integrating technology with compassionate care: Withdrawal of ventilation in a conscious patient with apnea. *American Journal Critical Care, 7,* 85–89.

Campbell, M. L., et al. (1999). Patient responses during rapid terminal weaning from mechanical ventilation: A prospective study. *Critical Care Medicine, 27,* 73–77.

Carlson, R. W., et al. (1996). Life support: The debate continues. *Chest, 109,* 852–53.

Chochinov, H. M., et al. (1997). "Are you depressed?": Screening for depression in the terminally ill. *American Journal of Psychiatry, 154*(5), 674–76.

Chochinov, H. M., et al. (1998). Depression, hopelessness, and suicidal ideation in the terminally ill. *Psychosomatics, 39*(4), 366–70.

Christakis, N. A., & Sachs, G. A. (1996). The role of prognosis in clinical decision making. *Journal of General Internal Medicine, 11,* 422–25.

Citron, M. L. (1984). Safety and efficacy of continuous intravenous morphine for severe cancer pain. *American Journal of Medicine, 77,* 199–204.

Cleary, J. F., & Carbone, P. P. (1997). Palliative medicine in the elderly. *Cancer, 80,* 1335–47.

Cleary, P. D., et al. (1991). Patients evaluate their hospital care: A national survey. *Health Affairs, Winter,* 254–67.

Cleeland, C. S., et al. (1986). Factors influencing physician management of cancer pain. *Cancer, 58,* 796–800.

Cleeland, C. S., et al. (1997). Pain and treatment of pain in minority patients with cancer: The Eastern Cooperative Oncology Group, Minority Outpatient Pain Study. *Annals of Internal Medicine, 127,* 813–16.

Cohen, M. H., et al. (1991). Continuous intravenous infusion of morphine for severe dyspnea. *Southern Medical Journal, 84,* 229–34.

Cohen, S. R., et al. (1995). Validity of the McGill Quality of Life Questionnaire, a measure of quality of life appropriate for people with advanced disease: A preliminary study of validity and acceptability. *Palliative Medicine, 9,* 207–19.

Collins, C. E., et al. (1994). Interventions with family caregivers of persons with Alzheimer's disease. *Nursing Clinics of North America, 29,* 195–207.

Costa, P. T., et al. (1996). Recognition and initial assessment of Alzheimer's disease and related dementias. Rockville, MD: U.S. Department of Health and Human Services, Public Health Service,

Agency for Health Care Policy and Research; AHCPR publication 97-0702.

Coyle, N., et al. (1990). Character of terminal illness in the advanced cancer patient: Pain and other symptoms during the last four weeks of life. *Journal of Pain Symptom Management, 5,* 83–93.

Crippen, D. (1992). Terminally weaning awake patients from life-sustaining mechanical ventilation: The critical care physician's role in comfort measures during the dying process. *Clinical Internal Care, 3,* 206–12.

Daly, B. J., et al. (1993). Withdrawal of mechanical ventilation: Ethical principles and guidelines for terminal weaning. *American Journal of Critical Care, 2,* 217–23.

Daly, B. J., et al. (1995). Procedures used in withdrawal of mechanical ventilation. *American Journal of Critical Care, 5,* 331–38.

Dartmouth Medical School. (1998). *The Dartmouth atlas of health care.* Chicago: American Hospital Publishing.

Davis, C. (1999). Lecture, Plenary on Chronic Disease, Second Learning Session, Breakthrough Collaborative to Improve Care of Patients with Advanced CHF and COPD, Atlanta, April 8, 1999.

Donadio, S., et al. *The New York Public Library book of twentieth-century quotations.* Boston: Warner Books.

Du Pen, S., et al. (1999). Implementing guidelines for cancer pain management: Results of a randomized controlled clinical trial. *Journal of Clinical Oncology, 17*(1), 361–70.

Emanuel, E. J., & Emanuel, L. L. (1998). The promise of a good death. *Lancet, 351*(Supplement 2), SII21–29. Review.

Faber-Langendoen, K. (1994). The clinical management of dying patients receiving mechanical ventilation. *Chest, 106,* 880–88.

Faber-Langendoen, K., & Bartels, D. M. (1992). Process of forgoing life-sustaining treatment: A university hospital: An empirical study. *Critical Care Medicine, 20,* 570–77.

Faber-Langendoen, K., et al. (1996). A prospective study of withdrawing mechanical ventilation from dying patients. *American Journal of Respiratory Critical Care Medicine, 153,* 45.

Fabiszewski, K. J., et al. (1990). Effect of antibiotic treatment on outcome of fevers in institutionalized Alzheimer patients. *Journal of the American Medical Association, 263*(23), 3168–72.

Ferrell, B. A. (1991). Pain management in elderly people. *Journal of the American Geriatrics Society, 39,* 64–73.

Fishman, B., et al. (1987). The Memorial Pain Assessment Card: A valid instrument for the evaluation of cancer pain. *Cancer, 35,* 279–88.

Fox, E., et al. (1999). Evaluation of prognostic criteria for determining hospice eligibility in patients with advanced lung, heart, or liver disease: SUPPORT investigators: Study to Understand Prognoses and Preferences for Outcomes and Risks of Treatments. *Journal of the American Medical Association, 282*(17), 1638–45.

George H. Gallup International Institute. (1997). Spiritual beliefs and the dying process: A report on a national study conducted for the Nathan Cummings Foundation and Fetzer Institute. Princeton, NJ.

Gianakos, D. (1995). Terminal weaning. *Chest, 108,* 1405–6.

Gift, A. G., & Pugh, L. C. (1993). Dyspnea and fatigue. *Nursing Clinics of North America, 28,* 373–84.

Gilligan, T., & Raffin, T. A. (1995). Rapid withdrawal of support. *Chest, 108,* 1407–8.

Greenlee, R. T., et al. (2000). Cancer statistics, 2000. *Ca: Cancer Journal for Clinicians, 50*(1), 7–33.

Greer, D. S., et al. (1984). National Hospice Study final report. Brown University, Providence, RI.

Grenvik, A. (1983). Terminal weaning: Discontinuance of life-support therapy in the terminally ill patient. *Critical Care Medicine, 11,* 394–95.

Health Care Financing Administration (HCFA) (1999). *Medicare managed care cost report,* Washington, DC.

Higginson, I. J., Wade, A. M., & McCarthy, M. (1992). Effectiveness of two palliative care support teams. *Journal of Public Health Medicine, 14,* 50–56.

Iezonni, L. I., et al. (1988). Paying more fairly for Medicare capitated care. *New England Journal of Medicine, 339,* 1933–38.

Innovations. (1999). Only connect: Promoting meaning in the lives of patients with advanced dementia. *Innovations in End-of-Life Care, 1*(4). Online. Available at http://www2.edc.org/lastacts/archives/archivesJune99/

Institute of Medicine (IOM). (1997). M. Field & C. Cassell (Eds.), *Approaching death: Improving care at the end of life.* Washington: National Academy Press.

Joranson, D. E., & Gilson, A. M. (1988). Regulatory barriers to pain management. *Seminars in Oncological Nursing, 14,* 158–63.

Kristjanson, L. J. (1993). Validity and reliability testing of the FAM-CARE scale: Measuring family satisfaction with advanced cancer care. *Social Science Medicine, 36,* 693–701.

Kuuppelomaki, M., & Lauri, S. (1998). Ethical dilemmas in the care of patients with incurable cancer. *Nursing Ethics, 5,* 283–93.

Langley, G. J., et al. (1996). *The improvement guide: A practical approach to enhancing organizational performance.* San Francisco: Jossey-Bass Publishers.

Lawton, M. P., et al. (1989). A controlled study of respite service for caregivers of Alzheimer's patients. *Gerontologist, 21,* 464–70.

Lubitz, J. D., & Riley, G. F. (1993). Trends in Medicare payment in the last year of life. *New England Journal of Medicine, 328,* 1092–96.

Lynn, J. (1997). Measuring quality of care at the end of life: A statement of principles. *Journal of the American Geriatrics Society, 45,* 526–27.

Lynn J., et al. (1997). Perceptions by family members of the dying experience of older and seriously ill patients. *Annals of Internal Medicine, 126,* 97–106.

Mainous, A. G., & Gill, J. M. (1998). The importance of continuity of care in the likelihood of future hospitalization: Is site of care equivalent to a primary clinician? *American Journal of Public Health, 88,* 1539–41.

McCracken, A. L., & Gerdsen, L. (1991). Sharing the legacy: Hospice care principles for terminally ill elders. *Journal of Gerontological Nursing, 17*(12), 4–8.

Melzack, R. (1983). The McGill Pain Questionnaire. In R. Melzack, *Pain measurement and assessment* (pp. 41–48). New York: Raven Press.

Melzack, R. (1987). The Short-Form McGill Pain Questionnaire. *Pain, 30*, 191–97.

Miller, R. H., & Luft, H. S. (1997). Does managed care lead to better or worse outcomes of care? *Health Affairs, 16*, 7–25.

Morycz, R. K. (1985). Caregiving strain and the desire to institutionalize family members with Alzheimer's disease: Possible predictors and model development. *Research on Aging, 7*(3), 329–61.

Moscicki, E. K. (1997). Identification of suicide risk factors using epidemiologic studies. *Suicide, 20*(3), 506.

Murphy, D., & Leighton, C. (Eds.) (1990). SUPPORT: Study to Understand Prognoses and Preferences for Outcomes and Risks of Treatment. *Journal of Clinical Epidemiology, 43*(supplement).

National Alliance for the Mentally Ill (NAMI). (1996). Depression in elderly fact sheet, September 29.

National Center for Health Statistics (NCHS). (1999). National vital statistics reports: Births, marriages, divorces, and deaths. *Provisional Data for 1998, 47*(21).

National Hospice Organization (NHO). (1998). Hospice fact sheet. On-line. Available at http://www.nho.org/facts.htm

National Hospice Organization (NHO). (1999). VA end-of-life initiative shows national leadership, openings for hospices. *NHO Newsline, 9*(21).

National Task Force on End-of-Life Care in Managed Care. (1999). *Meeting the challenge.* Newton, MA: Education Development Center.

Newhouse, J. (1998). Risk adjustment: Where are we now? *Inquiry, 35*, 122–31.

Nuland, S. B. (1994). *How we die: Reflections on life's final chapter.* New York: Alfred A. Knopf.

OPRR Reports. (1983). Protection of human subjects, code of federal regulations 45 CFR 46, revised March 8.

Pinkston, E. M., & Linsk, N. L. (1984). Behavioral family intervention with the impaired elderly. *Gerontologist, 24*, 576–83.

Pinkston, E. M., et al. (1988). Home-based behavioral family treatment of the impaired elderly. *Behavior Therapy, 19*, 331–44.

Portenoy, R. K. (1992). Cancer pain: From curriculum to practice change. *Journal of Clinical Oncology, 10*(12), 1830–32.

Pritchard, R. S., et al. (1998). Influence of patient preferences and local health system characteristics on the place of death. *Journal of the American Geriatrics Society, 46*, 1242–50.

Rabins, P. V., et al. (1982). The impact of dementia on the family. *Journal of the American Medical Association, 248*(3), 333–35.

Rader, J. (1996). Rader offers creative dementia care ideas. *Oregon Nurse, 61*(3), 16.

Rainey, T. G., et al. (1998). *Reducing costs and improving outcomes in adult intensive care.* Boston: Institute for Healthcare Improvement.

Remondet, J. H., and Hanson, R. O. (1987). Assessing a widow's grief—a short index. *Journal of Gerontology Nursing, 13*, 30–34.

Rich, M. W. (1999). Heart failure disease management: A critical review. *Journal of Cardiac Failure, 5*, 64–75.

Richie, K., & Kildea, D. (1995). Is senile dementia "age related" or "aging related"?: Evidence from a meta-analysis of dementia prevalence in the oldest old. *Lancet, 346*, 931–34.

Robinson, B. C. (1983). Validation of a Caregiver Strain Index. *Journal of Gerontology, 38,* 344–48.

Rushton, C., & Terry, P. B. (1995). Neuromuscular blockade and ventilator withdrawal: Ethical controversies. *American Journal of Critical Care, 4,* 112–15.

Scharlach, A., & Frenzel, C. (1986). An evaluation of institution-based respite care. *Gerontologist, 26,* 77–82.

Sloan, P. A., et al. (1998). Medical student knowledge of morphine for the management of cancer pain. *Journal of Pain Symptom Management, 15,* 359–64.

Sparks, N. (1996). *The notebook.* Boston: Warner Books.

Strother, A. (1991). Drawing the line between life and death. *American Journal of Nursing, 91,* 24–25.

Strouse, T. (1997). Identifying and treating depression in women with cancer: A primary care approach. *Medscape Women's Health, 2*(9), 3.

Stuart, B. (1994). *Medical guidelines for determining prognosis in selected non-cancer diseases.* Arlington, VA: National Hospice Organization (NHO).

Super, A. (1996). Improving pain management practice. *Health Progress, July–August,* 50–54.

SUPPORT Principal Investigators. (1995). A controlled trial to improve care for seriously ill hospitalized patients: The Study to Understand Prognoses and Preferences for Outcomes and Risks of Treatment (SUPPORT). *Journal of the American Medical Association, 274,* 1591–98.

Teno, J. M., & Lynn, J. (1996). Putting advance care planning into action. *Journal of Clinical Ethics, 7,* 205–13.

Tobin, D. R., & Lindsey, K. (1999). *Peaceful dying: The step-by-step guide to preserving your dignity, your choice, and your inner peace at the end of life.* Reading, MA: Perseus Books.

Tolle, S. W., et al. (1998). A prospective study of the efficacy of the physician orders for life-sustaining treatment. *Journal of the American Geriatrics Society, 46,* 1097–1102.

Truog, R. D., & Burns, J. P. (1994). To breathe or not to breathe. *Journal of Clinical Ethics, 5,* 39–42.

U.S. Department of Veterans Affairs. (1999). *Pain assessment: The fifth vital sign.* Veterans Health Administration, Acute Care Strategic Healthcare Group, Geriatric Extended Care Strategic Healthcare Group. Washington, DC.

Vachon, M. (1998). The emotional problems of the patient. In D. Doyle, G. Hanks, & N. MacDonald (Eds.), *Oxford textbook of palliative medicine* (p. 887). New York: Oxford University Press.

VandeCreek, L., et al. (1994). Where there's life, there's hope, and where there is hope, there is . . . *Journal of Religion and Health, 33*(1), 51–59.

Vogelzang, N. J., et al. (1997). Patient, caregiver, and oncologist perceptions of cancer-related fatigue: Results of a tripart assessment survey: The Fatigue Coalition. *Seminars in Hematology, 34,* 4–12.

Volicer, L., & Hurley, A. C. (1999). Assessment of behavioral symptom management in demented individuals. *Alzheimer's Disease and Associated Disorders, 13,* Supplement 1, S59–66.

Volicer, L., et al. (1999). Dimensions of decreased psychological well-being in advanced dementia. *Alzheimer's Disease and Associated Disorders, 13*(4), 192–201.

Von Gunten, C. F., et al. (1998). Prospective evaluation of referrals to a hospice/palliative medicine consultation service. *Journal of Palliative Medicine, 1,* 45–53.

Von Roenm, J. H., et al. (1993). Physician attitudes and practice in cancer pain management: A survey from the Eastern Cooperative Oncology Group. *Annals of Internal Medicine, 119,* 121–26.

Warner, S. C., & Williams, J. I. (1987). The meaning in life scale: Determining the reliability and validity of a measure. *Journal of Chronic Disease, 40*(6), 503–12.

Weissman, D. E. (1997). Consultation in palliative medicine. *Archives of Internal Medicine, 157,* 733–47.

Williamson, G. M., & Schulz, R. (1990). Relationship orientation, quality of prior relationship, and distress among caregivers of Alzheimer's patients. *Psychological Aging, 5*(4), 502–9.

Wilson, W. C., et al. (1992). Ordering and administration of sedatives and analgesics during the withholding and withdrawal of life support from critically ill patients. *Journal of the American Medical Association, 267,* 949–53.

World Health Organization (WHO). (1998). *Symptom relief in terminal illness.* Geneva: World Health Organization.

Zarit, S. H., et al. (1980). Relatives of the impaired elderly: Correlates of feelings of burden. *Gerontologist, 20*(6), 649–55.

Zech, D. F., et al. (1995). Validation of World Health Organization guidelines for cancer pain relief: Ten-year prospective study. *Pain, 63,* 65–76.

Zuckerman, C., & Mackinnon, A. (1988). *The challenge of caring for patients near the end of life: Findings from the Hospital Palliative Care Initiative.* New York, NY: United Hospital Fund.

# Index

bowel obstruction, 235
brain-death, 66
"breaking bad news" workshops, 84
breakthrough pain, 40
Breakthrough Series Collaborative on Improv-
     ing End-of-Life Care, 6–9
breast cancer, 236
breath, shortness of. *See* dyspnea
Breitbart, William, 253–54
Buckman, Robert, 84
burial plans, 79
"by next Tuesday" concept, 7, 18–19, 33, 274

cachexia, 245
California
     electronic data transfer program, 199
     end-of-life commission, 194
     life-sustaining treatment ruling, 192
Calvary Hospital (N.Y.C.), 186–87, 189, 243
cancer, 3, 235–43, 347
     advance care planning, 84, 237
     chemotherapy, 166, 235, 240, 348
     cultural issues and, 237, 241
     depression and, 245, 247, 251
     dyspnea and, 59, 235, 237
     final phases of, 5
     hospice care and, 235, 236, 237, 242
     "no action" as treatment option, 240–41
     oncologists, 37, 161–62, 351
     pain relief treatment, 37, 39, 40, 49–56
     palliative care improvements, 21–24, 25, 235
     palliative care services, 134, 135, 141
     patient hospitalization, 236, 237, 241–42
     quality of life considerations, 237, 241
     symptom management, 236, 237–39
     treatment plan checkpoints, 236, 239–40,
          242
Cancer Care Technicians, 186–87
Cancer Pain Algorithm, 49–50, 51, 52
capitation, 115, 121, 202, 347
     full risk, 152–53, 349
Cardiac Comfort Care Kits, 265
cardiac disease. *See* heart disease
cardiopulmonary resuscitation, 79, 88, 347
career advancement, for end-of-life workers,
          180, 186–87
caregivers
     Alzheimer's disease issues, 215, 216–17,
          219–32

confidence in care systems and, 96–98, 117,
          118
continuity of care and, 117
education programs for, 93
human resources issues, 179–89
Medicare reimbursement issues, 158
*See also* families
"Caregivers as Colleagues" project, 96–98
Care Plan Discussion Document, 84–85
case managers, 347
     heart patients and, 264
     management information services and, 174
     palliative care role of, 23
CCTs. *See* Cancer Care Technicians
Center to Improve Care of the Dying, 10
certified nursing assistants, 186
chambers of commerce, 194, 206
change concept, 348
changes, recommended
     development of, 17–18, 22–23
     feasibility and effectiveness of, 273–74
     pitfalls to avoid, 24–29
chapels, 106
chaplains and clergy, 348
     supportive care services by, 85–86, 92, 93,
          99, 106, 107
     ventilator withdrawal issues and, 64, 70
chemotherapy, 166, 235, 240, 348
Cherry, Kay, 204
CHF. *See* congestive heart failure
chlorpromazine, 251, 348
Chochinov, Harvey, 251
Choice in Dying, 89–90
chronic disease, 348
chronic obstructive pulmonary disease, 3, 195,
          257, 348
chronic pain, 57–58, 348
clergy. *See* chaplains and clergy
clinical pathways, 49
clinical social workers. *See* social workers
CNAs. *See* certified nursing assistants
codeine, 348
colon cancer, 236
Colorado, 194, 199–200
comfort care, 5, 8
     for Alzheimer's and dementia patients, 217,
          218–22, 224
     ventilator withdrawal and, 64, 70
comfort packs, 105

[drugs] (*continued*)

   Medicare coverage and, 155, 164, 165

   nursing home residents and, 37, 38, 39

   pain treatment practices, 40, 41, 56–57, 237,
      238, 239

   palliative care concerns, 136

   regulatory issues, 40, 192, 196–98, 199, 237

   sedative-hypnotics, 13, 59, 352

   side effects, 40, 245, 247–48

   transdermal delivery systems, 235

   *See also* opioids; sedation; *specific drugs*

durable medical equipment, 155, 164

dying, definition of, 4–5, 10. *See also* death;
   end-of-life

dyspnea, 8, 35, 59–71, 197, 349

   assessment practices, 41, 61, 62–64

   cancer and, 59, 235, 237

   delirium and, 245

   guidelines and standing orders, 64, 71

   heart patients and, 264

   management principles, 62–63

   supportive care and, 94

   ventilator withdrawal and, 59–60, 64–71

E&M services. *See* evaluation and management
   services

Eastern Cooperative Oncology Group, 198

ECG. *See* electrocardiogram

Edith Nourse Rogers Memorial Veterans Hospital (Mass.), 221–22, 223–24, 225, 231

EDT programs. *See* electronic data transfer
   programs

Education for Physicians on End-of-Life Care,
   9, 198, 209

education programs, 26–27

   advance care planning, 78, 80, 83–86, 88, 89

   advance directives, 74

   Alzheimer's disease, 222, 227, 229, 230

   "breaking bad news" workshops, 84

   cancer, 238, 239

   dyspnea management, 62–63

   family support, 100

   heart/lung patients, 262, 264

   interdisciplinary team training, 184–86, 189

   malpractice premium reduction and,
      199–200

   pain and symptom relief, 198, 237

   pain treatment issues, 40, 44, 47

   palliative care services, 135–36

   for physicians, 9, 198, 209, 237

   professional organizations and, 10, 209–11

   suicide risk factors, 253

   for supportive caregiving, 93

   whole-community care model, 116

Effexor, 248

EKG. *See* electrocardiogram

elderly people

   depression among, 247–48

   EverCare program, 121–22, 129, 154–55

   PACE initiative, 45, 115–16, 117, 121, 129,
      154–55, 224, 351

   pain management issues, 56–58, 237

   *See also* Medicare

electrocardiogram, 349

electronic data transfer programs, 199

Elements of Care Checklist (St. Thomas
   Health Services), 338–39

Elmhurst Hospital Infectious Disease Clinic
   (N.Y.C.), 81, 83

emergency medical services

   advance care planning issues, 77, 79, 80

   continuity of care concerns, 125, 126–27

emergency medical system, 349

   supportive care services, 106

emotional support, 91–111

emphysema, 141

EMS. *See* emergency medical services

end-of-life, 349

   changing assumptions about, 192–93

   and dying and home, 241–42

   state commissions on, 194

   *See also* death and dying

EPEC. *See* Education for Physicians on End-of-
   Life Care

equianalgesic cards/charts, 41, 55

equianalgesic conversions, 349

ethical issues

   Alzheimer's and dementia patients, 217,
      231–32

   continuous quality improvement and, 30–
      31, 33

   informed consent, 30, 64

   *See also* assisted suicide

ethics committee/consultant, 349

ethnic considerations, advance care planning
   and, 86–89

etiology, 349

euthanasia, active, 197. *See also* assisted suicide

guided imagery exercises, 94
"Guide to Hospice/Palliative Care" (booklet), 149
Gundersen Lutheran Medical Center (Wis.), 74–77
Gynecology Advance Planning consults, 84

hallucinations, delirium and, 249–50
haloperidol, 251
*Handbook for Mortals: Guidance for People Facing Serious Illness*, 206, 207
Harvard Geriatric Education Center (Mass.), 185–86
HCFA. *See* Health Care Financing Administration, U.S.
Health and Human Services Department, U.S., 198
Health Care Directive law (Minn.), 196
Health Care Financing Administration, U.S., 121, 161, 168, 200, 206
health care proxy, 86, 88
health care report cards, 193, 206
health care system
    continuity of care issues, 113–28, 202–3
    shortcomings of, 3–4, 10, 11
health insurance companies, 88, 89
health maintenance organizations, 122, 152, 349
    Social HMOs, 154–55
Health Partners (Minn.), 101, 103–5, 204
Health Plan Employer Data Information Set, 193
heart disease, 257–66
    Cardiac Comfort Care Kits, 265
    congestive heart failure, 3, 5, 141, 160, 166, 195, 257, 260–61, 348
    defibrillator devices, 348
    depression and, 247
    supportive services, 258–63
    symptom management, 258, 262, 264–65, 266
    tachycardia, 352
HEDIS. *See* Health Plan Employer Data Information Set
hemodynamic, 349
HHA. *See* home health agencies
HIV/AIDS
    advance care planning, 81, 83
    palliative care services, 131, 141

HMOs. *See* health maintenance organizations
home health agencies, 155, 156, 349
home health aides, 155, 165, 181, 349
home health care, Medicare reimbursement for, 155–57
homemaker services, 165
Hope Hospice (Fla.), 122–23, 169, 258–59, 262–63, 265
hopelessness, 248
hospice, 8, 9, 349
    access to health care providers, 122
    admission criteria, 5, 10, 164, 222, 257
    advance care planning issues, 76
    Alzheimer's and dementia patients and, 217, 219–23, 230–32
    bereavement programs, 107
    cancer patients and, 235, 236, 237, 242
    emotional and spiritual support, 92, 93
    heart patients and, 257–62
    Medicare benefits, 5, 140–41, 153, 162, 164–67, 192, 203, 217, 222–23, 232
    palliative care vs., 134
    Veterans Administration initiatives, 195, 196
Hospice Care of Rhode Island, 61–64
Hospice Foundation of America, 111
Hospice Interdisciplinary Clinical Competencies (Hospice of the Florida Suncoast), 344–45
Hospice of Michigan, 96–98
Hospice of the Florida Suncoast, 175–76, 178, 344–45
hospitality carts, 93, 100
hospitalization, during last year of life, 8
hospitals, 201, 349
    cancer patients and, 236, 237, 241–42
    emergency departments, 106
    heart patients and, 257, 258
    intensive care units, 93, 106, 350
    lung patients and, 257
    Medicare reimbursement and, 159–60
    palliative care consults and units, 131, 133–49, 162–63, 168, 203
    record-keeping systems, 169
    special care units, 106
    supportive care services, 105
human resources issues, end-of-life workers, 131–32, 179–89
    bereavement and counseling services, 180, 187–88, 189

career advancement, 180, 186–87
interdisciplinary teams, 180–86, 188–89
morale building, 183–84
palliative care staffing, 139
team-building strategies, 182, 189
team meeting effectiveness, 182–83, 185, 189
team training, 184–86, 189
hunches, as improvement dynamic, 13
Hurley, Ann, 221, 223
hydration, 79, 218, 349
hypersomnolence, 61, 349
hypnosis, 41
hypnotics. *See* sedatives/hypnotics
hypoxemia, 350

ICU. *See* intensive care unit
IHI. *See* Institute for Healthcare Improvement
Illinois, 194, 196
Illinois Coalition for Improving End-of-Life Care, 196
immediate t-bar placement, 65, 66, 350
improvement, initiation and acceleration of, 269–76
aim setting, 272, 273
change feasibility and effectiveness, 273–74
colleague participation, 271
institutional leadership and, 271–72
measure selection, 273
problem identification and definition, 269–71
solicitation of help, 275–76
testing of changes, 274–75
improvement teams
cancer patient issues, 237, 238, 239, 240
delirium assessment and treatment, 250–51
depression screening and treatment, 251–53
multidisciplinary conferences, 24
recruitment considerations, 14–16, 33, 271
individual counseling, 227
informed consent, 30, 64
innovation, 14, 20–24, 350
inpatient respite care, 350
inpatient symptom management care, 350
Institute for Healthcare Improvement, 6, 34, 114, 350
Institute of Medicine, 200–201, 202
Committee on Care at the End of Life, 116–17

institutional review boards, 30, 350
instruments, measurement and assessment, 278–326
intensive care units, 93, 106, 350
interdisciplinary teams, 14, 180–86, 188–89, 271
Interim Payment System, 156, 350
international organizations and agencies
clinical practice guidelines, 49
*See also specific groups*
Internet. *See* World Wide Web
intractable pain, 350
IPS. *See* Interim Payment System
IRBs. *See* institutional review boards

Jacob Perlow Hospice (N.Y.C.), 219–21, 225
Jastremski, Connie, 182
Joint Commission on Accreditation of Healthcare Organizations (JCAHO), 49, 53
*Journal of Palliative Medicine,* 149
journals, bedside, 105
"Journey Program" Process for Patients in the Final Stages of Life, 102
"Journey through the Dying Process" (booklet), 94
judicial rulings, 192–93, 231. *See also specific cases*

Kaiser Permanente (San Diego, Calif.), 45, 54–55, 125
Kaiser Permanente Bellflower (Calif.), 260–61, 264

language issues
advance care planning considerations, 86, 87
multilingual assessment tools, 47
speech/language pathology services, 155, 165
Last Acts Campaign, 9, 209–10
Last Acts Palliative Care Task Force, 134, 340–43
legal issues, 92, 191–94
advance directives, 74, 193, 194, 196
assisted suicide, 192, 193, 197, 200
decision-making authority, 191, 192
drug prescription, 40, 192, 196–98, 199
judicial rulings, 192–93, 231
life-sustaining treatment, 192
medical power of attorney, 350

"Packet, The: Communication Guide for Care of the Patient with Life Threatening Illness" (document collection), 98–99
pagers, caregiver use of, 96, 106
pain, 4, 7, 35, 37–58, 206
  advance care planning issues, 79
  alternative therapies for, 94, 95
  assessment of. *See* pain assessment
  assisted suicide issues, 192, 193, 197, 200, 237
  "best" and current management practices, 40–41
  biomedical research on, 10
  cancer patient issues, 237–39
  chronic, 57–58, 348
  clinical practice guideline use, 49–50, 51, 52
  controlled substance prescription registration, 7, 56
  delirium sufferer issues, 250
  diverse innovation implementation, 55–56
  elderly patient treatment, 56–58
  as fifth vital sign, 8, 12, 26, 48–49, 195–96, 238
  follow-up procedures development, 54–55
  institutional standards and priorities, 50–51
  intractable, 350
  medication underprescription, 198–99, 237
  negative effects of, 43
  oncologists' view of, 37
  opioid drug prescription, 40, 41, 56–57, 192, 196–98, 199, 235, 237, 238, 239
  palliative care issues, 133, 134, 136, 166
  patient and provider rights and responsibilities, 44
  patient definition of, 43, 45
  self-reporting of, 44, 45, 176
  supportive care and, 94
  treatment practices, 39–43, 53–54, 119
  ventilator withdrawal issues, 65, 66, 70
  *See also* suffering
Pain as a Fifth Vital Sign program, 48, 195–96, 238
pain assessment, 7, 8, 351
  cancer patients and, 237, 238
  culturally appropriate methods, 45–47
  frame of reference as important in, 43, 47–48
  measurement instruments, 287–90
  multilingual versions of tools, 47

palliative care improvements and, 23
patient self-reporting and, 44, 45, 176
practices related to, 40–43
protocol standardization, 44–45
Veterans Administration initiatives, 48, 195
pain rulers, 41, 45, 51, 351
Palliative Care Center of North Shore (Ill.), 185, 187, 265
palliative care kits, 94, 95
palliative care services
  for Alzheimer's and dementia patients, 217, 218–22
  billing codes for, 163
  for cancer patients, 21–24, 25, 166, 235, 237
  complementary therapies and, 94, 95
  consult key features, 136
  defined, 134–35, 351
  goals of, 134
  hospital-based consults and units, 131, 133–49, 162–63, 168, 203
  marketing of, 143–44
  Medicare reimbursement issues, 162–63, 166, 168
  model selection, 137–40
  patient enrollment, 140–42
  precepts of, 340–43
  response to provider concerns, 140
  satisfaction measurement, 141–43, 146
  settings for, 203
  standards and procedures implementation, 144, 146–48
  whole-community model, 116–17
  working models, 135–37
  *See also* hospice
paralytic agents, 65
paraprofessionals, interdisciplinary teams and, 180, 186–87, 189
parish nurses, 85–86
Parkland Health and Hospital System (Tex.), 21–24, 25, 141–43
pastoral companions, 100–101, 102
pastors. *See* chaplains and clergy
Patient Management System '98 (information system), 174
patients, 3
  advance care planning and, 73–83, 86–89
  advanced heart or lung failure, 257–66
  aim-setting considerations, 14
  Alzheimer's disease, 215–32

VITAS Healthcare of Miami (Fla.), 176–77
volunteers
    as interdisciplinary team members, 180, 181
    supportive care and, 93, 99, 100, 101, 123
von Gunten, Charles, 135

Walston, Beth, 196
Washington Home (D.C.), 225, 230–31
*Washington v. Glucksberg* (1997), 193
WHO. *See* World Health Organization

whole-community care model, 116–17
will to live, 38
Wisconsin, 199
Wishard Health Services (Ind.), 100
World Health Organization, 40, 59, 134, 239
World Wide Web, 174, 205, 207, 238
wrist bracelets, patient, 79, 125

Zoloft, 248